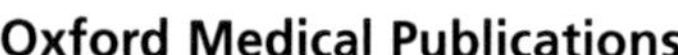

Oxford Medical Publications

Psychotherapy for borderline personality disorder

Psychotherapy for borderline personality disorder

Mentalization-based treatment

Anthony W. Bateman, MA, FRCPsych
Clinical Head and Research Lead of Psychotherapy Services,
Halliwick Unit, St Ann's Hospital,
North London

Honorary Senior Lecturer,
Royal Free and University College Medical School,
London

and

Peter Fonagy, PhD, FBA
Freud Memorial Professor of Psychoanalysis and Director,
Sub-Department of Clinical Health Psychology,
Univerity College London

Chief Executive of the Anna Freud Centre,
London

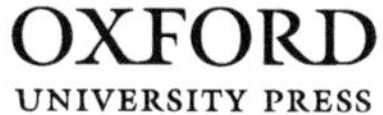

OXFORD
UNIVERSITY PRESS

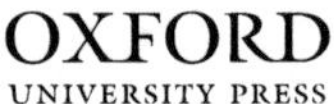

Great Clarendon Street, Oxford OX2 6DP

Oxford University Press is a department of the University of Oxford.
It furthers the University's objective of excellence in research, scholarship,
and education by publishing worldwide in

Oxford New York

Auckland Cape Town Dar es Salaam Hong Kong Karachi
Kuala Lumpur Madrid Melbourne Mexico City Nairobi
New Delhi Shanghai Taipei Toronto
With offices in
Argentina Austria Brazil Chile Czech Republic France Greece
Guatemala Hungary Italy Japan South Korea Poland Portugal
Singapore Switzerland Thailand Turkey Ukraine Vietnam

Published in the United States
by Oxford University Press Inc., New York

Reprinted 2009

ISBN 978-0-19-852766-4

Printed in the United Kingdom by
Lightning Source UK Ltd., Milton Keynes

Foreword

The prevailing views about the treatability and treatments for patients with borderline personality disorder have changed dramatically during the course of the thirty years in which this diagnosis has been used. Long-term individual psychoanalytic psychotherapy was considered the treatment of choice in the 1970s. The basis for this view was laid by the claims made for its effectiveness in a series of more than 50 books authored by psychoanalytic pioneers, who described the techniques, processes, and problems involved in conducting such therapies. After the diagnosis entered the official nomenclature of the American Psychiatric Association (APA) in 1980, its treatment received increasing attention from psychiatrists. During the decade of the eighties the rarity of success with psychoanalytic therapists and the potentially harmful effects of long-term or unstructured hospitalizations became widely recognized. In the same decade medication trials were begun, that, despite ambiguous results, established this modality as a standard of treatment for borderline patients. In the 1990s the social disabilities of borderline patients became central to therapeutics, and empirical evidence became a new standard for judging effectiveness. Family and group therapies both received support in preliminary trials. Without question, however, the major advance in the 1990s was the emergence of a behavioural therapy, DBT, directed at the self-destructive behaviour of these patients. Championed by empirical support and the tireless and charismatic advocacy of Marsha Linehan, DBT threatened to eclipse claims of benefit from all other therapies. It is in this context that the contribution of what in this book is called "Mentalization Based Therapy" (MBT) by Bateman and Fonagy appeared.

MBT has been shown to be effective in a randomized controlled clinical trial (Bateman and Fonagy, 1999). In that study, MBT was provided in a partial hospital setting for 18 months and was contrasted with usual psychiatric care. Like DBT, MBT showed dramatically effective results in diminishing hospitalizations, medication usage, and suicidal and self-injurious behaviours. In addition, and unlike DBT, it also showed significant benefits in symptoms of depression and anxiety, and in social and interpersonal function. Particularly impressive was that patients continued to improve during an 18-month period of follow-up (Bateman and Fonagy, 2001). In *Psychotherapy for borderline personality disorder*, the developers of this treatment provide a manual that will allow clinicians to understand and deploy it.

MBT is derived from a developmental theory advanced by Fonagy nearly a decade ago (Fonagy, 1991; Fonagy and Target 1997). This theory is based on systematic observations of infants with their caretakers, and is anchored within the growing science on attachment. It posits that a sense of self develops from observing oneself being perceived by others as thinking or feeling. The stability and coherence of a child's sense of self depends upon sensitive, accurate, and consistent responses to him and observations about him by his caretakers. By internalizing perceptions made by others about himself, the infant learns that his mind doesn't mirror the world, his mind interprets the world. This is termed a capacity to "mentalize", meaning the capacity to know that one has an agentive mind and to recognize the presence and importance of mental states in others. As applied to BPD, the authors assert that failures of parental responsiveness cause a failure in ability to mentalize, and thus an unstable and incoherent sense of self. The inability to mentalize and the consequent incoherence of self are reflected in the Borderline patient's typically inconsistent and often inaccurate perceptions of self and others, and in their inconsistent and inappropriate expressions of emotions. It is worth highlighting that the borderline patient's emotional volatility that is thought to be the core deficit (i.e. "emotional dysregulation") in borderline patients by Linehan, Livesley, and other major theorists, is in Bateman and Fonagy's theory reduced to a secondary phenomenon.

By promoting a theory in which the core deficit of BPD is an environmentally, and specifically parent-child, induced failure to develop a psychological function (i.e. mentalization), the authors are giving priority to once prominent etiologic factors that have faded in the face of growing evidence for biogenetic vulnerabilities, such as affective instability or behavioural dyscontrol (i.e. impulsivity). Prioritizing the environment and the interpersonal domain in interaction with genetic vulnerability offers a valuable and timely counterpoint to theories that propose biogenetic dispositions as the core of this disorder. At this point in our knowledge, contrasting theories are desirable stimuli to testable hypotheses and better understanding of borderline personality disorder. In this regard, Bateman and Fonagy are wonderfully forthright by repeatedly identifying differences between theory and knowledge, and when explicating their theory ask readers only to respect its plausibility. Such distinctions and modesty are usually absent when authors have a theoretical conviction.

As a manual, much of this book describes practical applications for the authors' developmental model of borderline psychopathology. The core and distinguishing characteristics of the MBT interventions are the attention given to identifying the mental state of others as the way to understand behaviour. Thus therapists focus on identifying (interpreting) here-and-now feeling states or thoughts in their BPD patients. Unlike usual psychoanalytic interventions, with MBT it is not the content of an interpretation that is thought to bring about change. Rather, change derives from the more generic lesson about the causal role of mental states in explaining or understanding behaviour. Moreover, in MBT, another focus is on having patients identify mental states in others, including that of the therapist, and to learn how they explain behaviour by others.

The emphasis on cognitive processes in the here-and-now is the level of therapist participation that bridges traditional cognitive and psychoanalytic techniques.

The application of MBT that has been empirically validated by Bateman and Fonagy took place in a partial hospital program, but the authors are clear that they believe it is the individual therapy and group therapy components that account for MBT's efficiency. This belief is now being tested, but their effort to sort out the effective components illustrates this book's larger purpose: MBT is a theory-based model of therapy whose possible applications are intended to be diverse — and certainly not confined to extended partial hospital services. This message is critically important and I expect that readers will find, as I have, that the attention to mental states given within MBT is a useful framework for thinking about what one is doing in all encounters with borderline patients. The attention and importance given to recognizing and labelling what a patient is thinking and feeling is an essential form of validation and self-building that cuts across all therapeutic modalities or paradigms.

This is a significant book written by two serious clinician-scientists. Beyond introducing readers to MBT and its theoretical background, the book contains multiple cogent and scholarly reviews of relevant BPD literature. The authors are not trying to simplify; they want readers to receive an education in a way of thinking about borderline patients that will modify currently prevailing conceptualizations and usual practices. It should become essential reading for all serious scholars and clinicians of borderline personality disorder.

John Gunderson
Dept of Psychiatry, McLean Hospital, Belmont MA, USA

Contents

About the authors xvii

Introduction xix

Aims xix
Organization of manual xx
Core component of treatment xxi
Who is this manual for? xxii
The authors xxiii

Chapter 1: Epidemiological and etiological research on borderline personality disorder 1

Definition of the problem 1
- Diagnostic procedures 2
- Thresholds for diagnosis 2

Epidemiology 3
Clinical picture 3
- Phenomenological picture 3
- Functional impairment 4
- Psychodynamic picture 5
  - BPO 5
  - Defence mechanisms 5
  - Object relations 5
- Co-morbidity 7
- Dimensional models of BPD 8

The natural history of BPD 9
- The stability of the diagnosis over time 9
- The course of BPD 10

Studies of mechanisms and aetiological factors 12
- Biological considerations 12
  - Biological markers 12
  - Genetic studies 12
  - Neurotransmitter abnormality 14
  - Candidate genes 14
  - Cortical localization 15
  - Attention and self-control 18
  - Conclusion 19

Psychosocial influences 19
Theoretical considerations 19
Parenting 21
Parental separation or loss 21
Family history 21
Abnormal parenting attitudes 22
Childhood trauma and maltreatment 23
Models of psychosocial aetiology based on neglect and trauma 26
The PTSD model 26
The stress-diathesis model 27
A multiple pathway model 28
Biological pathways of the impact of extreme stress 29
Childhood trauma as a risk factor for adverse brain development 29
Serotonin system 30
Endogenous opiate system 30
HPA axis 30
Anterior cingulate dysfunction 31
Psychological pathways linking BPD to the impact of extreme stress: the role of affect dysregulation 32
Attachment and BPD 34
Theoretical considerations 34
Empirical studies using the AAI 35
Empirical studies using self-report measures of attachment 35
Summary of empirical data 36
Problems with a simple attachment model 37
Conclusions 37

Chapter 2: Therapy research and outcome 39

Psychological treatments 40
Psychoanalytic psychotherapy 40
Empirical evidence for mentalization-based psychoanalytic treatment 43
Results 44
Cognitive analytic therapy 46
Cognitive therapy 46
Dialectical behaviour therapy (DBT) 47
Therapeutic community treatments 49
Drug treatments 50
Antipsychotic drugs 51
Antidepressant drugs 51
Mood stabilizers 51
Problems of outcome research 52
Randomization and personality disorder 52

Chapter 3: Mentalization-based understanding of borderline personality disorder 55

The developmental roots of borderline personality disorder 55
The relevance of the attachment theory perspective 56
Optimal self-development in a secure attachment context 57
Early stages of self-development 59
The infant's sensitivity to social contingency 59
The teleological stance 61
The self as an intentional and representational agent 62
Parental mirroring and the development of mental state concepts 64
Psychic equivalence and the pretend mode 68
Mentalization 70
Reflective function and attachment 75
Neurological basis of mentalization 79
The impact of an insecure base 82
The failure of mirroring 82
Lack of playfulness 83
Enfeebled affect representation and attentional control 85
Disorganization of attachment 87
Establishment of the 'alien self' 88
Controlling IWM 90
The impact of attachment trauma 91
Failure of mentalization 92
Changes to the arousal 'switch' 94
Psychic equivalence, shame, and the teleological stance 96
Failure of mentalization and the exposure of the 'alien self' 97
Interpersonal relating and the transference 99
Self-harm 100
Suicide 101
Impulsive acts of violence 101
Clinical illustration 103
Remembering trauma 104
Conclusion 109

Chapter 4: Current models of treatment for borderline personality disorder 111

Transference-focused psychotherapy (TFP) 112
Evaluation 117
Dialectical behaviour therapy 119
Dialectics 119
Emotional dysregulation 121
Mentalization and mindfulness 122
Practice 124

Cognitive behavioural therapy 126
Cognitive analytic therapy (CAT) 129
  Reciprocal roles 129
  Reformulation and interpretation 130
Psychodynamic-interpersonal 132
Therapeutic communities 134
Other North American approaches 135
Other European approaches 139
Mentalization: The common theme in psychotherapeutic approaches to borderline personality disorder 141
Conclusion 144

Chapter 5: Treatment organization 145

Introduction 145
Service models 145
  One-team model 146
  Treatment context 147
  Treatment guidelines 147
The treatment programmes 148
Staff 150
  The selection of staff 150
  Characteristics of training 152
  The team 152
  The key worker or primary clinician 153
  The responsible medical officer 154
Assessment 156
Engagement in treatment 158
  Pathway to admission 159
    Provision of information 159
      Clarification of key problems, as identified by the patient 160
      Explanation of the underlying treatment approach and its relevance to the problems 160
      Information about individual and group therapy and how it can lead to change 160
      An outline of confidentiality 161
    Clarification of some basic rules 161
      Violence 161
      Drugs and alcohol 161
      Sexual relationships 162
  Stabilizing social aspects of care 162
  Assuring the possibility of contact with the patient 162
  Clear-agreed goals 163
  Defining and agreeing roles of mental health professionals and others involved in the care of the patient 164

History taking 165
Interpersonal behaviour and intimate relationships 165
Previous treatments and their outcome 166
Formation of relational and working alliance 167
Empathy and validation 167
Reliability and readiness to listen 169
Dynamic formulation 169
Example of formulation 170
Expressive therapies 172
General strategic recommendations 173
Organization 173
Specific recommendations 173
Common problems 174
Drop-outs 174
In-patient care 174
Supporting the team 175
Team morale 175
Supervision 177
Care programme approach 179
Adherence 180
Conclusions 181

Chapter 6: Transferable features of the MBT model 183

Structure 183
Principle 183
Rationale 184
Boundary violations 184
Implementation 186
Consistency, constancy, and coherence 187
Principle 187
Rationale 187
Implementation 188
Relationship focus 189
Principle 189
Rationale 189
Implementation 190
Flexibility 191
Principle 191
Rationale 191
Implementation 191
Intensity 192
Principle 192
Rationale 193
Implementation 194

Individual approach to care 194
  Principle 194
  Rationale 194
  Implementation 195
Use of medication 195
  Principle 195
  Rationale 196
  Implementation 196
  Summary of guidelines for psychopharmacological treatment 199
Integration of modalities of therapy 200
Conclusions 201

Chapter 7: Strategies of treatment 203

Enhancing mentalization 203
Bridging the gaps 205
Transference 207
Retaining mental closeness 210
  Countertransference 211
Working with current mental states 212
Bearing in mind the deficits 214
Real relationships 216
  Working with memories 217
  Hyperactive mentalization and pretend mode 218
Conclusions 220

Chapter 8: Techniques of treatment 221

Identification and appropriate expression of affect 222
  General principles 222
    Rationale 222
    General strategic recommendations for identification of affects 222
    Individual session 222
    Group psychotherapy 223
  Impulse control 224
    General principles 224
      Rationale 224
      General strategic recommendations for dealing with problems of impulse control 225
      Suicide attempts and self-harm 225
        Suicide 228
        Self-harm 230
      Individual therapy 231
      Group therapy 232

Other challenging affect states 233
General principles 233
Rationale 233
General strategic recommendations 234
Aggression related to paranoid anxiety 234
Individual session 236
Group therapy 237
Passive aggression 238
Individual session 238
Group therapy 239
Envy 240
Individual session 240
Group therapy 241
Idealization 242
Individual session 242
Group therapy 243
Sexual attraction 244
Individual session 245
Group therapy 246
Hate and contempt 247
Individual session 248
Group therapy 249
Love and attachment 250
Individual session 250
Group therapy 251
Establishment of stable representational systems 252
General principles 252
Rationale 252
General strategic recommendations 253
Individual and group sessions 253
Identifying primary beliefs and linking them to affects 254
Identifying and understanding second-order belief states 256
Exploring wishes, hopes, fears, and other motivational states 257
Individual therapy 258
Group therapy 259
Formation of a coherent sense of self 260
General principles 260
Rationale 260
General strategic recommendations 261
Individual therapy 261
Group therapy 262
Development of a capacity to form secure relationships 263
General principles 263
Rationale 263
General strategic recommendations 265
Individual therapy 265
Group therapy 266
Conclusions 267

Chapter 9: Implementation pathway 269

Step 1: Consider the context in which you work, identify your skills and how you practice, and audit your resources 270
- Context 270
- Skills 271
- Audit of resources 272

Step 2: Apply organizational principles 272
- Structure 273
- Clarity 274
- Consistency 274
- Relationship focus 275
- Intensity 276
- Medication 277

Step 3: Modify the aims and techniques of your current practice 278
- Identify iatrogenic aspects of current practice 278
- Increase mentalization skill set incrementally to replace current iatrogenic techniques 279

Step 4: Implement procedures for dealing with challenging behaviours 281

Step 5: Constantly evaluate your practice 281
- Therapy adherence 281
- Systemic adherence 282
- Patient experience of treatment 282

Appendix 1: Suicide and self-harm inventory 287

Appendix 2: Training materials 301

Appendix 3: Crisis plan 313

Appendix 4: Rating of MBT adherence and competence 315

Appendix 5: Text of intensive out-patient programme (IOP) leaflet 319

Appendix 6: Admission feedback questionnaire 321

References 323

Index 373

About the authors

Dr Anthony Bateman is Clinical Head and Research Lead of Psychotherapy Services at Halliwick Unit, St Ann's Hospital, North London and Honorary Senior Lecturer Royal Free and University College Medical School, London. He is Clinical Tutor of Education for St Ann's Hospital, Deputy Chief Examiner of the Royal College of Psychiatrists, and holds other National positions including Chair of Psychotherapy Training Committee for the UK. His clinical and research interest is in personality disorder and attachment theory. He has authored several books, numerous chapters, and many articles on personality disorder. Recent books include *Introduction to Psychoanalysis* (with J. Holmes —published 1995 by Routledge), *Integration in Psychotherapy* (with J. Holmes —published 2000 by Routledge), and *Introduction to Psychotherapy* (with D. Brown and J. Pedder—published 2001 by Oxford University Press).

Peter Fonagy, PhD FBA is Freud Memorial Professor of Psychoanalysis and Director of the Sub-Department of Clinical Health Psychology at University College London. He is Chief Executive of the Anna Freud Centre, London. He is a clinical psychologist and a training and supervising analyst in the British Psycho-Analytical Society in child and adult analysis. His clinical interests centre around issues of borderline psychopathology, violence, and early attachment relationships. His work attempts to integrate empirical research with psychoanalytic theory. He holds a number of important positions, which include Chairing the Research Committee of the International Psychoanalytic Association, and Fellowship of the British Academy. He has published over 200 chapters and articles and has authored or edited several books. His most recent books include *Attachment Theory and Psychoanalysis* (published 2001 by Other Press), *What Works For Whom? A Critical Review of Treatments for Children and Adolescents* (with M. Target, D. Cottrell, J. Phillips & Z. Kurtz—published 2002 by Guilford), *Affect Regulation, Mentalization, Attachment and the Development of the Self* (with G. Gergely, E. Jurist and M. Target—published 2002 by Other Press) and *Psychoanalytic Theories: Perspectives from Developmental Psychopathology*. (with M. Target—published 2003 by Whurr Publications).

Introduction

The term personality remains one of the most confused and abstract ideas within psychiatry and psychology and there are frequent attempts to discard the concept altogether. Yet each generation of academics and practitioners seem to have to rediscover its significance in clinical practice (Livesley 2001) and over the last decade there has been increasing interest in the notion of personality disorder both in its own right (Rutter 1987; Clarkin and Lenzenweger 1996) and as a problem that interferes with treatment of other mental health problems. The result has been the development of multifaceted treatments which have led to a guarded optimism (Higgitt and Fonagy 1992*b*; Pilkonis *et al.* 1997) that personality is changeable and treatable.

This manual has been developed within this positive climate. Yet, despite the present zeitgeist, considerable problems remain in writing a manual for the treatment of borderline personality disorder. The aim of a manual is to help practitioners organize their thinking about a specific group of patients and to advise them what they need to do to treat them effectively. But even in short-term treatments lasting 12–16 sessions, no manual can cover all the clinical events that may occur during treatment. This is all the more so with this manual which is about a long-term treatment for patients with personality disorder. Manuals addressing long-term treatment are rare and cannot provide adequate detail about every clinical situation. This manual is no exception and you, the practitioner, will have to use discretion and ingenuity.

Aims

The overall aims of this manual are to:

- orientate the reader to our approach;
- ensure that the practitioner knows how to organize the programme;
- outline appropriate use of the strategies, tactics, and techniques;
- stimulate thinking about how to develop creative strategies consistent with the model in the many clinical situations that will arise.

It is important for a number of reasons that the manual is not followed slavishly. First, such an approach is likely to distort the interaction between the patient and therapist, which is itself central to treatment. Second, we describe how we have organized our programme but there is no reason to believe that our arrangement cannot be improved upon. Third, our core interventions focusing on mentalization can be modified to fit with therapeutic models other than the psychoanalytic approach and finally organization of treatment needs to suit the local pattern of services.

Our aim has been not to develop a therapy in its own right using prescriptive interventions which require extensive training but to create an approach to treatment that orientates the thinking of the practitioner and gives a framework in which to use his or her specialist skills. This allows a great deal of flexibility for the practitioner during treatment as long as his focus remains on our core therapeutic aim of increasing mentalization. Thus the manual should act as a learner-driven package to be used with local trainer and peer supervision and we do not anticipate that extensive support and supervision from a centre will be necessary to implement effective treatment. Indeed we trust that readers will recognize that the interventions we describe are things they already do but that we have packaged them more specifically to target the problems that define borderline personality disorder.

When reading the manual, three principal themes about treatment should be kept in mind:

- constantly attempt to establish an attachment relationship with the patient;
- aim to use this to create an interpersonal context in which understanding of mental states becomes a focus;
- attempt (mostly implicitly) to recreate a situation in which understanding the patient's self as intentional and real is a priority and ensure that this endeavour and aim is clearly perceived by the patient.

Organization of manual

The manual is organized into three main sections. The first section, Chapters 1 and 2, gives an overview of borderline personality disorder, including discussion of nosology, epidemiology, natural history, psychosocial aetiology, as well as summarizing the present state of our research knowledge about effective psychotherapeutic treatments and use of medication. The next section, Chapters 3 and 4, outlines our own theoretical approach and contrasts it with other well-known methods. It is in the final section that we outline our clinical approach starting in Chapter 5 with how we have organized treatment. In Chapter 6 we provide a detailed account of the transferable features of our model, before outlining in Chapters 7 and 8 the main strategies and techniques of treatment. The final chapter, Chapter 9, outlines a pathway to implementation in the hope that you, the clinician, can apply aspects of our treatment approach in your everyday practice, gradually extend your use of some of the techniques, and organize a framework around what you do so that patients with BPD will be treated more effectively and humanely.

Those readers who are more interested in the practicalities of treatment than the theoretical basis of our approach are advised to start at Chapter 5. The clinical chapters stand in their own right and there are frequent cross-references back to the theoretical sections of the book. However, the clinical interventions are more understandable if the reader has a grasp of the underpinning theoretical framework, so we recommend at minimum glancing at Chapter 3 before embarking on the rest of the book.

Core component of treatment

There is one concept, namely mentalization, that is a core component of treatment and we will have failed in our endeavours if any reader gets to the end of this book and fails to understand its centrality in how we think about borderline patients, how we organize treatment, and how we focus our interventions. We will therefore outline the concept here as simply as possible to orientate you, the reader, before you start on the manual itself.

Mentalizing is a new word for an ancient concept and bridges psychological and biological process. It is defined here as the mental process by which an individual implicitly and explicitly interprets the actions of himself and others as meaningful on the basis of intentional mental states such as personal desires, needs, feelings, beliefs, and reasons. It is a function of the pre-frontal cortex and is in effect a 'folk psychology' which every individual uses to interact with and to make sense of others as well as themselves. Borderline patients find mentalization hard and especially so in interpersonal and intimate situations because mentalizing interactively is one of the most complex of human tasks. It is at these times that we are all vulnerable to hyperarousal and we need a buffer to protect us against overwhelming affect, and it is mentalization that acts as this cushion. But for borderline patients hyperarousal throws a neurochemical switch which 'takes their pre-frontal cortex offline' and triggers fight and flight and freeze mechanisms. The result is panic responses and impulsive behaviour rather than mentalization. The question, then, for practitioners, is how to facilitate the development of mentalization in borderline patients to 'keep the pre-frontal cortex on line' at times of stress. That is the subject of this manual. We do not believe that we are saying something substantively new but that our mentalization-based treatment (MBT) offers a framework within which different types of models, including cognitive, supportive, and family interventions, can be accommodated as long as their aim is to increase mentalization.

We believe that the addition of mentalization to treatment will increase efficacy because some of the benefit which personality-disordered individuals derive from treatment comes through experience of being involved in a carefully-considered, well-structured and coherent interpersonal endeavour. What may be helpful is the internalization of a thoughtfully-developed structure, the understanding of the inter-relationship of different reliably-identifiable components, the causal interdependence of specific ideas and actions, the constructive interactions of professionals, and above all the experience of being the subject of reliable, coherent, and rational thinking. Social and personal experiences such as these are correlates of the level of seriousness and the degree of commitment with which teams of professionals approach the problem of caring for this group who may be argued on empirical grounds to have been deprived of exactly such consideration and commitment during their early development and quite frequently throughout their later life.

Who is this manual for?

The manual is intended for mental health practitioners who have wide experience of psychiatric treatments and have an interest in and some knowledge of psychoanalytical techniques. Professionals who have well-practised skills in assessing risk and de-escalating crises will have a head-start so clinical experience of working on in-patient wards and within community treatment services is helpful and, as a result, nursing staff are well-placed to be part of a treatment team implementing this manual. It is important that at least one practitioner is well-trained in both psychoanalytic techniques and the psychiatric care of patients with personality disorder and has the skills to take a leadership role. Other practitioners in the team do not need to be highly trained in individual and group psychotherapy but should have experience of organizing and running groups and seeing patients individually.

The treatment described in this manual integrates all aspects of the care of patients with borderline personality disorder. Psychiatric care is integrated with psychological treatment—a psychiatrist is part of the team, in-patient admission is organized through the treatment team when necessary, and medication is an integral aspect of the programme. Implementation requires the patient to be in reasonably stable social circumstances. Whilst unstable social circumstances would not prevent a patient being taken into treatment, it would mean that an urgent initial task would be to help the individual organize adequate and stable accommodation. This necessitates close links with social services and housing departments. The development of a stable internal sense of self, which borderline patients crave, is impossible without a stable external environment.

But it is equally important to say who this manual is not for. It is not for those who cannot work in a team, 'join in', share, and listen, or for those who want to work alone and form private, highly-protected, closed relationships with patients. In our view there is little evidence to suggest that working alone with patients with severe personality disorder is safe and effective. On the contrary it is probably dangerous.

Not all clinicians are able to treat borderline patients even with the help of a manual and extensive training. There is increasing evidence about the influence of therapist characteristics on outcome of psychotherapeutic treatment; they are likely to be highly significant in long-term treatment of personality disorder in which powerful countertransference feelings may stimulate disturbance in the therapist. A low level of generic psychotherapeutic skill and inadequate training will compound the problems. We do not yet know which therapist characteristics are best suited for safe and effective treatment of borderline personality disorder but some personal qualities seem better suited than others. Those who conduct therapy with 'high boundaries' do better than those who are high on 'anaclitic, depressive, and fusion tendencies' (Rosenkrantz 1992) and Gunderson has suggested that therapists who are 'effete, genteel, or controlling' (Gunderson 2001) (p. 253) are positively unworkable as therapists (see Chapter 5 for more discussion).

The authors

We are certainly not effete and controlling but we will leave it to others to bring an objective perspective on our positive and negative characteristics. Both of us are psychoanalysts but one a psychiatrist and programme director of a personality disorder service (AB) and the other an academic and research psychologist (PF). Between us we hope that we have managed to synthesize a treatment which makes sense to mental health professionals and contains within it our breadth of experience and academic rigour. We are only too aware of the many faults of omission and commission in the book and we have not tackled the issues of ethnicity, class, and gender as factors influencing treatment although both men and women from various ethnic groups and different socio-economic class have benefited from treatment within our unit. Apropos of gender, like many contemporary authors we have been stymied by the problem of pronouns, but, in the end, reluctantly have stayed (mostly) with the less obtrusive, but patriarchal 'he', despite the fact that statistically, female borderline patients outnumber males.

We have taken great care to develop clinical vignettes based on our real experiences which are illustrative rather than verbatim reports of events. To that extent they are fictitious and no single vignette represents a specific patient or corresponds precisely to a clinical situation. They are intended to illuminate the topics, to stimulate further discussion, and to guide the reader towards more effective intervention according to our model.

Over the years we have been fortunate to work with many compassionate, 'boundaried', thoughtful, therapists, without whom we would not have been able to write this manual. In their different ways they have all contributed, at times by asking difficult questions and at others by making constructive suggestions. In particular we would like to thank Jeremy Holmes, Catherine Freeman,

Rory Bolton, Kath Sutherland, Marina Gaspodini, Mary Target, Jon Allen, Efrain Bleiberg, George Gergely, and others too numerous to mention who were instrumental in developing the treatment and implementing it. They stuck with it through thick and thin and we can assure people that there were and still are many 'thin' times. Most of all, the patients have let us know, often with great clarity and directness, what is and is not useful, what makes sense and what is confusing, which interventions are helpful and which are singularly unhelpful, and, inevitably, they have pointed out our personal characteristics which have supported a therapeutic relationship and those which have disrupted it. We are grateful to them all and hope that this manual shows that we were listening and 'mentalizing' in a way that we hope many of them are now able to do.

Finally, without Dr. Liz Allison this book would not have been possible. In the writing of the book, her patience, her methodical approach, and her thoughtful attitude acted as an antidote to our moments of brash approximation whilst in the structuring of the chapters her logical mind brought order to chaos and rendered, we hope, our disparate ramblings into a coherent book.

Anthony Bateman
Peter Fonagy
London, August 2003.

1 Epidemiological and etiological research on borderline personality disorder

Definition of the problem

Borderline personality disorder (BPD) is a complex and serious mental disorder that is characterized by a pervasive pattern of difficulties with emotion regulation and impulse control and instability both in relationships and in self-image. (Skodol *et al.* 2002*b*). The current DSM-IV definition refers to: 'a pervasive pattern of instability of mood, interpersonal relationships, self-image and affects and marked impulsivity' (American Psychiatric Association 1994). The DSM-III definition of BPD (American Psychiatric Association 1980) was strongly influenced by a review by Gunderson and Singer (1975). The review emphasized features in areas of social maladaptation, psychotic-like cognitions, relationship difficulties, impulsive action, and dysphoric affect. The criteria changed over the years. For example while the DSM-III definition did not include impulsivity as an essential feature, this was introduced in DSM-IV. DSM-IV also included transient, stress-related paranoid thoughts and severe dissociative symptoms in the definition. Other criteria that have been present since the first systematic definition in DSM-III are a pattern of unstable relationships, affective instability, intolerance of being alone, self-harm, and chronic feelings of emptiness or boredom.

It has been pointed out that because there are nine criteria for BPD, of which only five need to be present to make the diagnosis, 151 different combinations of criteria for a BPD diagnosis are possible (Skodol *et al.* 2002*b*) although Karterud (personal communication) has suggested that this calculation is incorrect and there are in fact 256 combinations. It is possible for two individuals who receive the diagnosis to share only one of the nine criteria. Justifiably, some point to the degree of heterogeneity of presentation as a major barrier to effective research and progress in the field (Hyman 2002). Other shortcomings of the definition include the omission of the proneness to regression and the use of primitive defence mechanisms often seen in those with BPD.

Diagnostic procedures

Semi-structured clinical interviews are to be preferred to unstructured clinical assessment in the diagnosis of BPD, as they give more reliable results. Several instruments are available for this purpose. These include: the Diagnostic Interview for DSM-IV Personality Disorders (Zanarini *et al.* 1987, 2000*b*), the International Personality Disorder Examination (Loranger *et al.* 1994; Loranger 1999), the Structured Interview for DSM-IV Personality Disorder (Pfohl *et al.* 1997) and the Structured Clinical Interview for DSM-IV Axis-II Personality Disorders (SCID-II) (First *et al.* 1995*a,b*). There are no obvious differences between these instruments (Kaye and Shea 2000; Skodol *et al.* 2002*b*). The reliability of these interviews for diagnosing BPD has been high for interrater agreements (r=0.68 – 0.96) and only somewhat lower for test–retest agreements (r=0.40 – 0.85).

Instruments designed specifically for BPD diagnosis include Kernberg's Structural Interview, which aims to assess defences, reality testing, and identity issues (Kernberg 1977) but has no reported reliability, and Gunderson's Diagnostic Interview for Borderlines, which is the only one of the structured interviews to explore the history of the disorder along with the individual's current symptoms (Gunderson *et al.* 1981). Gunderson's instrument has been updated to include more detailed questioning concerning reality testing, cognitions, dysphonic affects, and types of impulse dyscontrol (Zanarini *et al.* 1989).

Thresholds for diagnosis

Borderline personality disorder, like other personality disorders (PDs), is most commonly diagnosed using a categorical approach (present vs absent) but personality in general is normally studied dimensionally assuming a more or less normally distributed set of underlying traits that best describe variation between individuals (Cloninger *et al.* 1993; Blais 1997; Wildgoose *et al.* 2001). There is no agreement that a categorical approach to the diagnosis of BPD is the most appropriate. Many favour a dimensional approach, which would do away with arbitrary thresholds, remove some of the heterogeneity that arises from categorical approaches, and limit the loss of information associated with categorical judgements of BPD (e.g. Clark *et al.* 1997). Empirical support for diagnostic thresholds is problematic at best as it is impossible to distinguish clearly between 'normal' and 'abnormal' personalities. DSM-IV suggests that 'when personality traits are inflexible and maladaptive and cause significant functional impairments or subjective distress do they constitute personality disorders' (American Psychiatric Association 1994, p. 630). The problem with the categorical approach is not that the wrong individuals are being identified, since the individuals identified by criteria as having BPD are indeed normally different from comparison groups, but that this method of diagnosis is insufficiently sensitive. Many of those not meeting criteria, say amongst a group of depressed patients, will have three or more features of BPD, and this is likely to have an impact on the course and outcome of their treatment (e.g. McGlashan 1987).

Epidemiology

Borderline personality disorder is a common condition with a prevalence of between 0.2% and 1.8% of the general population (Swartz *et al.* 1990) but most studies originate from North America and the situation may be different elsewhere. The most reliable study of the prevalence of the disorder in a community sample conducted in Oslo (Torgersen *et al.* 2001) suggested that the prevalence of BPD was not as frequent as commonly assumed; only 0.7% of patients from a representative community sample were diagnosed as borderline. Prevalence rates increase if patients within the mental health system are sampled. The highest prevalence rates are found in those patients requiring the most intensive level of care—out-patient rates range from 8% to 11%, in-patient from 14% to 20%, and forensic services from 60% to 80%. In a Dutch forensic psychiatric hospital, 80% of patients fulfilled criteria for at least one PD, with paranoid, antisocial, and borderline being the most common (Ruiter and Greeven 2000). Similar rates have been found in England and Sweden (Blackburn *et al.* 1990) with the most common being BPD and ASPD (Dolan and Coid 1993).

Clinical picture

Individuals with BPD display severe functional impairment (e.g. unemployment, failed interpersonal relationships). They are major utilizers of services and almost 10% commit suicide (Work Group on Borderline Personality Disorder, 2001).

Phenomenological picture

The DSM criteria do not yet include important aspects of the cognitive function in borderline patients. For example, cognitive therapists Beck and Freeman (1990) identified all-or-nothing, or 'black or white' thinking as typical of BPD. In addition, they suggested three disturbed cognitive schemata for BPD: (1) 'the world is dangerous and malevolent', (2) 'I am powerless and vulnerable' and (3) 'I am inherently unacceptable'. Mary Zanarini and colleagues (1998) suggested a further three typical cognitions: (1) 'I am endangered', (2) 'I am like a small child', and (3) 'I feel uncared for'.

Some patients with BPD under stress develop paranoid symptoms when they may have ideas of reference, display magical thinking and become suspicious of others. These may be termed mini psychotic episodes and are most likely to occur in the context of some interpersonal crisis that has made the patient feel that they have been abandoned. Prolonged psychotic episodes are unusual in BPD.

Several studies have attempted to identify the underlying dimensions of borderline phenomenology. One of these studies has found a single factor (Fossati *et al.* 1999*b*) but others tended to identify either two (Rosenberg and Miller 1989) or three factors (Clarkin *et al.* 1993*b*; Sanislow *et al.* 2000). The factors normally include a dimension of disturbed relatedness, emotional dysregulation, and impulsivity or behavioural dyscontrol.

Functional impairment

A large number of epidemiological studies speak indirectly to the functional impairment of borderline patients. Sociodemographic status variables are likely to reflect psychosocial function. Thus, epidemiological investigations commonly show those with PD diagnoses to be separated, divorced, or never married (e.g. Swartz *et al.* 1990) and to have had more unemployment, frequent job changes, or periods of disability (e.g. Reich *et al.* 1989). Studies looking directly at the quality of functioning have consistently shown poorer social functioning or interpersonal relations (e.g. Modestin and Villiger 1989) and poorer work functioning and occupational achievement (e.g. McGlashan 1983). Similarly, on global measures of functioning, BPD patients show substantial deficits (e.g. Paris *et al.* 1987). The most definitive findings come from the Collaborative Longitudinal Personality Disorder Study (Skodol *et al.* 2002*a*). In this study, 668 patients with at least one of four PDs or with major depressive disorder (MDD) and no PD was carefully diagnosed and assessed on the Longitudinal Interval Follow-up Evaluation Interview (Keller *et al.* 1987). Patients with borderline diagnoses were found to have more instances of severe impairment of functioning in the areas of employment, interpersonal relationships with parents and siblings, in global social adjustment, and on the GAF when compared to individuals with MDDs. Overall, patients with schizotypal PD and BPD were shown to have more impairments at work, in social relationships, and at leisure than patients with obsessive-compulsive PD and major depression. This is an important demonstration since these differences remain marked when Axis I symptoms have been taken into account. This suggests that PD per se undermines functioning in these areas.

Psychodynamic picture

BPO

The original descriptions of BPD were offered by Stern (1938) and Knight (1953). Kernberg (1967) was the first to systematize these features. He delineated borderline personality organization (BPO) and placed it between personality organizations to be found in psychotic and neurotic conditions. The four intrapsychic features pointed to by Kernberg were: (1) identity diffusion, (2) primitive defences of projection, projective identification, splitting, denial, (3) partially intact reality testing that is vulnerable to alterations and failures, and (4) characteristic object relations. A psychometric instrument, the Inventory of Personality Organization (Kernberg and Clarkin 1995) bears out Kernberg's assumptions in its latent structure. It yields three factors: primitive defences, identity diffusion, and reality testing (Lenzenweger *et al.* 2001).

Defence mechanisms

Empirical studies have demonstrated the value of characterizing defence mechanisms specific to BPD. For example, patients with BPD have been shown to use the defences of splitting and acting out more than, and the defences of suppression, sublimation, and humour less than non-BPD patients (Bond *et al.* 1994). In another study, hypochondriasis, projection, acting out, and undoing were found to discriminate patients with BPD from patients with other PDs (Zanarini *et al.* 1990). Those with a cognitive behavioural orientation have also noted that BPD patients engage in 'dichotomous thinking' (splitting) although it is claimed that such dichotomous thinking should not be characterized as simply seeing a person as 'all good' or 'all bad' but rather as a tendency to describe a person as possessing extreme qualities of character ("the most brilliant") but not necessarily all of the same valence (Veen and Arntz, 2000).

Object relations

A study comparing patients with BPD with those with either ASPD or bipolar II disorder (Perry and Cooper 1986) found greater anxieties about separation and abandonment, and greater conflict about the expression of emotional need and anger in borderline patients. BPD patients show a tendency to rely on transitional objects almost like children develop deep attachments to soft toys and teddy bears. A series of studies have documented that about 30% of adult patients with BPD use and rely upon transitional objects (Cardasis *et al.* 1997) although comparison figures for 'normal adults' are unavailable. This is suggested to reflect BPD patients' failed early attachment experiences (Modell 1963). It has been suggested that these experiences tend to be of the anxious-ambivalent sub-type (Fonagy *et al.* 1995*a*; Gunderson 1996).

At least seven studies have demonstrated extremely insecure attachments in patients with BPD, characterized by alternating fear of involvement and intense neediness (see summaries in Dozier *et al.* 1999; Bartholomew *et al.* 2001; pp 34–37, this volume). A questionnaire study of 1400 students found that those with high BPD ratings were distinguished by being significantly less secure and more fearful and more pre-occupied in their attachment styles (Brennan and Shaver 1998). Several studies have provided data on the relations between adult attachment styles, BPD, and maltreatment. For example, Salzman and colleagues (1997) reported that participants meeting diagnostic criteria for BPD can be classified as demonstrating ambivalent attachment and this feature is more helpful in identifying the group than other associated characteristics such as a history of abuse. In a convenience sample of 400 18-year-old university students screened for BPD features, parental bonding and attachment patterns were found to be related to BPD features (Nickell *et al.* 2002). The variables most strongly related to BPD features were lack of expressed care and over-protection by mother and an anxious and ambivalent attachment pattern. When gender, loss, physical and sexual abuse, and any other Axis I or Axis II diagnosis were adjusted for, the reports of parental bonding patterns and attachment patterns accounted for a significant additional variability in predicting borderline personality scores. In one study attachment, security and BPD features were shown to be related and in combination to predict response to treatment. In a naturalistic prospective study, 149 patients were assessed at the time of entering treatment (psychological, pharmacological, or both) (Meyer *et al.* 2001). They were assessed for both PD and attachment styles. Outcome at six months was predicted by both security of attachment and BPD symptom severity at intake. However, this applied only to clinician-assessed changes in functioning. A self-report measure of symptomatology (SCL-90) was not associated with either attachment or BPD.

The loose coupling of attachment representations and personality traits associated with BPD was demonstrated in a study of 44 BPD, 98 other Cluster B, 30 Cluster A and 70 non-PD patients and 206 non-clinical controls (Fossati *et al.* 2001). Patients were administered the Temperament and Character Inventory which measures Cloninger's trait dimensions assumed to link to PD and the Attachment Style Questionnaire and the Parental Bonding Instrument. BPD patients differed from all other groups on novelty-seeking and co-operativeness and this difference was not mediated by attachment style or parental bonding. This indicates that attachment representation disturbances are a separate and independent aspect of pathology from the temperament dimensions observed by Links and others (Links *et al.* 1999). Individuals with antisocial tendencies are well-characterized by their dismissiveness of attachment and attachment-related experiences (Frodi *et al.* 2001). In this latter study of 24 psychopathic criminal offenders, idealization of mother and a representation of father as rejecting (markers of dismissing-insecure attachment classification) were both correlated with scores on psychopathy.

Co-morbidity

Skodol et al. (2002*b*) reviewed 16 studies where structured or semi-structured diagnostic instruments were used to establish co-morbidity. The findings are consistent. In a series of 409 non-psychotic outpatients, 59 were diagnosed with BPD. Only one of these did not have a concurrent Axis-I diagnosis and over two-thirds had three or more Axis-I diagnoses (Zimmerman and Mattia 1999). Sixty-one percent were diagnosed with MDD while 29% had panic disorder with agoraphobia and 13% substance misuse. In the biggest study of subjects with PD comprehensively assessed for Axis-I and Axis-II disorders using both semi-structured interviews and self-rating scales, of 501 patients, 240 were diagnosed with BPD (Skodol *et al.* 1999). Almost 40% of the BPD cases met criteria for at least one mood disorder. 31% had major depression, 16% had dysthymia, 9% had bipolar-I and 4% bipolar-II. A patient's response to treatment of an Axis-I disorder is invariably worse if s/he also has BPD (e.g. Ilardi *et al.* 1997).

Co-morbidity may be an artefact of overlapping symptom sets used to define co-occurring disorders. Criteria for BPD include affective instability and recurrent suicidal threats or behaviours, both of which overlap with symptoms of MDD. Similarly, overlapping diagnostic criteria could account for the association of attention deficit hyperactivity disorder (ADHD) and BPD (Rey *et al.* 1995), as impulsivity, erratic behaviours, interpersonal problems, and moodiness are features of both disorders. Alternatively, co-morbidity may be the result of the presence of a third disorder. For example, it has been suggested that the co-occurrence of internalizing and externalizing disorder in young people may be the consequence of a characterological pre-disposition that makes young people vulnerable, perhaps in association with psycho-social stress (Gunderson and Elliott 1985). This would explain why Cluster B PD is so common in depressed conduct-disordered adolescents (Crawford *et al.* 2001*b*; Eppright *et al.* 1993).

The alternative hypothesis is that borderline and other Cluster B symptomatology is a complication that arises from a primary affective disorder (Akiskal 1983; Akiskal *et al.* 1983). Thus, interpersonal maladjustment may be a residue of depressive illness and chronic PD may result from recurrent depressive episodes. Consistent with this hypothesis, Crawford and colleagues (2001*b*) demonstrated that internalizing symptoms at age 10–14 predict Cluster B symptoms three years later in girls. Also in girls, externalizing symptoms in middle adolescence predict Cluster B symptoms in young adulthood. However, Cluster B symptoms in 10–14-year-old girls and boys were found to predict externalizing symptoms in adolescence. The results however speak most eloquently for the stability of Cluster B symptoms across development, which in turn is consistent with a genetic temperamental account (see below).

Dimensional models of BPD

Alternative to categorical descriptions of BPD are approaches that assume that PD is an amplification of normal personality traits (Paris 1998*b*). The best established is Cloninger *et al.*'s eight-factor model incorporated in the Temperament and Character Inventory (Cloninger *et al.* 1993). The dimensions suggested are: (1) novelty seeking, (2) harm avoidance, (3) reward dependence, (4) persistence, (5) self-directedness (autonomy), (6) co-operativeness, (7) compassion, and (8) self-transcendence (identity). More recently, Shedler and Westen proposed a clinician-oriented dimensional assessment procedure that asks the clinician to sort 200 personality characteristics into stacks of increasing applicability to an individual patient (Westen 1998; Westen and Shedler 1999*a*,*b*; Shedler 2002). The sort yields similarity scores to prototypes (profiles of characteristics) well-recognized by clinicians: (1) psychological health, (2) psychopathy, (3) hostility, (4) narcissism, (5) emotional dysregulation, (6) dysphoria, (7) schizoid orientation, (8) obsessionality, (9) thought disorder, (10) oedipal conflict, (11) dissociated, and (12) sexual conflict.

A range of studies reported BPD to be associated with temperament characterized by a high degree of neuroticism (i.e. emotional pain) and a low degree of agreeableness (i.e. strong individuality) (Clarkin *et al.* 1993*a*; Soldz *et al.* 1993; Trull 1993; Zweig-Frank and Paris 1995). BPD has also been shown to be associated with a high degree of harm avoidance (i.e. compulsivity) and novelty-seeking (i.e. impulsivity) (Svrakic *et al.* 1993). For BPD the key dimensions are likely to involve impulsive aggression and affective instability. In a factor analysis of 18 personality traits assessed in the general population (n=939), in patients with PD (n=656), and in twins (n=686 pairs) a four-factor solution was found (Livesley *et al.* 1992). The four factors were emotional dysregulation, dissocial behaviour, inhibitedness, and compulsivity. There seems to be a general consensus that impulsivity and negative affectivity/emotional dysregulation characterize BPD and possibly mediate the influence of psychosocial factors on BPD (Gurvits *et al.* 2000; Paris 2000; Silk 2000; Trull *et al.* 2000). It is the combination of impulsivity and negative affectivity that appears uniquely characteristic of BPD. Negative affectivity can be found in Narcissistic personality disorder (NPD) while impulsivity is evidently marked in ASPD.

Naturally, personality traits like affective instability or impulsive aggression are not unrelated to the putative intrapsychic disturbances such as identity disturbance or defense mechanisms such as passive aggression. In one study of 140 PD patients, degree of affective instability was found to be correlated with identity disturbance, chronic emptiness and boredom, defensive splitting, projection, acting out, and somatization (Koenigsberg *et al.* 2001). This kind of association is to be expected given that the phenomena upon which these apparently alternative modes of observation are made are the same.

However, the question of causality is moot. While dimensions such as affective instability and impulsiveness are known to be in part biologically-determined, the association with intrapsychic defenses may not be accounted for by the biological components of these traits. Nevertheless, the associations of trait and psychodynamic descriptions of BPD indicate the desirability of a multimodal approach to the aetiology of BPD.

The natural history of BPD

The stability of the diagnosis over time

This has been looked at in 13 studies. Some studies have found extremely low stability. For example, one study of 14 adolescents found 14% three-year-stability (Meijer *et al.* 1998), while at the other extreme 78% stability was found in a 18-months to 42-months follow-up of nine out of 30 in-patients. In general, the stability of BPD has a strong inverse relationship with the length of follow-up (McDavid and Pilkonis 1996). In a survey of 733 adolescents ranging in age from 11 to 21, Bernstein and colleagues (1993) found that adolescents with a severe diagnosis of BPD were 13 times more likely to have the same diagnosis two years later than participants without this initial diagnosis. However, when taken as a group, Cluster B disorders persisted for only 22% to 31% of those originally diagnosed with the same Axis II disorders. When assessed in a community sample of female adolescents, two-year stability estimates for Cluster B symptoms ranged between 0.51 and 0.65 depending upon the measurement instruments used (Daley *et al.* 1999). In a similar study of a community sample of 407 adolescents (Crawford *et al.* 2001*a*), Cluster B symptoms were found to be highly stable across an eight-year interval from early adolescence to early adulthood (from age 12 to age 20). Stability estimates were 0.63 in boys and 0.69 in girls. Interestingly, these stability coefficients are stronger than those observed for either internalizing (0.24) or externalizing symptoms (0.32) over the same period.

This suggests that Axis II symptoms are developmentally more stable than Axis I symptoms across this age group. By contrast, in a college student sample, the stability of borderline symptoms across two years ranged between 0.28 and 0.65 (Trull *et al.* 1998). It seems that when assessed as latent variables indicated by dimensional scales, dramatic-erratic personality traits are more stable from early adolescence into early adulthood than when measured as categorically-defined diagnoses. Cluster B personality dysfunction appears to diminish with age, but the odds of rediagnosis of BPD diminish less over time. Given the high stability of maladaptive personality traits from early adolescence into adulthood, sub-threshold but clinically significant Cluster B disturbances are likely to persist over time (Crawford *et al.* 2001*a*).

The course of BPD

There is surprisingly little information about the childhood precursors of adult PD. The Collaborative Longitudinal Personality Disorder Study suggests that a history of MDD with insidious onset in adolescence and recurrence, chronicity and progressive severity is particularly likely to be associated with adult PD (Skodol *et al.* 1999). A study of a random sample of 551 youths (Kasen *et al.* 2001) reported that the presence of MDD in adolescence increased the likelihood of the diagnosis of dependent PD, ASPD, passive-aggressive and histrionic PD, but not BPD. However, the odds ratios in this report were adjusted for childhood maltreatment and if MDD in BPD was principally a reaction to childhood abuse then MDD would not be observed to be associated with BPD in this analysis. A longitudinal study of 407 adolescents (208 boys and 199 girls) recruited from a community sample looked at the predictive significance of internalizing and externalizing symptoms for the development of Cluster B characteristics (Crawford *et al.* 2001*b*). The pattern for girls indicates that externalizing symptoms in adolescence (12–17) predict Cluster B symptoms at 17–24, even when earlier Cluster B symptoms are controlled for. However, early (10–14) internalizing symptoms (anxiety and depression) also predicted Cluster B symptoms in adolescence. The pattern for girls at least appears from this study to be that early internalizing symptoms predict adolescent Cluster B symptoms but adolescent externalizing symptoms predict adult Cluster B symptoms. The findings are intriguing because for boys there appears to be no forward prediction of Cluster B symptoms from either internalizing or externalizing symptoms. This finding complements the retrospective observation that antisocial behaviour in female adolescents is associated with BPD symptoms in early adulthood (Goodman *et al.* 1999). There are those who recommend the establishment of the diagnosis of BPD in childhood. A review of the literature (e.g. Ad-Dab'bagh and Greenfield, 2001) supports the creation of a new diagnostic label to describe a population of children whose symptoms are currently subsumed under the labels 'borderline' or 'multiple complex developmental disorder.' A full characterization of the syndrome, including its evolution, would require prospective studies and may differ from the known evolution for PD and/or pervasive developmental disorders.

There are a number of studies of the course of BPD although most have methodological problems. The studies tend to show reasonable stability for BPD, although less than one might expect for a PD (Paris 1998*a;* Grilo *et al.* 2000). The clinical course is somewhat heterogeneous even within samples. Borderline patients improve symptomatically over time. One exceptionally long (27-year) follow-up (Paris and Zweig-Frank 2001) showed that borderline patients continued to improve in late middle-age with only 8% of the BPD sample meriting diagnosis of BPD. Long-term outcome in this study was associated with severity of the disorder and the quality of adaptation (functioning) at the start of the study but not with parenting quality or child abuse or trauma (Zweig-Frank and Paris, 2002).

A definitive study (Zanarini *et al.* 2003) followed the syndromal and sub-syndromal phenomenology of 362 adult in-patients with PD over 6 years of prospective follow-up. The cohort was assessed with the Revised Diagnostic Interview for Borderlines (DIB-R) and BPD module of the Revised Diagnostic Interview for DSM-III-R Personality Disorders. Of these patients, 290 met DIB-R and DSM-III-R criteria for BPD and 72 met DSM-III-R criteria for other axis II disorders (and neither criteria set for BPD). Over 94% of the total surviving subjects were reassessed at 2, 4, and 6 years by interviewers blind to previously collected information. Of the subjects with BPD over one-third met the criteria for remission at 2 years, half at 4 years, and over two-thirds at 6 years. When the entire follow-up period was considered almost three quarters could be considered to have recovered at some stage and only 6% of those with remissions experienced recurrences. Importantly, the comparison subjects with other axis II disorders did not develop BPD over the course of the follow-up. The patients with BPD had declining rates of symptoms but remained symptomatically distinct from the comparison subjects. Comparing the rate at which categories of symptoms decline, the study found impulsive symptoms to resolve most quickly and affective symptoms to be the most chronic. Cognitive and interpersonal symptoms were intermediate in the rate of decline. The results suggest that symptomatic improvement is both common and stable, even among the most disturbed borderline patients, and that the symptomatic prognosis for most, but not all, severely ill borderline patients is better than previously recognized.

This contrasts with the relative stability of the disorder in late adolescence and young adulthood. In a study of the stability of Cluster B symptoms between the ages of 12 and 20, Crawford and colleagues reported higher stability for PD symptoms than for Axis I symptoms (internalizing and externalizing) (Crawford *et al.* 2001*a*). The stability for Cluster B symptoms was 0.63 for boys and 0.69 for girls whereas the stability for internalizing symptoms was 0.24 and 0.39 and externalizing symptoms 0.32 and 0.38 for girls and boys respectively. These findings underscore the persistence of normal and abnormal personality constellations. The lower stability of Axis I symptoms may be disguised by some developmental heterotypy (i.e. different manifestations of the same underlying disorder at different developmental stages). Nevertheless, the stability of Cluster B disturbance is striking and many might interpret this as supporting the link of Cluster B with biologically predetermined personality dispositions such as novelty seeking where genetic loadings are high (Livesley *et al.* 1998).

Borderline personality disorder patients who have been sexually abused in childhood (Paris *et al.* 1993; 1994*a*,*b*) or have been victims of incest (Stone, 1990) have a poor prognosis. If the patient's first psychiatric contact takes place at an early age (Links *et al.* 1993) and his/her symptoms are chronic, spontaneous recovery is less likely (McGlashan 1992). Phenomenological factors that predict poor outcome include higher levels of affective instability, magical thinking, and aggression in relationships (McGlashan 1992), impulsivity and substance abuse (Links *et al.* 1993), and greater severity of disorder (Links *et al.* 1998). Further, if the patients have co-morbid schizotypal (McGlashan 1986), antisocial (Stone 1993), or paranoid features, then the prognosis is likely to be poor (Links *et al.* 1998).

The evidence consistently suggests that even if the diagnosis of BPD ceases to be applicable, patients tend to remain functionally seriously impaired (Skodol *et al.* 2002*c*).

Studies of mechanisms and aetiological factors

Biological considerations

Biological markers

In the hope of identifying a mechanism for BPD, a number of studies have attempted to identify biological markers for BPD or traits related to the disorder. For example, a Finnish study reported low total serum cholesterol levels in a group of suicidal criminal offenders with early onset conduct disorder (Repo-Tiihonen *et al.* 2002). The search for a definitive biological marker has not so far been successful. As our understanding of the pathology of the disorder improves, definitive biological markers and more homogeneous descriptions of subtypes are bound to follow. We must remember that, as the brain is the origin of the mind, the identification of biological markers cannot be considered to imply a de-emphasis of psychosocial aspects of causation. The impact of these experiences will be as evident at biological as at psychological levels of observation.

Genetic studies

Original family studies of schizophrenia established the independence of BPD from schizophrenia and schizotypal PD (Nigg and Goldsmith 1994). This led to an alternative suggestion that BPD was linked to mood disorder (Stone *et al.* 1981). These findings were based on BPO rather than the BPD criteria. Further, co-morbidity with depression might reflect the high base rates of both BPD and depression in clinical samples. Studies that have reported depression in the relatives of individuals with BPD did not control in all cases for co-morbid mood disorder in the BPD probands (Schultz *et al.* 1989). When mood disorder is assessed blind to the PD diagnosis, depression is only found in the relatives of depressed borderlines (Zanarini *et al.* 1988) which suggests that family studies speak to the heritability of BPD rather than a link between depression and BPD.

The major twin study so far is the Norwegian study by Torgersen and colleagues (2000). Based on twin and patient registers 92 MZ and 129 DZ twin pairs were interviewed with SCID-II and contrasted with normal prevalence rates of more than 2000 individuals. The study found 38% concordance in MZ and 11% in DZ twins with a broad definition (three or more criteria met) and 35% and 7% with the narrow definition of BPD (i.e. five or more criteria met). Heritability for PDs generally was 0.60 with 0.37 for Cluster A, 0.60 for Cluster B, and 0.62 for Cluster C. Among the specific PDs narcissistic was 0.79, obsessive compulsive was 0.78, and borderline 0.69. Best fitting models never included shared environmental effects. The study could not model ASPD because of the low sample size. Unfortunately, the interviewers interviewed both twins and were not blind to zygosity, and this is known to inflate genetic effects. Nevertheless, there is a clear indication here that genetic factors are critical in the aetiology of BPD.

Trait or dimensional approaches are more appropriate for the study of the heritability of BPD, as we must assume that it is one of the brain mechanisms underlying personality differences that exist at extreme levels in BPD. The results of twin studies show that the heritability of traits delineating personality disorder is 35–56% (Jang *et al.* 1996). Phenotypic factor analyses look at the structure underlying a matrix of correlations derived from measures of multiple traits. Multivariate genetic analyses are applied to a matrix of genetic correlations. The data from MZ and DZ twins may be used to partition phenotypic correlations between two traits into genetic and environmental components. When this method is applied to the eight basic dimensions assessed (by the Dimensional Assessment of Personality Pathology Baseline Questionnaire) a four-factor structure of the inherited components of BPD emerges (Livesley *et al.* 1998). The large first factor contained: general tendency towards labile affects, unstable cognitive functioning, unstable sense of self, and unstable interpersonal relationships. This strongly resembles the clinical picture of BPD. The fact that the genetic structure strongly resembles the phenotypic structure suggests that the pattern of traits in BPD is highly heritable. A further study of 112 child twin pairs (70 MZ and 42 DZ) asked parents to assess features of PD and neuropsychological dysfunctional features (Coolidge *et al.* 2001). The median heritability for the 12 PD scales was 0.75 with the BPD scale yielding a heritability of 0.70. However, the sample was not recruited with representativeness in mind, and parents' ratings tend to yield higher heritability estimates than interview or self-rating studies as parents are not blind to zygosity.

Twin studies consistently show that aggressive antisocial behaviour is more heritable than non-aggressive antisocial behaviour (Eley *et al.* 1999). In a meta-analysis of twin and adoption studies (Rhee and Waldman 2002), moderate additive genetic, non-additive, shared environmental, and non-shared environmental influences on anti-social behaviour were found. Impulsive aggression is heritable in twin and adoption studies and can be measured in laboratory tests and has been consistently linked with biological indices, particularly serotonergic activity.

Neurotransmitter abnormality

Studies have repeatedly demonstrated that the metabolites of serotonin are altered amongst those who have attempted suicide (Asberg *et al.* 1976) or manifest externally-directed aggression (Coccaro 1998). Those who display impulsive aggression consistently show blunted neuro-endocrinal responses to agents that enhance serotonergic activities (Coccaro *et al.* 1996). It seems that impulsiveness, autoaggression, and outwardly-directed aggression are all associated with dysfunctions of the serotonergic system indicated by low 5-hydroxyindoleaceticacid levels in lumbar cerebro-spinal fluid (CSF) (Linnoila and Virkkunen 1992) and blunted neuroendocrine responses to fenfluramine (O'Keane *et al.* 1992; Herpertz *et al.* 1995; Cleare *et al.* 1996). There is some degree of cortical localization of these abnormalities to areas involved in inhibiting limbic aggression in the orbital-frontal cortex, ventral-medial cortex and cingulate cortex which show decreased activation in response to serotonergic probes (Siever *et al.* 1999; New *et al.* 2002). Reduced serotonergic modulation of these inhibitory areas may result in the disinhibition of aggression. It is consistent with this assumption that selective serotonin re-uptake inhibitors (SSRIs) appear effective in reducing impulsive aggression independent of depression when used in higher doses and/or for longer durations (Markovitz *et al.* 1991; Coccaro *et al.* 1997). The study of 5HT synthesis capacity using PET in medication-free BPD subjects (Leyton *et al.* 2001) provided evidence of reduced 5HT synthesis capacity in cortico-striatal sites, including the medio-frontal gyrus, anterior cingulated gyrus, superior temporal gyrus, and corpus striatum. Notably, the indication of 5HT synthesis capacity correlated with impulsivity scores.

There is some evidence of enhanced dopaminergic activity in association with psychotic-like thinking in PD, particularly schizotypal PD. Increased dopamine concentrations have been found in the CSF of schizotypal patients (Siever *et al.* 1999) including BPD patients with co-morbid schizotypal presentations. Psychotic symptoms are induced by amphetamines (a dopamine agonist) in BPD patients (Schulz *et al.* 1988). These findings are consistent with clinical reports that amphetamines benefit BPD patients with psychotic symptoms. Noradrenergic abnormalities have been noted in BPD associated with risk taking and sensation seeking.

Candidate genes

Potential serotonergic candidate genes have been investigated. These include tryptophan hydroxylase, the serotonin transporter, the 5-HT1b receptor, the 5-HT1a receptor and the 5-HT2a receptor. The serotonin transporter 'S' allele and the TPH 'L' allele have been associated with impulsivity and neuroticism (Lesch *et al.* 1996; New *et al.* 1998). The 5-HT1b receptor gene has been linked to suicide attempts (New *et al.* 2001). It is highly likely that at least some of these assumptions signal specific vulnerabilities to childhood environmental stressors (e.g. maltreatment, Caspi *et al.* 2002) or adult life stress (e.g. life events, Caspi *et al.* 2003).

Cortical localization

The methodology of neural imaging has only recently been brought to the study of BPD. In an early investigation of six female BPD patients without co-morbidity and six controls, Herpertz and colleagues (2001*b*) examined regional cerebral activity (haemodynamic changes) associated with emotional processing. They presented slides from the international Affective Picture System that include photographs of mutilated bodies, crying children, and scenes of violence and danger. In the BPD subjects, elevated blood oxygenation detected bilaterally in the amygdala and activation of the medial and infero-lateral-pre-frontal cortex were associated with the affect-inducing slides. Enhanced amygdala activation suggests intense and slowly subsiding emotions in response to even low-level stressors. The authors suggest that BPD subjects' perceptual cortex may be modulated through the amygdala leading to increased attention to emotionally salient environmental stimuli.

The frontal lobe is generally thought to be the location for the supervisory or executive functions of the brain, and many in addition suggest that this is not restricted to cognitive processes, but applies equally to affective responsiveness, social and personality development, self-awareness, and consciousness (e.g. Stuss and Alexander 2000). It has been suggested that a sub-group of BPD patients suffer from executive dysfunctions (Andrulonis *et al.* 1980; Swirsky-Sacchetti *et al.* 1993; van Reekum *et al.* 1993, 1996). However, some other studies failed to find any significant differences in developmental deficits or acquired brain insults between borderline patients and Axis II controls (Kimble *et al.* 1996). As pre-frontal brain injury is known to be associated with personality change, there may be a range of functions of the pre-frontal cortex and the sub-cortical-frontal connecting system that could account for the involvement of the frontal lobes in BPD. Luria (1966) suggested that there are three levels of frontal functions that interact with posterior basal functional domains: (a) the activation areas related to cingulated and medial regions; (b) anticipation, goal-selection, planning—collectively labelled executive functions, and (c) self-referential capacities such as self-awareness and self-consciousness. Neuro-imaging studies suggest that some executive processes such as goal management have effects in several cortical regions including posterior regions and not just the frontal lobes (Carpenter *et al.* 2000). Some have argued that the most important role of the frontal lobe may be for affective responsiveness, social and personality development, and self-awareness and consciousness (Stuss and Alexander 2000). This is consistent with Damasio's argument that subjectivity emerges during the process where the brain is generating an image of the organism in the act of perceiving and responding to an object (Damasio 1994).

Pre-frontal metabolic activity in the orbital and medial pre-frontal cortex has been reported to be reduced in association with impulsive aggression in patients with BPD and ASPD (Raine *et al.* 1998, 2000). A PET study of impulsive aggression found that compared with non-psychiatric controls, patients with PDs (ASPD, BPD, and NPD) showed a decreased anterior-medial and left anterior-orbitofrontal metabolism (Goyer *et al.* 1994). Impulsive aggression is associated with 'acquired sociopathy' after orbitofrontal cortex lesions which might disrupt the executive emotional systems that probably allow control over the brain stem systems that respond to threat (Blair 2001). Morphometric and functional neuroimaging studies of aggressive and violent subjects have consistently found frontal lobe abnormalities (Amen *et al.* 1996; Hirono *et al.* 2000). Compared with patients with non-aggressive dementia, those with aggressive dementia and the same degree of cognitive and psychiatric impairments had significant left anterior temporal and bilateral superior frontal hypoperfusion (Hirono *et al.* 2000).

A definitive systematic review of neuroimaging studies of antisocial behaviour found that findings were to some extent dependent on the methodology used (Bassarath 2001). Early computerized axial tomography (CT) studies yielded mixed results with about half the studies reporting no difference between controls and violent subjects. Those studies that reported differences tended to report temporal rather than frontal lobe differences. The early MRI studies implicated the temporal lobe in antisocial behaviour but recently this has extended to include amygdala atrophy or periamygdaloid lesions (van Elst *et al.* 2000), the frontal lobes (Raine *et al.* 1998, 2000) and bilateral hippocampal atrophy (Laakso *et al.* 2001). Early PET studies showed decreased cerebral blood flow to the temporal cortex but later studies have cast light on the role of serotonin in BPD (Soloff *et al.* 2000). In the latter study, five patients with BPD and no Axis-I MDD were compared with eight healthy controls. Patients had diminished response to serotonergic stimulation (with fenfluramine) in areas of the pre-frontal cortex associated with the regulation of impulsive behaviour. PET studies also showed murderers to have reduced pre-frontal glucose mechanism (Raine *et al.* 1998). SPECT findings tend to complement those of PET. In one study, 40 subjects with a history of person or property aggression were compared with 40 psychiatric control subjects. Aggressive patients had decreased activity in the pre-frontal cortex and increased activity in the anteromedial frontal lobes and in the left basal ganglia or limbic system or both and focal left temporal lobe abnormalities (Amen *et al.* 1996). Several studies suggest that the processing of input from the limbic system is dysfunctional, particularly in psychopathic ASPD individuals (Intrator *et al.* 1997; Kiehl *et al.* 2001).

Clinical observation consistently indicates that patients with BPD have difficulty in inhibiting behaviour and/or delaying responses. For example, in one study patients with BPD were observed to make significantly more punishment–reward commission errors on a go-no-go task than did healthy subjects (Leyton *et al.* 2001). Neuropsychological tests have implicated frontal lobe dysfunctions particularly in ASPD subjects (Brower and Price 2001). This result is consistent with observations of signs of frontal lobe dysfunction in violent impulsive individuals (Gorenstein 1982; Lapierre *et al.* 1995). In one study, psychopathic criminals appeared impaired on tasks believed to tap ventral-pre-frontal functioning, such as inhibiting a pre-potent response and following rules (Lapierre *et al.* 1995). A more recent study using the Cambridge Neuropsychological Test Automated Battery showed a marked impairment amongst violent offenders in an attentional set shifting task. In addition, their ability to alter behaviour in response to fluctuations in the emotional significance of stimuli appears to be compromised (Bergvall *et al.* 2001). Because neuropsychological symptoms of violent offenders and persons with pre-frontal lesions acquired early overlap, a number of workers have suggested that pre-frontal dysfunction contributes to the development of criminal behaviour by impairing the acquisition of social and moral knowledge (Anderson *et al.* 1999; Damasio 2000; Raine *et al.* 2000).

A recent meta-analytic review (Morgan and Lilienfeld 2000) identified 39 studies with a total of 4989 participants examining the relation between antisocial behaviour and performance on six reasonably well-validated measures of executive functioning. Overall, antisocial groups performed 0.62 standard deviation units worse than comparison groups (medium to large effect size). The effect sizes were largest for the Porteus Mazes task (a motor task). Almost all these studies used normal controls in comparison tasks. On measures sensitive to orbitofrontal dysfunction (such as object alternation tests which requires processing feedback information) ASPD subjects show marked deficits compared to normal controls (Dinn and Harris 2000). Children with psychopathic tendencies have been found to show similar deficits (Blair *et al.* 2001). In a particularly well-controlled study, 29 pure ASPD subjects who were contrasted with 20 normal controls matched for IQ were found to perform poorly on a go-no-go, attentional set shifting and the Tower of London task. It seems that ASPD subjects have particular problems in performing on tasks requiring shifting of attention between stimuli and higher order planning. Unmedicated ADHD children also perform poorly on tasks involving attention shifting and higher order planning. ASPD subjects appear to exhibit a range of deficits in a neural network that involves a variety of executive functions which cannot be accounted for by other potential confounds such as Axis-I disorders, organic brain disorders, or substance misuse.

It should be noted, however, that the findings of neuropsychological deficits largely pertain to ASPD rather than BPD samples. When samples are screened for neurological and substance use disorders and depressed rather than non-psychiatric controls are used neuro-behavioural differences are often not found (Sprock *et al.* 2000). Further, the studies that measure both neuro-psychological functioning and trauma often identify both as risk factors for borderline diagnosis, but they are largely independent. Thus in one study, (Zelkowitz *et al.* 2001), sexual abuse and witnessing violence accounted for 25% of the variance whilst neuro-psychological risk factors accounted for 33%. A combined model accounted for 48% of the variance and correctly classified 86% of the non-borderline children and 77% of the borderline children.

Attention and self-control

The term self-control has been defined as 'engaging in behaviours that result in delayed (but more) reward' (Logue 1995, p. 3). The concept relates closely to those of delay of or deferral of gratification, self-regulation, self-discipline, and conscience. All such concepts imply being able to engage in something that provides less immediate pleasure in the expectation of greater long-term benefit or the satisfaction of an ethical imperative. As borderline pathology entails impulsivity, and yielding to immediate demands, the possibility of a deficit in self-control is obviously of relevance. Conditions co-morbid with BPD centrally involve issues of self-control, for example, addiction problems, eating disorders, ASPD, and associated childhood disorders such as ADHD and conduct disorder. Insufficiency of self-control has been observed to emerge early in life and to show impressive consistency over contexts and time across studies (see, e.g. Block 1996). Kochanska and colleagues (1997) designed a number of ingenious tests of self-control for young children. Cortical localization of self-control invariably points to the pre-frontal cortex (Barkley 1997; Metcalfe and Mischel 1999). PET scan studies have shown that making choices between small likely rewards and large unlikely rewards entails activity in the right inferior and orbital pre-frontal cortex (Rogers *et al.* 1999). These pre-frontal regions are known to have rich interconnections with limbic structures likely to be involved in drives, rewards, and motivation. As these structures are also well-connected to dorso-pre-frontal cortical areas that serve a broad range of cognitive processes independent of social or emotional salience, the orbital and inferior pre-frontal cortex may be ideally suited to co-ordinate the probabilities of outcomes with their emotional reward value. Further, and once again in line with dysfunctions we have noted above, low serotonin activity is associated with impulsiveness (Linnoila and Virkkunen 1992) while enhanced serotonergic activity appears to enhance delayed gratification (Bizot *et al.* 1999).

There is considerable accumulating evidence that self-control and the capacity to direct attention are linked (Posner and Rothbart 1998, 2000). For example, in one study a laboratory measure of the ability to suppress attention to irrelevant stimuli was correlated with self-report of success in college students (Diefendorff *et al.* 1998). Attention may be just one component of self-control but it is likely to be an extremely important one (Cousens and Nunn 1997). Strong arguments have been advanced to suggest that self-control is a feature of temperament and therefore genetically determined. There is also good evidence that the quality of mother–child relationship is a further important predictor of the growth of self-control skills (Olson *et al.* 1990; Silverman and Ragusa 1990;

Jacobsen *et al.* 1997; Mauro and Harris 2000; Strayhorn 2002). Stable relationships with individuals with whom a powerful affective bond is retained, outside of relationships with the primary caregiver, turn out to be important (Lewis 2000) because relationships serve as the context for the development of several aspects of emotion regulation (Bell and Calkins 2000). We will return to the issue of developmental influences on self-control in Chapter 3.

Conclusion

In a review of biological factors in PD, Silk (2000) concludes that exploration of biology of neurotransmitters and polymorphic genes that influence behaviour will increase the understanding of the complexity of PD but not to the exclusion of environmental effects. The findings suggest that the association between low serotonin and impulsive aggression may in part be genetic. It is most frequently suggested that low serotonin levels create a deficit in inhibitory capacity. Cloninger, however proposed that what is seen clinically as impulsive aggression is a combination of high novelty seeking and low harm avoidance (Cloninger *et al.* 1993). He postulates that harm avoidance is associated with serotonergic activity. Thus low harm avoidance would be linked to reduced serotonergic activity, as has been noted above. Clinical implications of either of these propositions include the need to differentiate and assess separately impulsive aggression, suicide attempts and traits of neuroticism, and novelty seeking in patients with BPD. However, as even this brief overview has clearly indicated, there is as yet no question that a genetic-molecular biological model of BPD can provide a comprehensive account of what is known about the disease. Perhaps the current state of the field is best summarized in the words of the geneticists Reiss *et al.* (1991):

> "Psychiatry has been forced into the chronically uncomfortable position of straddling biomedicine and the social sciences and seems always to hunger for relief… [yet] the data simply do not permit a conception of the future centred on a straightforward biomedical answer to the fundamental question of the pathogenesis of major disorders. Indeed, a balanced image of the future contains a growing and equal partnership of the social sciences and molecular biology" (p. 290).

Psychosocial influences

Theoretical considerations

Psychological theories of BPD historically arose from the clinical rather than the research context. Accordingly, they will be described in Chapters 3 and 4. However, to orientate the reader to research concerning psychological influences on the origins of BPD, it may be helpful to briefly consider the dominant psychological approaches to aetiology.

One orientation influentially advanced by Otto Kernberg and his colleagues (1975) suggests that excessive early aggression in the young child leads to excessive splitting, i.e. the separate representation of positive and negative aspects of images of the self and mother. The cause of the excessive aggression may be environmental (frustration) or constitutional, but in either case children who are to become borderline are assumed to have considerable difficulty in integrating the positive and negative relationship images and affects that correspond with them. They, therefore, never achieve a realistic and balanced view, but oscillate between unmitigated extremes of goodness and badness. A second approach to psychosocial causation places the responsibility for the development of BPD on failures of early mothering, which in turn creates a failure of object constancy (Adler and Buie 1979). The mothering of borderline children is considered excessively insensitive and non-empathic, leading to a failure to evolve a consistent self-image and an image of the caregiver that would be available to comfort and sustain them at times of stress. A third influential theory arose out of Margaret Mahler's developmental theory (Mahler 1971). On the basis of observations of children's behaviour in the second and third year of life, Masterson (Masterson and Rinsley 1975) suggested that fear of abandonment is the organizing conflict of borderline pathology. It was assumed that mothers of pre-borderline children somehow undermined their child's natural strivings for autonomy by selectively withdrawing emotional support at a moment when the child acted in an independent manner. This was thought to be particularly crucial in Mahler's separation–individuation phase in the second year of life. Subsequent experiences that called for autonomy or independence were assumed to trigger abandonment panic and depression. Consequently, individuals with BPD remain dependent and will go to excessive lengths to retain emotional support.

There are many other psychodynamic formulations of borderline pathology (e.g. Green 1977; Steiner 1992, 1993) but none that have such clear implications for the likely quality of early psychosocial experience. The views advanced in this volume may be considered to build on these classical ideas and integrate them with considerations drawn from attachment theory (Bowlby 1969, 1973, 1980; Gunderson 1996). However, psychodynamic ideas suffer from an adult-centred focus on child development—they make sense and add much meaning to discourse with adult patients but the developmental experiences they point to remain hypothetical. Indeed, non-psychoanalytic clinicians have found it difficult to credit that severe disorders of character such as BPD could arise out of relatively subtle early difficulties which are, in any case, likely to have higher prevalence than the 2% of the population normally considered to be affected by the disorder (e.g. Swartz *et al.* 1990).

A number of psychosocial factors supposed to be related to aetiology of BPD have been investigated. Zanarini and Frankenburg presented a comprehensive review of these (Zanarini and Frankenburg 1997; Zanarini 2000). The factors listed by these authors included: (1) studies of prolonged early separations and losses confirming the high prevalence of these in the histories of individuals with BPD; (2) studies of disturbed parental involvement confirming the perception of individuals with BPD that their relationship with both their parents is highly conflictual; (3) childhood histories of physical or sexual abuse confirming the high prevalence particularly of sexual abuse and parent–child incest; (4) the high prevalence of affective disorder in first degree relatives of borderline probands. Data in all these areas is fraught with methodological problems including bias from retrospective accounts, early studies with uncertain diagnostic criteria, poorly established criteria for psychosocial adversity and lack of blindness to diagnosis in judgements of adversity as well as inevitable confounds of genetic and psychosocial explanations of psychiatric morbidity in first-degree relatives. The two most empirically robust aspects of the psychosocial aetiology of BPD are family history of psychopathology and childhood trauma or abuse.

Parenting

Parental separation or loss

One of the early studies (Walsh 1977) identified high rates of parental loss through divorce, parental illness, or death in the history of those individuals with BPD. In all, almost 80% came from families with at least one of these three disruptions. This result was confirmed by other investigations (Bradley 1979; Soloff and Millward 1983; Akiskal *et al.* 1985) where the family disruption of those with BPD was observed in most cases to exceed those of psychotic, depressed, or other PD controls. In more recent retrospective studies (Links *et al.* 1988; Zanarini *et al.* 1989*c*) early separations of one to three months or more were found to characterize the BPD group. There is thus some indication of prolonged childhood separation characterizing this group.

Family history

Family history of mood disorders and substance use disorders are more common in BPD patients than would be expected by chance (e.g. Widiger and Trull 1992). A positive history of psychopathology is more commonly found in one or both biological parents than would be expected by chance (Shachnow *et al.* 1997; Paris 2000). For example, Goldman and colleagues (1993) reported that 71% of outpatient youngsters with BPD had at least one parent with an Axis I disorder versus 30% of non-BPD youngsters. Another study (Shachnow *et al.* 1997) of female in-patients found that in 82% of these cases both parents met criteria for parental psychopathology, and severity of parental psychopathology was associated with BPD severity. These findings, while consistent with a genetic model, indicate a heterogeneity in parental pathology that points to the influence of an unstable home environment that could foster the development of BPD features. It appears that controlling for both childhood abuse and Axis I diagnoses in the young person does not remove the influence of parental psychopathology on BPD scores (Trull 2001*a*). None of these studies, however, points to the specific features of parenting that create a vulnerability for BPD. A study based on undergraduates screened for borderline features found that, when 197 individuals with borderline features were contrasted with 224 without, parental mood disorder correlated 0.3 with DIB-R (Trull 2001*b*).

Abnormal parenting attitudes

Classically, parents of borderline patients were considered to be overinvolved in and overprotective of the patient's welfare. The first empirical investigation (Grinker *et al.* 1968) found only a minority to be overinvolved and overprotective, with families most commonly manifesting a high degree of discord between family members or pervasive denial of problems. In a second look at these data, Walsh (1977) reported that 57% of the BPD cases believed that they were overinvolved with one of their parents. This was considered a reaction to the parent's need to be needed. In almost all the cases surveyed, patients reported that one or both of the parents were remote and lacking in feelings of attachment. Two-thirds of the cases mentioned highly conflictual relationships with their parents, which included hostility, devaluation, or frank abuse.

A better controlled investigation by John Gunderson and colleagues (1980) failed to identify overinvolvement in families of patients with BPD and suggested that a more common pattern was for the parents to be involved with one another to the exclusion of their children. A similar retrospective study (Frank and Paris 1981) compared BPD with neurotic and normal controls and found all three groups to commonly report disturbed attitudes in their mothers. The unique identifier was the father's attitude that appeared specifically less approving of the child than in the other groups. This finding echoes that of an investigation of BPD in-patients with schizophrenic and depressed controls (Soloff and Millward 1983) where all patient groups were reporting maternal over-involvement, but only the BPD group reported their fathers as likely to be over-involved. In a subsequent investigation (Paris and Frank 1989) women with BPD were shown to perceive their parents as significantly less caring than the control group. In a final study by this group, with a mixed gender sample, the recollections of BPD patients characterized both parents as having been less caring and more protective or controlling than non-psychotic psychiatric controls (Zweig-Frank and Paris 1991). The finding of low parental care combined with high overprotection is echoed in other questionnaire-based investigations (Goldberg *et al.* 1985; Torgersen and Alnaes 1992).

These findings suggest that in retrospective investigations, the parents of BPD individuals emerge as seeing their relationships with their mothers as conflictual, distant, or overprotective, their fathers as less involved and more distant suggesting that problems with both parents are more likely to be the common pathogenic influence in this group than problems with either parent alone.

Childhood trauma and maltreatment

Trauma is frequently noted in the history of those with BPD, although it is important to note that this association is also true of many other disorders on Axis-I and Axis-II. Numerous studies with good diagnosis and coding of retrospective experience methodology have found that a substantial percentage of patients with BPD report that they were sexually abused as children (e.g. Zanarini *et al.* 1997). These studies also report prevalence figures for sexual abuse that are higher for patients with BPD than for comparison subjects. Links and colleagues (1988) and Zanarini and colleagues (1989*c*) were the first to report significant elevation of accounts of sexual abuse by a caregiver in the childhood experience of BPD in-patients and out-patients respectively. Importantly, other trauma such as physical abuse and various forms of neglect appeared not to discriminate the BPD group from an Axis II control in the Zanarini study, but reports of physical abuse were elevated in the Links report. Herman and colleagues (1989) found evidence for physical and sexual abuse both being more common amongst patients with BPD than in Axis II controls. Ogata and colleagues (1990) also reported elevation of sexual abuse, but while physical abuse was high it was not significantly different from an Axis II comparison group. Finally, in another in-patient investigation Westen and colleagues (1990) reported significantly elevated sexual abuse but not physical abuse in BPD patients. These findings continue to be reported in more recent studies (Zlotnick *et al.* 2001). In a study of students, those reporting a history of sexual abuse or physical abuse were significantly more likely to score highly on the DIB-R (Trull 2001*b*). When specific Axis I diagnostic groups are studied, those with a history of sexual abuse are often found to have BPD co-morbidity. For example, in a study of 235 treatment-seeking out-patients with major depression, patients reporting sexual abuse were more likely to have the diagnosis of BPD (29% vs 10%) and PTSD (41% vs 11%) (Zlotnick *et al.* 2001). Research also indicated that ASPD is more prevalent among victims of childhood abuse or neglect (Silverman *et al.* 1996).

Across these studies, about a quarter of patients described having been sexually abused by their fathers, about 5% by their mothers, up to about a quarter by their siblings and the largest group by non-relatives (40–50%). These classical studies taken together suggest that while physical and sexual abuse are both common in the self-reported histories of BPD patients defined according to diagnostic criteria, it is only sexual abuse that is consistently reported more often by BPD patients than other Axis II groups. As physical and sexual abuse frequently co-occur, it is hard to judge without multivariate statistics if one or both are necessary or sufficient for the development of BPD. Two detailed Canadian reports have cast further interesting light on this picture (Paris *et al.* 1994*a*,*b*). The first study was restricted to the pathological childhood experiences of women with BPD contrasted with Axis II female control subjects and confirmed that sexual abuse was the only significant multivariate predictor of the diagnosis of BPD. The reported rate of sexual abuse in childhood was 71% versus 46%, but abuse involving penetration was over five times more common in the BPD group and the involvement of relatives other than caregivers or siblings was three times more frequent. Multiple perpetrators were two and a half times more frequent. However, for the majority of both samples reporting sexual abuse this was a one-off occurrence and the involvement of the caregiver was more common in the control than the BPD group. The second report concerned men with a diagnosis of BPD and confirmed that in a multivariate analysis, sexual abuse makes a unique contribution, although in this sample separation and loss added to diagnostic specificity. Almost half the male sample report sexual abuse, twice as many as controls, and nine times as many report penetration. The involvement of caregivers was also more common.

A retrospective study that underscores the importance of neglect in BPD was reported by Zanarini and colleagues (1997, 2000*a*). The study is based on the childhood experiences of 358 in-patients with BPD and 109 Axis II controls. The study found that 91% of patients with BPD reported some kind of sexual abuse and 92% reported some kind of childhood neglect. 27% experienced abuse from the caregiver and 56% sexual abuse by a non-caregiver. 62% of BPD versus 32% of controls report childhood sexual abuse. Patients with BPD are more likely to report physical and emotional neglect. Those with childhood sexual abuse histories were more likely to report other kinds of abuse and all kinds of neglect. The most common pattern associated with BPD in this study was biparental failure, present in 84% of the BPD sample but only 60% of the other PD sample. The combination of female caretaker neglect and male caretaker abuse was most clearly characteristic of the female BPD diagnostic group. About half the patients reported biparental denial of the validity of their feelings and thoughts.

Most of the evidence indicating that PDs are associated with a history of childhood abuse or neglect is based on retrospective reports of childhood maltreatment by psychiatric patients (Rutter 2000). There is genuine concern that the presence of PDs impacts on the interpretation and the quality of recall of childhood experiences (Loftus 1993). Although there is good evidence supporting the validity of retrospective reports (Bifulco *et al.* 1997), prospective studies are required to demonstrate that individuals who have experienced childhood maltreatment are at elevated risk for subsequent PDs. This has become a key issue in the field as a relatively small group of clinicians refuse to give credence to accounts of molestation and maltreatment regardless of the details and emotional content of the accounts. Requests for corroborative evidence are voiced by researchers and clinicians alike, yet all can appreciate the complexity of such requests for both patient and family. A far better research strategy entails following-along known cases of childhood sexual or physical maltreatment and estimating the increase in the likelihood of BPD emerging as a sequel to it.

There are longitudinal studies that suggest a link between PDs and childhood neglect. Drake and colleagues (1988) reported that lack of parental affection and supervision and family instability appeared to increase the risk for dependent and passive-aggressive PDs. The definition of environmental failure in this study, however, was too global. An important study reported by Luntz and Widom (1994) reported that young adults who experienced childhood abuse or neglect had a higher prevalence of ASPD than the comparison groups. The study, however, did not report on neglect as either a moderator or as a risk factor in its own right.

The New York Children in the Community Study (Johnson *et al.* 1999) included 738 youths recruited from upstate New York and assessed repeatedly between 1975 and 1993, and reported that childhood abuse substantially increased the risk of Cluster B PD in general and BPD in particular. In a follow-up report to this study (Johnson *et al.* 2000), these researchers demonstrated that emotional, physical, and supervision neglect were all associated with increased risk for PDs. The emphasis on neglect is consistent with the higher prevalence of neglect compared to either physical or sexual abuse but has been relatively ignored by aetiological theories. It appears that supervision neglect is particularly likely to be associated with borderline, paranoid, and passive-aggressive PDs. Interestingly, cognitive neglect was not associated with any PD symptoms. Supervision neglect includes items such as allowing the child to go out as he or she pleases, being tolerant of the child using cannabis, and so on. The prevalence of supervision neglect among parents of any Cluster B PD was 30% and the odds ratio for BPD was 7.3. The contribution of neglect remained significant after abuse was controlled for. The study was unique in exploring the onset of abuse associated Cluster B disorder symptoms (Cohen *et al.* 2001). After the general effect of neglect and sexual abuse was controlled for, two significant interactions with age emerged in the prediction of Cluster B symptoms: physical abuse record and neglect. Both had non-linear (quadratic) interactions with age, suggesting that while neglect cases had a partial remission in adulthood, physical abuse cases showed an increasingly consolidated pattern of antisocial and impulsive behaviour. These differences may be argued to underpin the relatively better prognosis of BPD compared to ASPD. ASPD and physical maltreatment tend to be associated and physical maltreatment, it seems, has longer-lasting effects.

Another longitudinal design recruits subjects from records of documented court cases of child abuse and neglect. The subjects are then followed up sometimes decades later. In one study (Horwitz *et al.* 2001), 641 male members of an abuse and neglect group were matched with a control group of 510 persons in a 20-year follow-up. 27% of those abused and neglected met ASPD diagnoses compared to 17% of controls. They also had significantly more lifetime symptoms of ASPD and dysthymia. A particular intriguing result in this report was the apparent mediating effect of life events. If life events were introduced into the logistic regression, the impact of abuse and neglect either totally or almost totally disappeared on symptoms and diagnoses. This study is consistent with follow-ups of children with childhood psychological problems where the adult outcome is often increased risk of life events rather than adult disorder itself (Champion *et al.* 1995). One way of interpreting such results is that neglect and abuse in childhood impact on the development of relationship representational systems. These individuals are then more vulnerable to adverse interpersonal encounters, which are the direct causes of adult disturbance, including PD. In a review of studies of interpersonal functioning of women with a history of childhood sexual abuse, DiLillo (2001) concluded that the abuse most commonly had its impact via interpersonal dysfunction that generated problems in partner relations and difficulties in the parental role. Both of these are likely to generate events that could trigger severe and enduring mental health problems. Adult female survivors are at greater risk of being revictimized in the context of couple relationships. Their peer relationships appear to be less markedly impaired although their relationships with their own mothers are too poor for them to benefit fully from maternal social support in the face of life events. There is extensive evidence of difficulties in maintaining appropriate boundaries with children as well as discomfort with the emotional demands of parenting (Cohen 1995).

Models of psychosocial aetiology based on neglect and trauma

The PTSD model

Fifteen years ago the suggestion emerged that BPD could be considered a trauma spectrum disorder (Herman and van der Kolk 1987). In clinically referred samples of children, post-traumatic stress disorder (PTSD) rates resulting from sexual abuse range from 42% to 90% (McLeer *et al.* 1994; Dubner and Motta 1999; Lipschitz *et al.* 1999). In non-clinically referred samples, the prevalence rates are somewhat lower (McLeer *et al.* 1998). PTSD rates for domestic violence referrals are between 50% and 100% (Pynoos and Nader 1989; Dubner and Motta, 1999). Childhood victims of physical and sexual abuse as well as physical neglect are reported to be at increased risk for developing a lifetime history of PTSD when assessed prospectively in young adulthood (Widom 1999). These rates are similar to the rate of PTSD in children traumatized by war and homicide (De Bellis 2001). In a meta-analysis of studies examining the relationship between BPD and childhood sexual abuse, only a moderate relationship (ES = 0.28) was found despite the fact that 90% of studies used clinical samples (Fossati *et al.* 1999*a*). 'The moderate pooled effect size for the association between childhood sexual abuse (CSA) and BPD, as well as the fact that larger effect sizes are strongly linked to smaller, less representative samples, does not seem to support the theoretical formulations considering CSA as a major psychological risk factor or a causal antecedent of BPD' (Fossati *et al.* 1999*a*, p. 276). Thus the role of CSA in BPD is at this time still an open question.

It cannot be claimed that sexual abuse is a necessary or sufficient condition for BPD as not all patients with BPD report sexual abuse and known cases of abuse do not inevitably result in BPD. In Zanarini's review, 40–70% of BPD patients and 19–46% of controls are identified as sexually abused in childhood or adolescence (Zanarini 2000). A complication of the PTSD account is that childhood sexual abuse almost invariably occurs in the context of biparental failure rather than in response to a single traumatic event or series of events (Zanarini *et al.* 1996). Some reported experiences of abuse are severe while others appear to be relatively mild (Paris *et al.* 1994*a*). Dividing borderlines along the lines of severe versus less severe reported experiences is probably clinically unhelpful and theoretically hard to justify. Further, it appears that BPD patients with or without co-morbid PTSD have almost identical sub-syndromal phenomenology (Zanarini and Frankenburg 1997).

The clinical risk of overemphasizing trauma from our point of view will be made clear in Chapter 3. We will argue that borderline individuals may have a specific vulnerability in understanding their own states of mind. Consequently, they are particularly eager to identify a coherent account of the pain they experience and they are in a poor position to critically appraise persuasive suggestions put to them. A psychotherapist who is overconfident concerning the aetiological significance of a vaguely remembered or even unremembered account of maltreatment places his or her client at risk in a number of ways: (1) by paying insufficient attention to other aetiologically possibly more significant psychosocial experiences; (2) by suggesting to the client that their abuse experience was graver than it was, distorting the client's experience of reality and potentially undermining the client's relationship with the individuals concerned; (3) given the insubstantial nature of the claim, generating a dependence on the person of the therapist through whose 'superior knowledge' the client's discomfort may be diminished, even at the expense of generating new instances of maltreatment experience; and (4) because the clinician is dictating the topic, the client is forced to adopt a passive position in relation to their own experience and an agentive sense of self will be hard to recover. The complexity of aetiological models required to take account of known evidence concerning trauma suggest a need for a far more cautious attitude as far as technical recommendations for therapeutic work are concerned.

The stress-diathesis model

This is not to say that we consider trauma an insignificant aspect of our model of borderline disturbance. There are many models that incorporate traumatic childhood experience alongside constitutional neurological and biochemical dysfunction.

Michael Stone (1980) was the first to advance a diathesis-stress model of BPD. The model suggests that constitutional vulnerability interacts with environmental stress so that the more vulnerable an individual, the less stress may be needed for BPD to develop. There is an accumulating body of evidence that genetics plays a crucial role in the development of PTSD. For example, in one twin study of Vietnam Veterans with combat-related PTSD it was found that genetic factors accounted for about a third of shared variance in PTSD symptoms (True *et al.* 1993). The Stone model would account for the variable degree of stress reported by patients with BPD. However, as there is no agreement as yet about how to assess constitutional vulnerability, the model is explanatory but has no predictive power.

A multiple pathway model

Zanarini and Frankenberg (1994) advanced a multi-factorial model for BPD, suggesting BPD to be a final common pathway to a complex admixture of innate temperament, challenging childhood experiences and neurological and biochemical dysfunction, the latter being possible consequences of a combination of early adverse experiences and innate vulnerabilities. For example, sexual or physical abuse may 're-set' stress systems such as the HPA axis (e.g. Yehuda 1998, and see below). Traumatic experiences may provide content for chronic unhappiness called borderline temperament and lead through a kindling process to subtle biochemical changes or changes in neurological functioning (Zanarini 2000). Alternatively, the temperament of individuals with BPD may place them at increased risk of exposure to childhood experiences of abuse and neglect. The model also proposed that different combinations of risk factors may help to define sub-groups within the BPD population.

The multiple pathway model offered a helpful categorization of environmental impingements. They distinguished Type 1 trauma that was made up of childhood experiences that could be considered unfortunate but not unexpectable from Type 2 trauma and Type 3 trauma that represent psychosocial challenges of increasing severity. Thus Type 1 trauma includes early separations, chronic insensitivity to the child's feelings, and serious emotional discord in the family. Type 2 includes experiences of verbal and emotional abuse, neglect of physical needs, and parental psychiatric illness. Type 3 might include frank physical and sexual abuse, chronic psychiatric illness of the caretaker, particularly severe PD or substance abuse.

In addition to the trauma, Zanarini and colleagues suggest that a 'hyperbolic temperament' (Zanarini and Frankenburg 1997, p. 99) leads BPD patients to insist that attention be paid to the enormity of the subjective pain they have experienced which they genuinely feel is worse than anything anyone has felt. Additionally, Zanarini proposes a triggering event that may be normative or traumatic, that brings their condition to attention for the first time. The trigger separates individuals who are pre-borderline, for example intense and demanding but not impaired, from those who are impulsive, and no longer initially capable of undertaking collaborative therapeutic work. The triggering event reminds the pre-borderline person of the earlier trauma and acts as a catalyst for the full borderline condition with chronic intense dysphoria, transient paranoid dissociative experiences, impulsivity in a number of self-destructive areas, troubled interpersonal relations, extreme dependency, manipulativeness, etc.

While fully integrative of clinical knowledge concerning BPD, the multiple pathways model has limited clinical utility. As the authors point out: 'there are as many pathways to the development of BPD as there are borderline patients' (Zanarini and Frankenburg 1997, p. 100). This may indeed be the case but this formulation does not offer a clear intervention strategy or a hierarchy of goals to be addressed with patients depending on the pathways they followed to the acquisition of the disorder.

Biological pathways of the impact of extreme stress

Childhood trauma as a risk factor for adverse brain development

There is increasing interest in a life-course developmental approach to psychopathology (Munir and Beardslee 1999; Rapaport 1999). The upsurge of interest is rooted in longitudinal epidemiological studies that have pointed to the prediction of adult psychiatric problems from childhood (Hofstra *et al.* 2002). Further, across a number of disorders, the identification of different developmental trajectories has been found to yield insights relevant to the course and prognosis of a range of disorders. For example, juvenile onset forms of a number of disorders are known to be associated with more severe prognoses in adulthood (e.g. Moffitt *et al.* 2002).

The impressive findings from the Dunedin Prospective Longitudinal Cohort Study are clearly also suggestive of a developmental continuum. Of those diagnosed with ASPD (n=39), 60% had a diagnosis of conduct disorder (CD) or oppositional defiant disorder (ODD) by age 11–15 years compared to 18% of those without ASPD. Only 15% did not have a diagnosis before 18 years of age. In this study, of those at 26 years with eating disorder (n=26), 84% had some kind of childhood diagnosis, 45% had conduct disorder by age 11–15. This was compared to 19% of those without eating disorder. Of those diagnosed with depression at 26 (n=172), over 30% had an anxiety diagnosis at 11–15, 15% had a diagnosis of depression and 24% had a diagnosis of CD or ODD. Between 50% and 60% of diagnoses at 26 years were anticipated by some diagnosis of psychiatric disorder at 11–15 years of age. Although data from BPD is not included in this report, findings from these co-morbid conditions offer a clear indication that most, if not all, psychiatry is developmental psychiatry and in the case of BPD we must assume that early experience and associated changes to the brain are critical to our understanding of the unfolding of later psychopathology.

Studies of brain development have demonstrated in longitudinal studies that there are regionally specific non-linear pre-adolescent increases followed by post-adolescent decreases in cortical grey matter, which reflects reductions in synaptic density and pruning at much later stages of development than traditionally thought (Giedd *et al.* 1999; Thompson *et al.* 2000). For example, sub-cortical grey matter and limbic system structures increase in volume non-linearly and peak at age 16.6 (Giedd *et al.* 1999). These findings underscore the potentially formative nature, at least in terms of brain development, of experiences of early adolescence. Findings from De Bellis and colleagues, using similar MRI methodology suggest that maltreated children and adolescents have smaller intracranial volumes, cerebral volumes, and larger lateral ventricles than controls after adjustment for intracranial volumes and SES (De Bellis *et al.* 1999*b*). Neuronal loss may account for this finding and underpin the pervasive problems of maltreated children and adolescents.

Serotonin system

The serotonin system is a stress response system but it also plays a major role in the regulation of emotions and aggressive and impulsive behaviour, including suicidal behaviour (Siever and Trestman 1993). Animal studies of stress have shown serotonin levels to decrease in the brains of animals subjected to inescapable shock (Southwick *et al.* 1992). Long-term stress or high doses of glucocorticoids induce 5-HT_{1A} and 5-HT_{1B} receptor alterations in the hippocampus and the cortex. The onset of major depression is associated with a history of childhood PTSD (Breslau *et al.* 2000) and may be accounted for by the dysregulation of the serotonergic system. There is direct evidence that severe and sustained traumatic stress in childhood affects the 5-HT system and especially 5-HT_{1A} receptors (Rinne *et al.* 2000). The cortisol and prolactin responses to meta-chlorophenylpiperazine (m-CPP) challenge in BPD patients were significantly lower compared to those of healthy controls. Within this small group ($n=12$) of patients the net prolactin response to the challenge showed a high inverse correlation with the independently-rated severity of both physical and sexual abuse. This suggests that the blunted prolactin response to m-CPP may be independent of BPD diagnosis and is the result of severe early traumatization.

Endogenous opiate system

Dissociative symptoms are commonly seen in both traumatized individuals and individuals with BPD. These symptoms are usually defined as disruptions in the normally integrated functions of consciousness, memory, and identity (Putnam 1997). It has been suggested that dissociative symptoms are mediated by dysregulation of the endogenous opiate system (Bremner *et al.* 1993*a*).

HPA axis

The hypothalamic–pituitary–adrenal (HPA) axis is the pathway that connects the adrenal cortex, where stress hormones are secreted, to the brain. Results from baseline and challenge studies of the HPA axis of individuals with trauma histories suggest a complex picture. Lower levels of urinary free cortisol are found in many studies of victims of adult trauma and some studies of childhood trauma (e.g.Yehuda *et al.* 1995*a*). Other studies found raised levels of urinary free cortisol, including in women sexually abused in childhood with current symptoms of PTSD (Lemieux and Coe 1995). It has been suggested that a long-term consequence of trauma experience is to prime the HPA axis so that ACTH and cortisol secretion are set at lower 24-h levels as a compensatory adaptation (De Bellis *et al.* 1999*a*). Such a system will hyper-respond during acute stress but have lower resting levels. Consistent with this suggestion was the observation of augmented plasma cortisol levels in sexually abused girls recruited within six months of disclosure (Putnam *et al.* 1991). By contrast, sexually abused girls studied several years after abuse disclosure show attenuated plasma ACTH (De Bellis *et al.* 1994).

Elevated gluco-corticoids may have neuro-toxic effects and cause hippocampal degeneration. Smaller hippocampal volumes have been reported in adult PTSD sufferers, and in female adult survivors of childhood sexual abuse (Bremner *et al.* 1997; Stein 1997). In the developing brain, elevated levels of catacholamines and cortisol may lead to adverse brain development through the mechanism of accelerated loss of neurons (Smythies 1997), inhibition of neurogenesis (Gould *et al.* 1997), or delays in myelination (Dunlop *et al.* 1997). Sapolsky (1997) appropriately summarized the correlation between excess stress, cortisol, and damage to the hippocampus in humans in the title of his paper: 'Why is stress so bad for your brain'.

While it is tempting to make a simple link between early maltreatment and abnormalities in the HPA-axis as an account of BPD symptomatology, there are also troubling aspects to this model. Silk (2000) argues that the way HPA-axis functioning interacts with symptomatology is different in patients with BPD from those with MDD. While 50% of persons with BPD seem to have non-suppression on a test of the efficacy of the functioning of the HPA-axis (the Dexamethasone Suppression Test) and this is close to the figure for this abnormality among MDD patients, in BPD patients (unlike MDD patients) no correlation is observed between severity of depression and this measure of HPA-axis dysfunctionality.

The complexity is also well-illustrated in McEwen's (1999) discussion of the long-term physiological effects of stress on the HPA axis (see an excellent and comprehensive review of research on the impact of abuse on the brain field by Glaser 2000). As we have seen when faced with chronic stress, suppression of the stress response can lead to a restoration of cortisol levels to normal limits.

Anterior cingulate dysfunction

The anterior cingulate cortex is a region of the medial pre-frontal cortex. It is part of an executive attention system that is activated during decision-making and novel or dangerous situations (Posner and Petersen 1990). In a PET study, comparing sexually abused women who had PTSD with those with a similar history who did not, the women with PTSD were found to have lower levels of anterior cingulate blood flow during traumatic imagery (Shin *et al.* 1999).

A similar observation was reported as women were asked to recollect memories of sexual abuse (Bremner *et al.* 1999*a*). This suggests that some BPD symptoms may be connected to an impairment of medial-pre-frontal cortical functioning (Zubieta *et al.* 1999). It has been argued that exposure to stress impairs pre-frontal-cortical function (Arnsten and Goldman-Rakic 1998) and the impairment may be catecholamine-mediated (Arnsten 1998). In line with this suggestion is the observation that *N*-acetyl-aspartate (NAA), a marker of neural integrity, is lowered in the anterior cingulated region of the medial-pre-frontal cortex of maltreated children and adolescents (De Bellis *et al.* 2000).

Psychological pathways linking BPD to the impact of extreme stress: the role of affect dysregulation

Recent research on the impact of childhood trauma on psychological and neuro-development may help to explain the association of BPD and childhood trauma. Maltreatment in children and adolescents is known to disrupt the developmental process, cause delays, deficits or failures in multi-system developmental achievements in motor, emotional, behavioural, language, psychosocial, social, and cognitive skills (Cicchetti and Lynch 1995; Pynoos *et al.* 1995; Trickett and McBride-Chang 1995). Symbolic function has also consistently been shown to be lowered in maltreated children. A well-controlled prospective study of early onset abuse and neglect has shown significant changes in IQ (Perez and Widom 1994). Space does not permit a comprehensive review of the extensive literature on the psychological dysfunctions associated with maltreatment, many of which indicate potential links to BPD. In Chapter 3 we shall consider pathways that we consider most relevant from the standpoint of our treatment approach. Here we shall only consider one potential pathway where psychosocial and biological mechanisms triggered by maltreatment might be seen to combine to bring about aspects of the clinical problems presented by BPD.

Affect dysregulation or the absence of emotion regulation skills is well-established as a common sequel of child maltreatment. The capacity for emotion regulation and behavioural self-control may suffer as a consequence of maltreatment and lead to symptoms such as explosive anger, suicide attempts, suicidal ideation, and mood disorder (Pynoos *et al.* 1995; Thompson and Calkins, 1996). Emotion regulation skills of maltreated children have been shown to be less adaptive and culturally and age appropriate than non-maltreated controls (Shields *et al.* 1994; Shields and Cicchetti 1997). Sexually-maltreated girls, for example, demonstrate lower levels of emotion understanding for both anger and sadness as compared to their non-maltreated peers (Rogosch *et al.* 1995; Shipman *et al.* 2000). Part of the explanation for this might lie not simply in the child's reaction to the stress (see below) but in the socialization characteristics of families where maltreatment is present. There is evidence that maltreated children grow up in families characterized by high degrees of negative affect (e.g. Crittenden 1981), difficulties in the production and recognition of emotion expression (e.g. Camras *et al.* 1996), less support for and less recognition of the reasons for a child showing emotion (Shipman and Zeman 2001), and decreased discussion of emotion in the parent–child relationship (Beeghly and Cicchetti 1994; Shipman and Zeman 1999). Not only do maltreating mothers engage in emotion socialization practices that differ from those of non-maltreating mothers but that the extent of the distortion of socialization processes corresponds to the children's ability to regulate their emotional expression and arousal (Shipman and Zeman 2001). In particular, the extent to which mothers were able to generate effective coping strategies when their child was distressed, explained the association between child maltreatment and children's regulation of emotional arousal.

We have seen that BPD rarely occurs in isolation. Those with BPD often present with mood, anxiety, or substance use disorders, see above. Trull (2001*a*) demonstrated that Axis I disorders are also relevant amongst non-clinical subjects with significant borderline features. It has been suggested that this association is a consequence of the central relationship between BPD and syndromes characterized by disinhibition or emotion dysregulation (Trull *et al.* 2000). It is possible that childhood maltreatment may be the causal aetiological factor in bringing about affect dysregulation and the consequent clustering of Axis I disorder.

Drawing upon parallels in the phenomenology of groups of Axis I and Axis II disorders as well as genetic and physiological data, Siever and Davis (1991) proposed that affective instability was the psychobiological dimension of PDs most closely linked with BPD. Neurochemical studies reviewed in the previous section lent support to this view (see Gurvits *et al.* 2000). It is not clear from the general affect instability assumption whether the affective instability of BPD patients reflects a rapid shifting of emotions, abnormal intensification of certain emotions, dyscontrol over specific emotions (e.g. anger, depression), or whether the abnormality entails all emotions or only selected ones. In a direct test of this hypothesis, in one study (Cowdry *et al.* 1991) in-patients were asked to rate their general mood twice each day. BPD patients were distinguished from depressed psychiatric controls and normal controls by greater random distribution of morning moods and greater morning to evening variability of mood. Another study, specifically aimed at illuminating the nature of affective instability drew participants from a number of PD groups although most of the patients met criteria for BPD (Woyshville *et al.* 1999). While the mood variation of normal subjects from day-to-day appeared to follow a random model, the affective variability of BPD patients was non-random. The authors argued that the process that brought about the affective instability was responsible for this underlying systematic variability. A study of 41 patients with BPD contrasted with 104 patients with other PDs, (Koenigsberg *et al.* 2002) found more self-reported lability in the anxiety and anger but not in elation or depression of BPD patients. BPD patients also reported more depression/anxiety oscillations but no greater affect intensity in the BPD group. Thus, if affective instability is a core dysfunction of BPD, it does not appear to involve all affects and does not entail differences in the experience of affect intensity. Further, the differences between index and control groups were small ($p<0.05$) indicating that either the measure of lability was insensitive or affective lability is secondary to some other as yet unspecified process which effects a range of PDs. We shall propose our own model linking affect lability and BPD in Chapter 3 in the context of a broader hypothesized disturbance of subjective experience.

Attachment and BPD

Theoretical considerations

Clinicians and theoreticians involved with BPD have consistently pointed to attachment difficulties as a core phenomenological characteristic of this group. John Bowlby's theory of the development of the attachment system (Bowlby 1969, 1973, 1980) could, but does not, speak to the complete disorganization of the attachment system which clinicians working with borderline patients encounter daily. It is self-evident that an overarching framework that could incorporate the evidence on psychosocial influences with the clinical observations of failures of intimate relationships would be helpful in advancing clinical and theoretical understanding of BPD.

A number of theorists have drawn on Bowlby's ideas in explanation of borderline pathology. Most specifically Gunderson (1984, 1996) suggested that intolerance of aloneness was at the core of borderline pathology and the inability of those with BPD to invoke a 'soothing introject' was a consequence of early attachment failures. He carefully described typical patterns of borderline dysfunction in terms of exaggerated reactions of the insecurely-attached infant, for example clinging, fearfulness about dependency needs, terror of abandonment, and constant monitoring of the proximity of the caregiver. Lyons-Ruth and colleagues (Lyons-Ruth 1991; Lyons-Ruth and Jacobovitz 1999) focused on the disorganization of the attachment system in infancy as predisposing to later borderline pathology. Notably, she identified an insecure, as opposed to a secure, disorganized pattern as predisposing to conduct problems. Crittenden (1997) has been particularly concerned to incorporate in her representation of adult attachment disorganization, the specific style of borderline individuals deeply ambivalent and fearful of close relationships. Fonagy and colleagues (Fonagy 2000; Fonagy *et al.* 2000) have also used the framework of attachment theory but emphasize the role of attachment in the development of symbolic function and the way in which insecure disorganized attachment may generate vulnerability in the face of further turmoil and challenges. All these, and other theoretical approaches, predict the representations of attachment (Main and Hesse 2001) to be seriously insecure and arguably disorganized in patients with BPD.

Empirical studies using the AAI

To our knowledge there have been five studies using the Adult Attachment Interview (AAI) with BPD (Patrick *et al.* 1994; Stalker and Davies 1995; Fonagy *et al.* 1996; Rosenstein and Horowitz 1996; Frodi *et al.* 2001). All these studies report that individuals with BPD diagnoses according to structured interview or diagnostic criteria are more likely to be classified as pre-occupied on the AAI. AAI transcripts that are classified as pre-occupied tend to be long, confusing, incoherent, angry, passive or fearful accounts of childhood attachment experiences. In addition, in one study (Patrick *et al.* 1994), almost all BPD subjects were classified as the somewhat unusual E3 (fearful of losing attachment sub-category). The AAI permits the assignment of an unresolved (U) for experiences of trauma or loss on the basis of subtle signs of cognitive disorganization as experiences of maltreatment or loss of attachment figures is described. In these studies, individuals with BPD diagnosis were more likely than Axis I or Axis II controls to receive U classifications. In the Frodi *et al.* study (2001) psychopathic criminal offenders were contrasted with AAI norms. This study showed that the offenders were more likely to be categorized as dismissing or unresolved but not pre-occupied. This is consistent with the results of an unpublished study from our laboratory (Levinson and Fonagy, in preparation).

Empirical studies using self-report measures of attachment

Several measures of attachment have been used and to make matters worse, many of these measures are versions of each other but offer slightly different classifications or dimensional scoring indicators. Two studies have used the Attachment Rating Scale (ARS) (Sack *et al.* 1996; Nickell *et al.* 2002). The ARS (Hazan and Shaver 1987) employs a three-category scheme of secure, pre-occupied, and dismissing. The BPD group emerge from these studies as more likely to be anxious-ambivalent or avoidant than a normal sample or those with other psychiatric disorders. Ambivalent on the ASR is a self-description of an individual who is lonely in romantic relationships, craves intimacy, fears dependency. The Nickell study is particularly important because it controlled for adverse childhood events as well as Axis I and non-BPD Axis II pathology. Thus the ambivalent attachment style predicted BPD scores after physical or sexual abuse, Axis I and Axis II symptoms and perceived abnormal parenting attitudes were controlled for.

Two studies have used the Relationship Questionnaire (RQ) or Relationship Scales Questionnaire (RSQ) (Dutton *et al.* 1994*a*; Brennan and Shaver 1998). The RQ (Bartholomew and Horowitz 1991) and the RSQ (Griffin and Bartholomew 1994) use a four-category attachment typology that includes secure, pre-occupied, fearful, and dismissing. In this scheme fearful is an individual longing for intimacy but mistrustful and fearful of rejection. In both these studies, the BPD group emerged as fearful relative to normals and also pre-occupied relative to other PD groups. The Attachment Styles Questionnaire (ASQ) (Fossati *et al.* 2001) and the Relationship Attachment Questionnaire (RAQ) (Sack *et al.* 1996) were used in one study each. The ASQ (Feeney and Noller 1990) is a derivative of the ARS and the RQ and has five factors: confidence, discomfort with closeness, need for approval, pre-occupation with relationships, and relationships as secondary. BPD patients relative to normals, other PDs and those with no PD were more insecure but were not distinguished by a specific pattern. The investigation reported by Fossati *et al.* is unusually well-controlled. While showing differences in attachment style in the directions indicated, controlling for attachment styles did not reduce the difference between BPD and other groups in terms of impulsiveness-related traits. The authors suggest that, given that in at least one longitudinal study impulsiveness-related traits turned out to be significant and substantial predictors of BPD diagnosis at a seven-year follow-up, the independence of attachment classification from this important dimension questions the centrality of the attachment construct (Links *et al.* 1999). Another well-controlled study with a far more appropriate measure of attachment (Meyer *et al.* 2001) found that changes in psychosocial functioning over a six-month period were uniquely predicted by attachment classifications at intake using Pilkonis's attachment prototype interview assessment (Pilkonis 1988), particularly in clinician-rated scales of depression and anxiety, rather than self-report scales. This finding highlights the particular problems associated with using self-report measures of attachment in BPD. Further, the Meyer *et al.* study confirmed the close association between BPD features and prototypes for pre-occupied and insecure attachment and the stability of attachment styles over a one-year period. The associations between attachment prototypes and treatment success were also reported in other studies using the Pilkonis prototype method and was replicated by a large-scale-German investigation (Mosheim *et al.* 2000).

Summary of empirical data

Studies using varying and mostly quite limited methodologies are nevertheless quite consistent in showing borderline patients as seeking intimate relationships at the same time as being alert to signs of rejection and undervaluation. The ambivalent pre-occupied dysfunctional attachment pattern perhaps reflects difficulties in managing anxiety and distress that arise from interpersonal challenges and may be manifested in emotional instability, extreme rage, and suicidal behaviour aimed at achieving one's interpersonal needs (Bartholomew *et al.* 2001). It should be noted, however, that not all studies find an association between BPD and ambivalent pre-occupied attachment patterns. For example, Salzman and colleagues (1997) found that all participants meeting diagnostic criteria for BPD demonstrated ambivalent attachment in their first study but in their replication study, BPD participants were classified as demonstrating avoidant attachment. The fearful sub-type of pre-occupied attachment in the AAI appears to coincide with the diagnosis in some studies (Patrick *et al.* 1994) and not others (Fonagy *et al.* 1996). It should be noted that sub-categories of the AAI are not normally part of reliability tests for coders. Nevertheless, there is a clear indication that BPD diagnosis is linked with insecure, pre-occupied, ambivalent, and perhaps fearful attachment patterns.

Problems with a simple attachment model

To the extent we assume that abnormal patterns of attachment arise as a consequence of abnormalities in child rearing, it is somewhat of an embarrassment that prospective studies of maltreatment often fail to yield powerful personality effects beyond the contextual (e.g. life-events, Widom, 1999).

A more important problem is that all adult attachment measures are hopelessly confounded with symptoms and traits. Thus, for example, in Meyer *et al.*'s study (Meyer *et al.* 2001) of Pilkonis' Borderline Attachment Prototype, the correlation between the attachment prototype and symptomatology was so high that only one of these variables could be used in the regression because of co-linearity problems. Similarly, the AAI coding for fearful pre-occupied categories calls for statements about fear of loss which are also symptomatic of a diagnosis of BPD.

The model of attachment in use by attachment theorists places greatest importance on early experience, yet the social experiences of individuals with BPD are likely to be distorted by later rather than earlier social encounters. It is unclear in most theories proposing attachment as an explanatory variable how early attachment and later maltreatment might interact.

As we have seen, controlling for attachment styles does not account for temperamental and characterological differences between BPD and non-BPD patients. Impulsivity and negative affectivity/emotional dysregulation characterize BPD best (Gurvits *et al.* 2000; Paris, 2000; Silk 2000; Trull 2001*a*).

Many attachment measures such as the AAI rely on autobiographical memory. In fact in the AAI, specific memories are coded as indicators of insecurity. Studies of autobiographical memory of borderline patients suggest that they have a tendency to produce over-general memories (Startup *et al.* 2001) which again underscore the difficulty of establishing independent measures of BPD status and attachment.

Conclusions

In this chapter we have considered current empirical research on BPD. Major problems remain in relation to defining the condition and identifying related biological and psychosocial correlates. Enormous progress has been made in this field over the past fifteen years. Earlier controversies concerning the legitimacy of the diagnosis and its relationship to other conditions appear far less pertinent. It has also become clear that the psychosocial pathways to BPD are extremely complex and there is no one-to-one relationship between particular trauma such as childhood sexual abuse and BPD. So far no model has been advanced that is able to integrate all the available data. The best we can hope for is that new models should be broadly compatible with available evidence. This includes considerations of the role of genetics and constitutional vulnerabilities, new information concerning the neurophysiological dysfunctions of affect regulation and the stress response, evidence concerning executive and attentional control and frontal cortex dysfunction, emotional lability and dyscontrol, psychosocial histories of childhood maltreatment and abuse in a significant proportion of cases and the disorganization of aspects of the affiliative behavioural system, most particularly the attachment system, in almost all individuals with the diagnosis of this disorder.

2 Therapy research and outcome

Treatment of personality disorder (PD) continues to be governed by clinical opinion, whim and dogma rather than being based on evidence. Although psychotherapy has long since considered PD as its domain and attempted to help individuals modify socially and personally-damaging behaviours (Bateman and Holmes 1995), this clinical zeal has not been matched by enthusiasm for research. It was our concern about the gap between passion for psychoanalytic therapy as a treatment for PD on the one hand and absence of 'hard data' on the other that stimulated us to design a psychoanalytically-oriented treatment based on 'best clinical evidence' and to subject it to scientific scrutiny.

If we assume that PD is akin to other mental disorders that have a long-time course then scientific requirements include: studying robustly-defined populations, carefully defining treatment and assessing its specificity, ensuring treatment is superior to no treatment since personality disorders show gradual improvement over time (McGlashan 1986; Paris *et al.* 1987; Stone 1993), demonstrating that treatment impacts on personality rather than merely causing a change in mood, incorporating an adequate follow-up, and addressing cost-effectiveness relative to other alternative interventions. In brief, studies should show that personality change is both measurable and clinically meaningful. Research into PD singularly fails to meet these requirements and our research fulfilled only some of the criteria.

Despite these problems, a number of reviews of treatment of PD have been published, all of which conclude that further studies are necessary to examine specific forms of psychotherapy for specific types of PDs (Perry 1999; Bateman and Fonagy 2000). In a recent meta-analysis (Leichsenring and Leibing 2003) psychodynamic therapy yielded a large overall effect size of 1.46 with effect sizes of 1.08 for self-report measures and 1.79 for observer-rated measures. For cognitive behavioural therapy, the corresponding values were 1.00, 1.20, and 0.87. In addition, the effect sizes for psychodynamic therapy indicated long-term rather than short-term change in PD. The purpose of this chapter is to summarize some of this research and to review critically the available data, including our own, on the effectiveness of different treatments for PD, and to place our mentalization-based psychoanalytic treatment within a broader therapy research context.

Psychological treatments

Psychoanalytic psychotherapy

Most of the therapeutic interest for psychoanalytic psychotherapy has been with borderline personality disorder (BPD) (Higgitt and Fonagy 1992), which differs from almost all other types of PDs in frequent help-seeking behaviour and wish to change. This makes it more amenable to interventions. However, with a few notable exceptions, the literature is dominated either by descriptive papers or cohort studies.

One of the first and most detailed naturalistic, cohort studies of out-patient treatment for PD was the Menninger project (Wallerstein 1986). The study began in 1954 as a prospective study and spanned a 25-year period looking at assessment, treatment, and outcome in patients referred to the Menninger Clinic. Forty-two patients were selected for intensive study. Many would now be classified as borderline and were referred because of failure of standard psychiatric treatment. Patients, their families, and their therapists were subjected to a battery of tests, and process notes and supervisory records were kept, charting the course of therapy. Not surprisingly, the mass of data has led to some disagreement about interpretation (see Kernberg 1972; Horwitz 1974; Wallerstein 1986). Nevertheless, the data have been used to compare classical psychoanalysis with psychoanalytic psychotherapy in the treatment of BPD. Wallerstein classified 22 cases as having received psychoanalysis, 20 as in psychotherapy, but there was a clear spectrum from classical psychoanalysis, modified psychoanalysis, expressive-supportive psychotherapy (probably equivalent to the way psychoanalytic psychotherapy is delivered in departments in Britain), supportive-expressive psychotherapy to supportive psychotherapy. Full follow-up data were available for 27 patients. Good outcomes were obtained in 11 and a partial improvement in seven. Outcomes were generally better for patients with greater ego-strength.

An important finding was the absence of a difference between psychoanalysis and supportive psychotherapy with this group of patients. Forty-six percent of psychoanalytic cases and 54% of psychotherapy cases did well, with good or moderately good outcomes. Improvements brought about by supportive therapy were just as stable, as enduring, as proof against subsequent environmental vicissitudes, and as free (or not free) from the requirement for supplemental post-treatment contact, support, or further therapeutic help as the changes in those patients treated via psychoanalysis. Nevertheless, there was a trend for patients with relatively good ego-strength and interpersonal relationships to do better with psychoanalytic or expressive therapy whilst those with low ego-strength responded best to supportive psychotherapy.

An important aim of the study was to elucidate the controversy about the 'widening scope' of psychoanalysis (Stone 1993)—the use of psychoanalytic techniques to treat much more severely disturbed patients than had previously been thought possible. Kernberg's (1972) contribution to the Menninger project suggested that a modified analytic approach including the use of 'psychodynamically guided hospitalization', early interpretation of negative transference, and a focus on here-and-now interactions rather than reconstructions, enabled severe patients to be successfully treated. Wallerstein looked in detail at this group of 'heroic indication' patients and identified 11 such patients with paranoid features, major alcohol or drug addiction, or borderline pathology. The overall results were not good. Six of these were in the psychoanalysis group: three died of mental illness-related causes, two from alcoholism, one by suicide; three dropped out of analysis, of whom two did badly, and one well. Five were in the psychotherapy group, of whom two had mental illness-related deaths, four were total failures, and one did moderately well.

The conclusions about this group of patients were that the best form of therapy is 'supportive-expressive' for however long it is necessary; that periods of hospitalization will be required alongside long-term therapy; and that a network of informal support, often centred around the sub-culture associated with a psychiatric unit is also an important ingredient if these patients are to survive at all, let alone thrive. Finally: 'even if they had little chance with psychoanalysis, they might have had no chance at all with other forms of treatment' (Wallerstein 1986, p. 671).

It is important not to underestimate the importance of this study in the development of treatment of PD since other studies of treatment and long-term follow-up seemed to confirm the results that some patients did well whilst others did spectacularly badly (McGlashan 1986).

Stevenson and Meares (1992) and Meares *et al.* (1999) were amongst the first to report on a different approach in which 48 borderline patients were treated with twice-weekly psychoanalytic psychotherapy that focused on a psychology of the self. Significant improvements were observed in the 30 patients who completed the therapy. Subjects made considerable gains compared to wait list controls in number of episodes of self-harm and violence, time away from work, number and length of hospital admissions, frequency of use of drugs, and self-report index of symptoms. Thirty percent of patients no longer fulfilled the criteria of BPD at the end of treatment. Improvement was maintained over 1 year. Further follow-up at 5 years has confirmed the enduring effect of treatment and demonstrated a substantial saving associated with health care costs (Stevenson and Meares 1999). The therapy concentrated on the development of a therapeutic alliance and a relative or close friend was seen at the start of treatment. Both these factors may account for the low drop-out rate of 16% since other out-patient naturalistic studies of psychodynamic therapy, both prospective and retrospective, have shown high drop-out rates of 23–67%, particularly early in treatment (Skodol *et al.* 1983; Gunderson *et al.* 1989). Smith and colleagues (1995) have analyzed factors associated with such attrition, finding that younger patients and those with high initial hostility were most likely to withdraw, and the same group (Yeamans *et al.* 1994) showed that the therapist's investment in the initial treatment contract and maintenance of an alliance were important factors in continuation of treatment.

Other naturalistic studies have indicated the utility of psychoanalytically-based treatments for BPD. Høglend (1993) studied the outcome of manualized psychodynamic focal therapy which lasted an average of 27.5 sessions and Monsen *et al.* (1995) used a form of psychodynamic therapy that focused on object relations and self-psychology in a treatment that lasted for an average of 25 months. Both studies showed promising results for patients with Cluster B PD when applied to an out-patient population. Tucker *et al.* (1987) and Antikainen and colleagues (1995) studied in-patient treatment of severe borderline personality organization for an average of 8.4 months and 3 months respectively, again finding positive results, but none of these trials were randomized and so the possibility remains that the benefits are the result of time or other factors.

The only randomized evaluation of psychoanalytic psychotherapy before our trial showed no difference between short-term dynamic psychotherapy and brief adaptational psychotherapy but both were superior to a waiting-list control (Winston *et al.* 1991). This study specifically excluded patients with borderline and narcissistic features although a later study including some Cluster B disorders produced similar results (Winston *et al.* 1994).

Studies of Transference-Focused Psychotherapy (TFP) (see p. 112) are now becoming available and give promising results although the outcome of a randomized controlled trial comparing TFP, DBT, and supportive psychotherapy is not yet known. TFP relies on the techniques of clarification, confrontation, and transference interpretation within the evolving relationship between patient and therapist. The primary focus is on the dominant affect-laden themes that emerge in the therapeutic relationship in the here-and-now of the transference. At the beginning of treatment, a hierarchy of issues is established: the containment of suicidal and self-destructive behaviours, the various ways of destroying the treatment, and the identification and recapitulation of dominant object relational patterns as they are experienced and expressed in the here-and-now of the transference relationship. In a cohort study (Clarkin *et al.* 2001) 23 female borderline patients were assessed at baseline and at the end of 12 months of treatment with diagnostic instruments, measures of suicidality, self-injurious behaviour, and measures of medical and psychiatric service utilization. Compared with the year prior to treatment, the number of patients who made suicide attempts significantly decreased, as did the medical risk and severity of medical condition following self-injurious behaviour. In addition, patients during the treatment year had significantly fewer hospitalizations as well as number and days of psychiatric hospitalization compared with the year before. The drop-out rate was 19%. When patients were compared with an untreated sample, significant differences on the same measures were reported in favour of the treated group.

Other studies of dynamic therapy have used control groups and some have reported on day-hospital treatment. Karterud *et al.* (1992) studied prospectively 97 patients treated in a psychodynamically orientated day-hospital of whom 76% had an axis II DSM-III-R diagnosis. After a mean treatment time of 6 months, outcome on measures of global symptoms and overall mental health was best for anxious-avoidant PD with only modest gains for BPD. Dick and Woof (1986), using a similar programme, found that after 12 weeks of treatment a small sub-group of patients diagnosed retrospectively as BPD increased their use of services possibly indicating that longer-term treatment was necessary for this group. A feminist, psychodynamically-informed programme with a sociopolitical dimension was effective in reducing symptoms and health service usage in 31 personality disordered patients treated in day and semi-residential facilities. Gains were sustained over a 2-year follow-up (Krawitz 1997). Use of a sociopolitical dimension may be highly pertinent given the breadth of social adaptational difficulties of most patients.

In a prospective study using a design of treatment-versus-control (delayed treatment), Piper *et al.* (1993) found significant treatment effects of 18 weeks day-hospital treatment for 79 patients with both affective disorder and long-standing PD. Interpersonal functioning, symptoms, self-esteem, life satisfaction, and defensive functioning all improved after 4 months treatment when compared with the control group and gains were maintained at 8-month follow-up.

Finally the relative effectiveness of three psychoanalytically-orientated treatment models for a mixed group of personality disorders—(a) long-term residential treatment using a therapeutic community approach; (b) briefer in-patient treatment followed by community-based dynamic therapy; and (c) general community psychiatric treatment—has been studied (Chiesa *et al.* in press). The results are discussed on p. 49 under therapeutic communities although it is unclear whether the treatment model used was based on therapeutic community principles or specific treatment interventions founded on a psychoanalytic theory.

Empirical evidence for mentalization-based psychoanalytic treatment

Our research demonstrates a trade-off between internal and external validity. On the positive side, firstly, the programme was developed and implemented by a team of generically-trained mental health professionals with an interest in psychoanalytically-orientated psychotherapy rather than by highly-trained personnel within a university research department. Secondly, the research took place within a normal clinical setting and in a locality and healthcare system in which patients were unlikely to be able to obtain treatment elsewhere. The latter allowed effective tracing of patients within the service and accurate collection of clinical and service utilization data. Thirdly, patients were treated at only two local hospitals for medical emergencies such as self-harm, enabling us to obtain highly accurate data of episodes of self-harm and suicide attempts requiring medical intervention. On the negative side, the programme was complex, leading to difficulty in identifying any effective ingredients should this be the result. However, the programme was designed so that it could be dismantled at a later date to determine the therapeutic components. At present a randomized controlled trial is underway of an out-patient treatment package made up of only group and individual therapy—the elements that we consider to be the effective components of the programme.

Our initial task in setting up the treatment programme was to review the literature, to consider the evidence for effective interventions, and to match those to the skills within the team. From the evidence discussed above we concluded that treatments shown to be effective with BPD had certain common features. They tended (a) to be well-structured, (b) to devote considerable effort to the enhancing of compliance, (c) to be clearly focused, whether that focus was a problem behaviour such as self-harm or an aspect of interpersonal relationship patterns, (d) to be theoretically highly coherent to both therapist and patient, sometimes deliberately omitting information incompatible with the theory, (e) to be relatively long term, (f) to encourage a powerful attachment relationship between therapist and patient, enabling the therapist to adopt a relatively active rather than a passive stance, and (g) to be well-integrated with other services available to the patient. While some of these features may be those of a successful research study rather than those of a successful therapy, we concluded that the manner in which treatment protocols were constructed and delivered was probably as important in the success of treatment as the theoretically-driven interventions.

With these general features in mind, we set about developing a programme of treatment and organizing a research programme to test the effectiveness of the intervention. From the outset it was clear that this was to be 'effectiveness research' rather than 'efficacy' research—we would investigate the outcome of BPD treated by generically-trained but non-specialist practitioners within a normal clinical setting. In this way, the treatment was more likely to be translatable to other services without extensive and expensive additional training of personnel.

Results

The details of our studies can be found in published papers (Bateman and Fonagy 1999, 2001). Our first study compared the effectiveness of the psychoanalytically-oriented partial hospitalization programme with routine general psychiatric care for patients with BPD. Thirty-eight patients with BPD, diagnosed according to standardized criteria, were allocated either to partial hospitalization or to general psychiatric care (control group) in a randomized control design. Treatment which included individual and group psychoanalytic psychotherapy was for 18 months. Outcome measures included frequency of suicide attempts and acts of self-harm as evaluated using a suicide and self-harm inventory (see Appendix 1), number and duration of in-patient admissions, use of psychotropic medication, and self-report measures of depression, anxiety, general symptom distress, interpersonal function, and social adjustment. Data analysis used repeated measures analysis of covariance and non-parametric tests of trend. Patients in the partial hospitalization programme showed a statistically significant decrease on all measures. This was in contrast to the control group which showed limited change or deterioration over the same period. Improvement in depressive symptoms, decrease in suicidal and self-mutilatory acts, reduced in-patient days and better social and interpersonal function began after 6 months and continued to the end of treatment at the 18th month. Replication is needed with larger samples.

Our most important overall finding was shown in our second study. The aim of this study was to determine whether the substantial gains made by treated patients were maintained during 18-month follow-up. Forty-four patients who participated in the original study were assessed at 3-month intervals after completion of the earlier trial. Outcome measures included frequency of suicide attempts and acts of self-harm, number and duration of in-patient admissions, service utilization, and self-report measures of depression, anxiety, general symptom distress, interpersonal function, and social adjustment. Data analysis again used repeated measures analysis of covariance and non-parametric tests of trend. Patients who had received partial hospitalization treatment not only maintained their substantial gains but also showed a statistically significant continued improvement on most measures in contrast to the control group of patients who showed only limited change during the same period. This suggests that 'rehabilitative' changes had occurred in association with partial hospital treatment enabling patients post discharge to negotiate the stresses and strains of everyday life without resorting to former ways of coping such as self-harming activity.

Health care utilization of all patients who participated in the trial was assessed using information from case notes and service providers (Bateman and Fonagy 2003). Costs of psychiatric, pharmacological, and Emergency Room treatment 6 months prior to treatment, during 18-months treatment, and at 18-months follow-up were compared. There were no differences between the groups in the costs of service utilization pre-treatment or during treatment. The additional cost of day-hospital treatment was offset by less psychiatric in-patient care and reduced emergency room treatment. The trend for costs to decrease in the experimental group during 18-months follow-up was not apparent in the control group suggesting that day-hospital treatment for BPD is no more expensive than general psychiatric care and shows considerable cost-savings after treatment.

Cognitive analytic therapy

This form of therapy postulates that a set of partially dissociated 'self-states' account for the clinical features of BPD and the treatment has been manualized (Ryle 1997) (see p. 128). It is claimed that BPD patients typically experience rapid switching from one state of mind to another, and in the process undergo intense uncontrollable emotions alternating between feeling muddled and emotionally cut off. Although many are enthusiastic about the effectiveness of this approach there is no evidence supported by controlled trials to date (Margison 2000) although there are some indications that the treatment method may be of help in some patients (Ryle and Golynkina 2000). In this study, 27 patients who entered treatment were followed-up at the sixth month and eighteenth month. At the sixth month, 14 of the 27 patients no longer met criteria for BPD and, of the 18 who attended the 18-month follow-up, most showed improvement on psychometric measures. However, using a primary outcome measure of no longer meeting criteria for BPD may simply be measuring instability of diagnosis rather than a positive effect of treatment. Naturalistic longitudinal follow-up of BPD shows 43% of patients no longer meet criteria for BPD for at least two consecutive months within the first 12 months of diagnosis. In a small, as yet unreported, randomized controlled trial comparing patients treated either with CAT or alternative psychological treatment, all patients showed significant improvement over time on a range of clinical measures. There was no difference between people receiving CAT and other psychological treatments so the effects may be non-specific. However, there was some indication that CAT was judged more helpful than other psychological treatments by borderline patients.

Cognitive therapy

Cognitive therapy is a goal-directed problem solving therapy that focuses on teaching specific cognitive and behavioural skills to improve current functioning. The therapeutic aim is to define the patient's presenting problems, to set goals, and to modify dysfunctional thinking and associated behaviours, which prevent adaptive functioning. The clinician's role is to teach the patient to identify and modify dysfunctional thoughts and beliefs.

In cognitive therapy for PDs, more emphasis is placed on changing core beliefs than dysfunctional thoughts and on maintaining a collaborative therapeutic alliance. This is based on the assumption that the patient's maladaptive beliefs are consistent across a wide range of settings, and therefore are also likely to manifest in the therapeutic relationship. Thus the therapeutic relationship is used as a 'relationship laboratory' as the patients are helped to learn new and more adaptive ways of relating to others.

Davidson and Tyrer (1996) in an open study, have used cognitive therapy for the treatment of two Cluster B PDs, viz. antisocial (ASPD) and BPD. They evaluated a brief (10-session) cognitive therapy approach using single-case methodology, which showed improvement in target problems. The approach is now currently being evaluated in a three-centre randomized controlled trial. Another small ($n=34$), randomized controlled trial has recently been carried out using a mixed cognitive therapy and dialectical behaviour therapy protocol for treating Cluster B personality difficulties and disorders (Evans *et al.* 1999). Self-harm repeaters with a parasuicide attempt in the preceding 12 months were randomly allocated to Manual Assisted Cognitive Behaviour Therapy (MACT) ($n=18$), and the rest ($n=16$) to treatment as usual (TAU). The rate of suicide acts was lower with MACT (median 0.17/month MACT; 0.37/month TAU; $p=0.11$) and self-rated depressive symptoms also improved ($p=0.03$). The treatment involved a mean of 2.7 sessions and the observed average cost of care was 46% less with MACT ($p=0.22$). A further multi-centre study (Tyrer *et al.* 2003) on patients who self-harm, not all of whom had PD, compared the same clinical application of CBT with treatment as usual but found no difference on most measures between the two groups at either the sixth or twelfth month. It is possible that a longer period of treatment or greater engagement in face-to-face treatment, where this is achievable in routine health care settings, would show more favourable results. However, when those patients with PD were separated out a significant delay was observed to the next episode of self-harm. There was also some evidence of cost-effectiveness of MACT compared with routine treatment (Byford *et al.* 2003).

Dialectical behaviour therapy (DBT)

This is a special adaptation of cognitive therapy, which was originally used for the treatment in a group of repeatedly parasuicidal female patients with BPD and which led to a marked reduction in the frequency of self-harm episodes compared with treatment as usual (Linehan *et al.* 1991). Although dialectical behaviour therapy (DBT) reduces episodes of self-harm initially, it is less effective in the longer term. DBT is a manualized therapy (Linehan 1993*b*) (see p. 119) which includes techniques at the level of behaviour (functional analysis), cognitions (e.g. skills training) and support (empathy, teaching management of trauma). Patients were admitted to the trial if they met DSM-III-R criteria and had made at least two suicide attempts in the previous five years, with one in the preceding eight weeks. Twenty-two women patients were assigned to DBT and 22 to the control condition. Assessment was carried out during and at the end of therapy, and again after one year-follow-up (Linehan *et al.* 1993). Control patients were significantly more likely to make suicide attempts (mean attempts in control and DBT patients, 33.5 and 6.8 respectively), spent significantly longer as in-patients over the year of treatment (mean 38.8 and 8.5 days respectively), and were significantly more likely to drop out of those therapies they were assigned to (attrition 50% vs 16.7% respectively).

Follow-up was naturalistic, based on the proposition that the morbidity of this group precluded termination of therapy at the end of the experimental period. At 6-month follow-up, DBT patients continued to show less parasuicidal behaviour than controls, though at one year there were no between-group differences. While at one year DBT patients had had fewer days in the hospital, at the 6-month assessment there were no between-group differences. Treatment with DBT for one year compared with treatment as usual led to a reduction in the number and severity of suicide attempts and decreased the frequency and length of in-patient admission. However, there were no between-group differences on measures of depression, hopelessness, or reasons for living. Later dismantling studies suggest that individual elements of the DBT programme are not enough to effect change.

A Dutch research project (Verheul *et al.* 2003) investigated standard DBT treatment in 58 women with BPD who were randomly assigned either to 12 months of DBT or treatment as usual using a randomized controlled design. Participants were clinical referrals from both addiction treatment and psychiatric services. Outcome measures included treatment retention, and of course suicidal, self-mutilating, and self-damaging impulsive behaviours. The results showed that DBT resulted in better retention rates and greater reductions of self-mutilating and self-damaging impulsive behaviours than treatment as usual, especially among those with histories of frequent self-mutilation. This suggests that DBT enhances treatment retention, reduces severe dysfunctional behaviours (e.g. parasuicide and binge eating), and reduces psychiatric hospitalization for both substance using and non-substance using BPD patients. A 6-month follow-up showed that gains were maintained but there was no difference in parasuicide attempts or substance abuse between the two groups and the differences at the end of treatment were becoming smaller suggesting that DBT for 1 year is inadequate for this group of patients (personal communication).

Across studies, the effect of DBT on levels of depression, hopelessness, and survival and coping beliefs, and overall life satisfaction is inconclusive. Although originally designed for the out-patient treatment of suicidal individuals with BPD, DBT has been applied to many more populations, including co-morbid substance dependence and BPD, and juveniles with antisocial behaviours, and in different contexts such as in-patient wards. The studies are discussed in two reviews (Koerner and Dimeff 2000; Koerner and Linehan 2000). Barley *et al.* (1993) evaluated the effectiveness of dialectical behaviour therapy for treatment of BPD in an in-patient setting. They found that during and following implementation of a DBT programme there was a significant fall in rates of parasuicide when compared to a period before implementation of DBT. There was no significant difference, however, between the reported rates of parasuicide on the specialized DBT unit and another unit offering the hospital's standard treatment (treatment as usual control). The results suggest that DBT may have made a successful contribution to reducing parasuicide but it is not unique in preventing parasuicidal behaviour. Confirming this argument is a study reported by Springer *et al.* (1996). These workers randomly assigned personality-disordered patients either to a modified DBT programme or to a wellness and lifestyles group during a short in-patient stay. Patients in both groups improved significantly on most measures and there were no between-group differences.

Overall DBT is associated with better retention rates and is more effective than TAU in reducing self-mutilating behaviours and self-damaging impulsive acts than TAU, especially among those with histories of frequent self-mutilating behaviours, but it may not be a treatment for the PD itself.

Therapeutic community treatments

A therapeutic community (TC) may be defined as an intensive form of treatment in which the environmental setting becomes the core therapy in which behaviour can be challenged and modified, essentially through group pressure. Although they have been in existence in the United Kingdom and Denmark for over 50 years, they have only recently been subjected to direct controlled evaluation and although the treatments and patient populations treated are so varied that the results are difficult to interpret, the consensus is generally favourable. A recent systematic review of the literature (Lees *et al.* 1999) concluded that studies of TCs demonstrated a positive outcome. However, there are considerable difficulties in interpreting the results of this meta-analysis due to the heterogeneous nature of the treatments, the participants in the trials, the control conditions, the outcome measures, and the length of follow-up. Only eight of the 29 studies qualifying for inclusion were randomized controlled trials and half of these were from the same US facility for drug-involved offenders with a work release scheme. The most positive results came from those TCs that offered treatment for substance misuse and all of these were from secure (predominantly prison) settings.

In a recent study, Chiesa and Fonagy (2000) compared two models of psychosocial intervention for PD. Two groups of people with PD were allocated (but not randomly) to a one-stage treatment model (in-patients with no specialist after care) and to a two-stage model (shorter in-patient admission followed by outreach treatment), and were prospectively compared. It was found that the subjects in the two-stage sample did significantly better on global assessment of mental health and in social adjustment at 12 months. Subjects with BPD allocated to the two-stage model improved significantly more than such patients in the one-stage model at 36-month follow-up (Chiesa and Fonagy 2003). These two models have, in turn, been compared with treatment within the general psychiatric service (Chiesa *et al.* in press). The results suggest that the brief in-patient therapeutic community treatment followed by out-patient dynamic therapy is more effective than both long-term residential therapeutic community treatment and general psychiatric treatment in the community on most measures including self-harm, attempted suicide, and readmission rates to general psychiatric admission wards and more cost-effective (Chiesa *et al.* 2002*b*).

It may be expected that the more severe patients would be treated within in-patient settings and yet a recent comparison of data suggested that severity was not the main factor in determining who was treated as an in-patient or day-patient. Chiesa *et al.* (2002*a*) compared data on personality-disordered patients from an in-patient unit (Cassel Hospital) with two day-hospitals (Halliwick in England and Ulleval in Norway) on a number of demographic, diagnostic, and other key clinical variables. Outcome in the areas of symptom severity (Symptom Chek-List-90-R) and social adaptation (Social Adjustment Scale) was evaluated by comparing admission with discharge scores. Treatment costs for each sample were also estimated and compared. Significant differences were found on most baseline variables across the three sites. In general, with regard to severity of psychopathology, the Halliwick sample was the most disturbed, Ulleval the least with Cassel somewhat in-between. No significant differences in improvement were found amongst the three sites, but treatment costs were considerably higher at Cassel than in the two day-centres. The differences found in the three samples bear no clear relationship to context of treatment. These results suggest that referral of PD for in-patient or day-hospital treatment is less influenced by severity of problem than had been previously supposed and may depend more on availability of treatment facility.

Drug treatments

A review of drug treatment is included here because we have integrated medication into our treatment (see p. 195). We view medication as useful in the treatment of PD. Indeed, occasionally, it is essential if patients are to be able to participate in psychotherapy. To this extent we firmly differentiate ourselves from those treatment programmes that either refuse patients who are on medication as being unsuitable for treatment or consider the medication as an intervention separate from psychotherapy. The former simply serves to exclude those patients who are the most ill and appears to deny the evidence base for the use of medication in PD whilst the latter does not allow prescription of medication to take into account transference and countertransference processes. Although there are no trials exploring this question, we suspect that a combination of psychotherapy and medication may be better than either alone.

Antipsychotic drugs

Although antipsychotic drugs are perhaps the most widely used in the treatment of PD there is considerable confusion about their value. Two studies published in 1986 showed that in randomized-placebo-controlled trials low doses of haloperidol and thiothexene were effective in reducing typical borderline and schizotypal symptoms, and it was of special interest that they were more effective than amitriptyline in reducing the symptoms of depression (Soloff *et al.* 1986*a*,*b*). However, this level of efficacy has not been replicated. Recent studies suggest the utility of atypical antipsychotic medication. In an open-label trial of olanzapine for 8 weeks in 11 patients with BPD, treated patients showed an improvement in symptoms of psychoticism, depression, interpersonal sensitivity, and anger (Schulz *et al.* 1999*a*). In a further 6-month double-blind placebo-controlled trial of 28 female subjects, patients treated with olanzapine showed significant improvement in anxiety levels, paranoia, anger and hostility, and interpersonal sensitivity (Zanarini and Frankenburg 2001). A controlled study of risperidone for BPD in 27 patients showed a reduction of interpersonal sensitivity, anger-hostility, psychoticism, and paranoid ideation in patients taking the active drug although those taking placebo also made some symptomatic gains (Schulz *et al.* 1999*b*). Clozapine may also reduce severe self-mutilation and aggression in psychotic patients with BPD (Chengappa *et al.* 1999). It is important to note that in all these studies drop-out rates are around 50% or more by 12 weeks.

Antidepressant drugs

Both tricyclic antidepressants and selective serotonin reuptake inhibitors (SSRIs) have been used in the treatment of PD and, although the most positive finding has been in BPD in which the results are difficult to interpret as depression is a feature of this condition, there is good evidence that SSRIs reduce impulsiveness. Venlafaxine with noradrenergic reuptake properties has also been shown to reduce symptoms, somatic complaints, and self-injurious behaviour in an open-trial (Markovitz and Wagner 1995). There are also suggestions that abnormal personality may itself be improved by SSRIs (Ekselius and von Knorring 1998) but this problem has to be studied in patients with abnormal personality alone if the effects of mental state contamination are to be discounted.

Mood stabilizers

Lithium, carbamazepine, and sodium valproate have all been used to treat PD, and the borderline variant in particular. Results with lithium have been inconsistent, apart from one old study that showed clear reduction of anger and impulsiveness in those with ASPD which has not been replicated.

Sodium valproate is a well-tolerated medication with possible efficacy in the treatment of agitation and impulsive aggression seen in patients of BPD. Hollander *et al.* (1996) and his colleagues have reported the results of a preliminary double blind, placebo-controlled trial of valproate in the treatment of BPD. Although the number of patients treated with divalproex sodium was 12 and those on placebo were only four, the authors concluded that divalproex sodium (sodium valproate and valproic acid) was more effective than placebo for improvement in the global symptomatology, level of functioning, aggression, and depression, but added that this could only be confirmed by carrying out further trials using a larger sample size.

Problems of outcome research

This brief review of the present literature reveals several serious problems that need to be addressed if future research is to be fruitful. These include problems of case identification, the presence of co-morbidity, specificity of psychotherapies, use of outcome measures, and randomization of patients to treatment. The specificity of approaches is discussed in Chapter 4 in which the common components and key distinguishing features of different treatments are outlined. Other problems of PD research are reviewed in detail elsewhere (Bateman and Fonagy 2000). However, the difficulties associated with randomization are often underestimated, particularly by those people who have never tried to randomize patients with BPD!

Randomization and personality disorder

Borderline patients do not take kindly to randomization. Although their lives may be dominated by apparently random behaviour, their search is for stability, certainty, and control. Offering them referral into a research project quickly stimulates hope of effective help but when they realize that their allocation to treatment appears to be dependent on the toss of a coin, they are confronted with uncertainty, loss of control, and anxiety about rejection. Both randomization in and randomization out can cause problems. Borderline patients at the severe end of the spectrum have usually had years of psychiatric treatment and psychotherapy. For those accepted into treatment, early expectations may not be met. When confronted with the reality of hard therapeutic work, the result may be, at best, a feeling of demoralization and, at worst, rage and aggression and refusal to participate in any further aspect of research. Randomization out of treatment into a control group can lead to refusal to co-operate, yet the researcher needs patients who are randomized out of the treatment programme to agree to further interviews and to fill out questionnaires. This can become progressively difficult over time leading to 'holes' in the data due to the high attrition rate in a control group. Some patients may even take pleasure in ensuring that researchers do not get the information they ask for at the time that it is needed leading to further sampling problems. A reasonable way around these problems is to ensure that randomization is only done when two active treatments are offered. Most of the studies discussed above were conducted comparing specialist treatment with routine care and the one thing that borderline patients do not like is to be considered routine.

Associated with these personal and practical problems of randomization are other factors that may interfere with interpretation of any outcome data. Difficulties in implementing randomized controlled trials (RCTs) of long-term treatment are extensive. First, there is an accumulating literature on the importance of patient expectations for therapy outcome (Horowitz *et al.* 1988, 1993). Strict randomization may lead to treatment allocations incongruent with patient expectation and this may be particularly problematic for patients whose lack of flexibility is almost a defining feature of their disorder (Bleiberg 1994). Second, given the relatively small cell sizes of RCTs, attrition represents a serious threat to internal validity. PD patients tend to show relatively high attrition rates in treatment trials (Tyrer *et al.* 1990) although this varies according to PD diagnosis (Shea *et al.* 1990) and treatment approach (Rosser *et al.* 1987; Linehan *et al.* 1991). Third, RCTs, with notable exceptions (Shapiro *et al.* 1995), do not randomize therapists to patients even though it is known that the personality, skills and training of the therapist have significant effects on outcome (Beutler *et al.* 1994). This potential confound is likely to be even greater for psychotherapeutic treatments of PD given that interpersonal relationship problems are undoubtedly at the core of personality disturbance. Fourth, investigator allegiance (Robinson *et al.* 1990) has been shown to strongly affect outcome and unbiased, blind evaluations are even harder to achieve in long-term than in short-term treatments.

There is a trade-off between the internal validity (Cooke and Campbell 1979) of well-controlled trials, which ensure that causal inferences may be appropriately drawn from experimental manipulations, and the external validity of naturalistic research designs which are limited in terms of causal inference but which generate findings more readily generalisable to everyday practice (Hoagwood *et al.* 1995; Jensen *et al.* 1996). In our outcome research we used a population of patients seen in everyday practice which on the one hand resulted in a reduction in internal validity due to confounds such as co-mobidity but on the other ensured that the patients being scrutinized represented individuals seen by practising clinicians thereby increasing the external validity and generalisability. But there remains a long way to go before we can be sure about which patients are best suited to psychoanalytic, behavioural, or supportive therapy, and who should be treated within what context and with what intensity.

3 Mentalization-based understanding of borderline personality disorder

The developmental roots of borderline personality disorder (BPD)

Underpinning our approach is the assumption that understanding borderline personality disorder (BPD) depends on an understanding of *normal human development*. In thinking about self-development, rather than focusing on the content of the mental representation of self, which has been the focus of psychological investigation for much of the century (for a review see Harter 1999), we are instead concerned with the process that allows the representation of self to come into being: that is, the evolution of the 'self as agent'. The development of the self as agent (for convenience often referred to here as the 'agentive self') has historically been a neglected topic, because of the dominance of the Cartesian assumption that the agentive self emerges automatically from the sensation of the mental activity of the self ('I think therefore I am'). The influence of Cartesian doctrine has encouraged the belief that the conscious apprehension of our mind states through introspection is a basic, direct, and probably pre-wired mental capacity, leading to the conviction that knowledge of the self as a mental agent (as a 'doer' of things and a 'thinker' of thoughts) is an innate-given rather than a developing or constructed capacity. If we understand the acquisition of knowledge of the self as a mental agent to be the result of a developmental process, which can go wrong in certain circumstances, we can gain a new perspective on the origins of BPD. In order to gain this new perspective, we must first go back to consider our earliest days, reviewing self-development in the context of the individual's early attachment relationships.

The relevance of the attachment theory perspective

There have been many past attempts to illuminate the symptomatology of BPD using attachment theory. Implicitly or explicitly, Bowlby's (1973) suggestion that early experience with the caregiver serves to organize later attachment relationships has been used in explanations of psychopathology in BPD. For example, it has been suggested that the borderline person's experiences of interpersonal attack, neglect, and threats of abandonment may account for their perception of current relationships as attacking and neglectful (Benjamin 1993). Others have suggested that individuals with BPD are specifically characterized by a fearful and pre-occupied attachment style reflecting 'an emotional template of intimacy anxiety/anger' (Dutton *et al.* 1994*b*). In studies of adult attachment interview (AAI) narratives of BPD patients, the classification of pre-occupied is most frequently assigned (Fonagy *et al.* 1996) and, within this, the confused, fearful, and overwhelmed sub-classification appears to be most common (Patrick *et al.* 1994). Past attempts at linking work on attachment with theories of borderline pathology have stressed the common characteristic shared by the ambivalently attached/pre-occupied and borderline groups 'to check for proximity, signaling to establish contact by pleading or other calls for attention or help, and clinging behaviors' (Gunderson 1996). Borderline patients also tend to be unresolved with regard to their experience of trauma or abuse (Patrick *et al.* 1994; Fonagy *et al.* 1996).

There is no doubt that borderline individuals are insecure in their attachment, but descriptions of insecure attachment from infancy or adulthood provide an inadequate clinical account for several reasons. (1) Anxious attachment is very common; in working class samples the majority of children are anxiously attached (Broussard 1995). (2) Anxious patterns of attachment in infancy correspond to relatively stable adult strategies (Main *et al.* 1985), yet the hallmark of the disordered attachments of borderline individuals is the absence of stability (Higgitt and Fonagy 1992). (3) In both delinquent and borderline individuals there are variations across situations or types of relationships. The delinquent adolescent is, for example, aware of the mental states of others in his gang and the borderline individual is at times hypersensitive to the emotional states of mental health professionals and family members. (4) The clinical presentation of borderline patients frequently includes a violent attack on the patient's own body or that of another human being. It is likely that the propensity for such violence must include an additional component that predisposes such individuals to act upon bodies rather than upon minds. An adequate account of the relationship between the individual's early attachment environment and their later manifestation of the symptoms of BPD requires that *the way the individual experiences that environment* be taken into account, and that the mere fact of experiencing it, which in Cartesian fashion has historically been viewed as an unproblematic given, be viewed as an achievement determined by developmental factors.

Optimal self-development in a secure attachment context

John Bowlby, a major Darwin scholar, (Bowlby 1991) was impressed by the obvious selection advantages of infant protest at separation, i.e. protection from predation (Bowlby 1969). Given that phylogenetically and ontogenetically, infancy is a period of extreme risk, it is unarguable that natural selection would favour individuals with a capacity for making attachments. The generally recognized components of attachment behaviours that serve to establish and maintain proximity are: (1) signals that draw the caregivers to their children (e.g. smiling), (2) aversive behaviours (such as crying) which perform the same function, and (3) skeletal muscle activity (primarily locomotion) that bring the child to the caregiver. But there is a fourth component that provides a better evolutionary rationale for the entire enterprise of human attachment, going beyond the issue of physical protection. According to Bowlby, at about the age of three behaviours signifying a goal-corrected partnership begin to emerge. The central psychological processes for mediating goal-corrected partnerships are the *internal working models* (IWMs).

Bowlby's original concept has been thoughtfully elaborated by some of the greatest minds in the attachment field (Main *et al.* 1985; Crittenden 1990, 1994; Sroufe 1990, 1996; Bretherton 1991; Main 1991; Bretherton and Munholland 1999) and no attempt to duplicate this will be undertaken here. However, it might be helpful to summarize the four representational systems that are implied in these reformulations: (1) expectations of interactive attributes of early caregivers created in the first year of life and subsequently elaborated; (2) event representations by which general and specific memories of attachment-related experiences are encoded and retrieved; (3) autobiographical memories by which specific events are conceptually connected because of their relation to a continuing personal narrative and developing self-understanding; (4) understanding of the psychological characteristics of other people (inferring and attributing causal motivational mind states such as desires and emotions and epistemic mind states such as intentions and beliefs) *and differentiating these from those of the self.* Thus a key developmental attainment of the IWM is the creation of a processing system for the self (and significant others) in terms of a set of stable and generalized intentional attributes, such as desires, emotions, intentions, and beliefs inferred from recurring invariant patterns in the history of previous interactions. The child becomes able to use this representational system to predict the other's or the self's behaviour in conjunction with local, more transient intentional states inferred from a given situation.

Classically, in attachment theory this phase change from behaviour to representation has been regarded as a modification of the attachment system propelled by cognitive development (Marvin and Britner 1999). Our contention here will be the reverse. We propose that a major selective advantage conferred by attachment to humans was the opportunity it afforded for the development of social intelligence and meaning making: *attachment also propels cognitive development*. The capacity for 'interpretation', which Bogdan (1997) defined as 'organisms making sense of each other in contexts where this matters biologically' (p. 10), becomes uniquely human when others are engaged 'psychologically in sharing experiences, information, and affects' (p. 94). The capacity to interpret human behavior—to make sense of each other—requires the intentional stance: 'treating the object whose behavior you want to predict as a rational agent with beliefs and desires' (Dennett 1987, p. 15).

The capacity for interpretation in psychological terms—let us call this the interpersonal interpretive function (IIF)—is not just a generator or mediator of attachment experience; we contend that it is also a product of the complex psychological processes engendered by close proximity in infancy to another human being, the attachment figure. The IIF should not be identified with Bowlby's IWM; it does not contain representations of experiences and is not a repository of personal encounters with the caregiver. Rather, it is a means of processing new experiences. Emotion regulation, the establishment of attentional mechanisms and the development of mentalizing capacities may be usefully considered under a single heading as components of the interpersonal interpretative function, acting together to ensure that the individual collaborates productively with others. In order to be able to exercise this function, the individual needs a symbolic representational system for mental states and also needs to be able to selectively activate states of mind in line with particular intentions (attentional control). Close proximity in infancy to another human being is seen as a necessary condition for the development of these capacities. It follows that disruption of early affectional bonds not only sets up maladaptive attachment patterns but also undermines a range of capabilities vital to normal social development. We suggest that BPD can be understood in terms of the absence or impairment of the capacity for emotion regulation, attentional control, and mentalization, all of which are normally acquired in the context of attachment relationships. Mentalizing, which is at the pinnacle of these self-regulatory capacities, entails making sense of the actions of oneself and others on the basis of intentional mental states, such as desires, feelings, and beliefs. Mentalization entails the recognition that what is in the mind is in the mind. It reflects the recognition of one's own and others' mental states as mental states. In effect, mentalizing refers to making sense of each other and ourselves, implicitly and explicitly in terms of mind states and mental processes. Of course as psychodynamic clinicians we mentalize continually when we endeavour to understand the seemingly anomalous actions we construe as psychopathology and when we take the lead in psychotherapeutic conversations intended to ameliorate that psychopathology. This makes it particularly challenging for us to understand individuals whose capacity for mentalization is limited, who do not make use of their capacity to understand others as mental entities, or who create confused and confusing inaccurate representations of the mental states of others and themselves. As we will see, such individuals are then particularly vulnerable in the face of trauma.

Let us begin by reviewing the processes by means of which the capacity for interpersonal interpretation is acquired in an environment where closeness to the caregiver is available in infancy.

Early stages of self-development

As a child normally develops, he gradually acquires an understanding of five increasingly complex levels of agency of the self: physical, social, teleological, intentional, and representational (Gergely 2001; Fonagy *et al.* 2002). We shall describe the normal developmental stages before speculating about the deviations in the development of the agentive self that might constitute the roots of BPD. Physical agency involves an appreciation of the effects of actions on bodies in space. The child begins to understand that he is a physical entity with force that is the source of action and that he is an agent whose actions can bring about changes in bodies with which he has immediate physical contact (Leslie 1994). Developing alongside this is the child's understanding of himself as a social agent. Babies engage from birth in interactions with their caregivers (Meltzoff and Moore 1977; Trevarthen 1979; Stern 1985). In these exchanges the baby's behaviour produces effects on his caregivers' behaviour and emotions. Early understanding of the self as a social agent, therefore, involves at least knowing that one's communicative displays can produce effects at a distance, in the social environment (Neisser 1988).

The infant's sensitivity to social contingency

Watson's extensive studies of infants (Watson 1979, 1985, 1994) have led Gergely and Watson (1999) to propose that the earliest forms of self-awareness evolve through the workings of an innate mechanism which they call the *contingency detection module*. This mechanism enables the infant to analyze the probability of causal links between his actions and stimulus events. Watson (1994, 1995) proposed that one of the primary functions of the contingency detection module is self-detection. While our own actions produce effects that are necessarily perfectly response-contingent (e.g. watching our hands as we move them), stimuli from the external world typically correspond less pefectly to our actions. Detecting how far the stimuli we perceive depend on our actions may be the original criterion that enables us to distinguish ourselves from the external world. Our bodies are by far the most action contingent aspects of our environments.

Numerous studies have demonstrated that young infants are highly sensitive to the relationship between their physical actions and consequent stimuli (e.g. Watson 1972, 1994; Papousek and Papousek 1974; Field 1979; Lewis and

Brooks-Gunn 1979; Bahrick and Watson 1985; Lewis *et al.* 1990; Rochat and Morgan 1995). For example Watson (1972) has shown that two-month-olds increase their rate of leg kicking when it results in the movement of a mobile, but not when they experience a similar, but non-contingent event. Sensitivity to contingency thus explains how we learn that we are physical agents whose actions bring about changes in the environment.

In a seminal study Bahrick and Watson (Bahrick and Watson 1985; see also Rochat and Morgan 1995; Schmuckler 1996) have demonstrated that infants can use their perception of perfect contingency between actions and their consequences for self-detection and self-orientation as early as 3 months of age. In a series of experiments, 5- and 3-month-old infants were seated on a high-chair in front of two monitors so that they could kick freely. One monitor showed a live image of the child's moving legs, providing a visual stimulus that corresponded perfectly. The other monitor showed a previously recorded image of the infant's moving legs, which was unrelated to his present movements. Five-month-olds clearly differentiated between the two displays, looking significantly more at the *non-contingent image*. A number of other preferential looking studies (Papousek and Papousek 1974; Lewis and Brooks-Gunn 1979; Rochat and Morgan 1995; Schmuckler 1996) in which the live image of the self was contrasted with the moving but non-contingent image of another baby indicate that 4–5-month-old-infants can distinguish themselves from others on the basis of response-stimulus contingencies and prefer to fixate *away* from the self.

Interestingly, Bahrick and Watson found that among 3-month-olds some preferred the perfectly contingent image, while others were more interested in the non-contingent image. Field (1979) also reported that her sample of 3-month-olds were more inclined to look at their own images. Piaget's (1936) observation that during the first months of life babies perform the same actions on themselves over and over again also suggests that babies are initially preoccupied with perfect contingency. Watson and Gergely (1999), (see also Watson 1994, 1995) have therefore proposed that during the first 2–3 months of life, the contingency detection module is genetically set to seek out and explore perfectly response-contingent stimulation. Watson hypothesizes that this initial bias enables the infant to develop a *primary representation of his bodily self* as a distinct object in the environment, by identifying what he has perfect control over. Watson (1995) suggests that an initial phase of self-seeking behaviour may be necessary to prepare the baby to cope with the environment. At around three months, the target value of the contingency analyzer in normal infants is 'switched' to prefer *high-but-imperfect contingencies*—the kind of responses that are characteristic of children's caregivers. This change reorients infants after 3 months away from self-exploration (perfect contingencies) and towards *the exploration and representation of the social world*. The infant is now ready to identify regularities in the external world that are clearly linked to its actions but are not perfect reflections of it.

The teleological stance

The types of causal relations that connect actions to their agents on the one hand, and to the world on the other, go far beyond the level of physical description, and we grow to understand much more about both of these relations as we develop. Thus, around 8–9 months of age (Tomasello 1999) infants begin to differentiate actions from their outcomes and to think about actions as means to an end. This is the beginning of their understanding of themselves as *teleological agents* (Leslie 1994; Csibra and Gergely 1998) who can choose the most efficient way to bring about a goal from a range of alternatives. The limitation of this stage of experiencing the agentive self is one of physicality. Experimental studies of infants towards the end of their first year of life clearly indicate that they expect the actors in their environment to behave reasonably and rationally given physically apparent goal state and constraints which are also physically evident to the self (Gergely and Csibra 1996, 1997, 1998, 2000, 2003; Csibra and Gergely 1998; Csibra *et al.* 1999). Imagine an object which has repeatedly followed a path that included a deviation to get around an obstacle. Then the obstacle disappears. The nine-month-old infant observing this shows surprise if the object continues to follow the path that includes the deviation around the obstacle that is no longer present. The infant shows no surprise when the object modifies its path to take account of the changed circumstance, the disappearance of the obstacle. In the latter case the object behaved 'rationally' while in the former the infant could not understand why the object was apparently 'inconveniencing itself'.

The reader should note that there is no implication here that the infant has an idea about the 'mental state' of the object. He/she is simply judging rational behaviour in terms of the physical constraints that prevail and that which is obvious in terms of the physical end-state which the object has reached. This albeit quite advanced mode of thinking on the part of a 9-month-old does not go beyond that which is apparent on the surface. Later on, we will suggest a connection between the focus on understanding actions in terms of their physical as opposed to mental outcomes, which is characteristic of the teleological stance, and the mode of experience of agency we often see in the violent acts of some individuals with BPD. Expectations concerning the agency of the other are present but these are formulated in terms restricted to the physical world. We would argue that this is not because a representation of the internal (the mental) does not exist. It exists, but with highly significant developmental constraints. Thus, it may be enough for a patient with BPD to note a slight shift in the body position of his or her treater or note an incidental physical circumstance such as a door being shut for that individual to impute complex and elaborate states of mind, which most of us would fall short of considering. These instances give us hints that that individual may be functioning predominantly in a teleological mode, where physical appearance rather than what might lie beyond in terms of intentional states provide the foundation for complex interpersonal judgment. Even more telling are instances when patients cannot accept anything other than a modification in the realm of the physical as a true index of the intentions of the other. Thus, the therapist's benign disposition, her motivation to be helpful, has to be demonstrated by increasingly heroic acts, such as availability on the telephone, extra sessions at weekends, physical touching, holding, and ultimately in some sad instances serious violations of therapeutic boundaries.

Under circumstances where the use of the intentional stance (mentalization) is only partially accessible because of either biological deficits or social experiences beyond the normal range, the clinician frequently finds the client falling back on an understanding of agency based on the teleological stance when he/she interprets interpersonal behavior. This is most marked in relation to actions of others in attachment contexts. It is in these contexts that early adverse experience was most likely to generate a stance where an individual would deliberately stop engaging in mentalization in order to avoid the trauma of having to conceive of malevolent intent in the other. This re-emergence of teleological principles is thought to be more likely in those individuals in whom the ability to take the intentional stance and form second-order representations of emotional constitutional self-states was not firmly established in the first place.

The self as an intentional and representational agent

Sometime during their second year infants develop an understanding of agency that is already mentalistic: they start to understand that they are intentional agents whose actions are caused by prior states of mind, such as desires (Wellman and Phillips 2000). At this point, they also understand that their actions can bring about change in minds as well as bodies: for example, they clearly understand that if they point at something, they can make another person change their focus of attention (Corkum and Moore 1995). Developmentally, this point is prototypically marked when the two-year-old child becomes able to distinguish his own desires from those of the other person. Repacholi and Gopnik (1997) demonstrated that when 18-month-olds were asked to give the experimenter something to eat, they provided her with the particular food item (broccoli vs gold fish crackers) that she had previously expressed a liking for (by saying 'yuk' or 'yummy' when first facing the food item). Thus, they modulated their own action by considering the specific content of the desire they had attributed to the other previously, even when that desire was different from their own preference. In contrast, 14-month-olds gave the experimenter the item they themselves liked, basing their choice on their own preference without being able to consider the other's relevant prior intention. The younger children had assumed an identity between their experience of their own desire and the likely experience of the other. Around three-to-four years of age this understanding of agency in terms of mental causation also begins to include the representation of so-called 'epistemic mind states' concerning knowledge about something (such as beliefs) (Wimmer and Perner 1983). At this stage, we can say that the young child understands himself as a representational agent: that is, his intentional mental states (desires and beliefs) are representational in nature (Wellman 1990; Perner 1991).

Still later, perhaps as late as the 6th year, emerge related advances such as the child's ability to relate memories of his intentional activities and experiences into a coherent causal-temporal organization (Povinelli and Eddy 1995) leading to the establishment of the (temporally) 'extended' or 'proper' self (James 1890). Consider this simple variation on the famous 'rouge' studies of mirror self-recognition. A five-year-old child is videoed playing with an experimenter. In the course of the play, the experimenter places a sticky label on the child without his knowledge. The sticky label remains on when the experimenter and child watch the video together. The child, who has absolutely no difficulty recognizing himself, notices the sticky label but fails to check if it is still on him. When asked to comment he says: 'That child has a label on him' and not 'In the video I have a label on me'. A few months later, aged six, he clearly experiences himself as the same person as the child on the video and immediately removes the label and smiles with the experimenter at the trick perpetrated on him. In other words, the autobiographical self has come into being.

As this brief overview indicates, the development of understanding self and agency entails increasing sophistication in awareness about the nature of mental states. A full experience of agency in social interaction can emerge only when actions of the self and other can be understood as initiated and guided by assumptions concerning the emotions, desires, and beliefs of both. This complex developmental process must start with the emergence of concepts for each mental state. In order to be able to think about mental states, say fear, we have to develop concepts that correspond to and integrate the actual internal experiences that constitutes that state. The concept of fear is a 'second order representation of fear' that relates physiological, cognitive, and behavioural experiences, just as the concept of 'table' labels and thus integrates our actual experiences of tables.[1] Most psychodynamic developmental models, perhaps including Freud's, have assumed that second-order representations of internal states emerged simply on the basis of cumulative experience of such things.

[1]The role that language plays in the development of mentalization has been a subject of controversy for many years. Here we are suggesting that representations for internal states may in the case of emotions for example antedate the acquisition of a verbal label. The signifier in the case of primary emotions is perhaps the expression of the caregiver as it contingently and congruently mirrors the infant's expression.

The implication of this would be that the child suddenly became aware of himself as a thinking being. Taking a somewhat Cartesian view, it could be suggested that the repeated experience of fear will inevitably give rise to this concept in the child's mind just like the experience of tables generates the linguistic label (this view is no longer tenable—see Carpendale and Lewis, in press). Yet, mental states are private and by definition opaque while physical objects have a socially shared quality. Of course, even concepts concerning the physical world are profoundly socially conditioned. So how do we understand the influence of social experience upon the emergence of mental state concepts? Although in the Cartesian view that is implicit to much of our thinking, the spontaneous emergence of internal state concepts is rarely questioned, recent advances in developmental theory suggest a clear role for social experience in the development of mental state concepts. We have to assume a dialectic model of self-development (Hegel 1807) where the child's capacity to create a coherent image of mind is critically dependent on an experience of being clearly perceived as a mind by the attachment figure. Carpendale and Lewis (in press) make a strong case that assumes that social understanding is an emergent property of the child's experience of certain regularities in interaction with others. The 'epistemic triangle', referential interactions between infant and caregiver about the object, is assumed inevitably to generate the discovery that others sometimes have different beliefs about the world from one's own. If we, taking the point of view of the infant, assume the existence of a stable external world, the actions of others in communicative interactions can only be understood given the supposition that they have different beliefs about aspects of the world. Children achieve comparable levels of development at similar ages simply because of the commonalities of their experience. The corollary of this is that differences in the acquisition of social understanding are to be understood in terms of crucial differences in their experience of triadic interactions between the infant, the caregiver, and the object. The remainder of this section is an elaboration of the processes entailed and of the possibilities of their dysfunction in the childhood of individuals with BPD.

Parental mirroring and the development of mental state concepts

A large body of evidence indicates that from the beginning of life babies can tell people apart (Stern 1985). From a very early age they are sensitive to facial expressions (Fantz 1963; Morton and Johnson 1991), they get used to their mothers' voice *in utero* and recognize it after birth (DeCasper and Fifer 1980), and can imitate facial gestures from birth (Meltzoff and Moore 1977, 1989). Young babies' interactions with their caregivers have a 'protoconversational' turn-taking structure (Brazelton *et al.* 1974; Trevarthen 1979; Brazelton and Tronick 1980; Beebe *et al.* 1985; Stern 1985; Tronick 1989; Jaffe *et al.* 2001). The currently dominant biosocial view of emotional development holds that mother and infant are engaged in affective communication from the beginning of life (Bowlby 1969; Sander 1970; Brazelton *et al.* 1974; Stern 1977, 1985; Trevarthen 1979; Tronick 1989; Hobson 1993) in which the mother plays a vital role in modulating the infant's emotional states to make them more manageable.

Mothers are generally very good at telling what their babies are feeling, and sensitive mothers tend to attune their responses to modulate their children's emotional states (Malatesta *et al.* 1989; Tronick 1989). During these interactions, the mother will often mimic her baby's displays of emotion with the apparent intention of modulating or regulating the infant's feelings (Malatesta and Izard 1984; Stern 1985; Papousek and Papousek 1987; Gergely and Watson 1996, 1999). The caregiver's mirroring of the infant's subjective experience has been recognized as a key phase in the development of the child's self by a wide range of psychoanalytic developmental theorists (e.g. Winnicott 1967; Kohut 1971; Pines 1982; Kernberg 1984*b*; Tyson and Tyson 1990) as well as developmental psychologists (Meltzoff 1990; Schneider-Rosen and Cicchetti 1991; Mitchell 1993; Legerstee and Varghese 2001). But why should the mere replication of the outward manifestation of the infant's putative internal experience lead to a moderation of affect expression, and how does it lead to the creation of a sense of self?

Contrary to the classical Cartesian view, and following Gergely and Watson's 'social biofeedback theory of parental affect-mirroring' (Gergely and Watson 1996, 1999), we assume that at first we are not introspectively aware of our different emotion states. Rather, our representations of these emotions are primarily based on stimuli received from the external world. Babies learn to differentiate the internal patterns of physiological and visceral stimulation that accompany different emotions through observing their caregivers' facial or vocal mirroring responses to these. The 'switch' that takes place in the contingency detection module at about 3 months predisposes them to pay attention to *high-but-imperfect contingencies*—the kind of responses that are characteristic of their caregivers when they are in mirroring interaction with them. Contingent mirroring succeeds at downregulation because it generates a sense of 'agency' and control in the infant that is inherently pleasurable. Social biofeedback in the form of parental affect mirroring enables the infant to develop a second-order symbolic representational system for his mind states. The internalization of the mother's mirroring response to the infant's distress (caregiving behaviour) comes to represent an internal state. The infant internalizes the mother's empathic expression by developing a secondary representation of his emotional state with the mother's empathic face as the signifier and his own emotional arousal as the signified. The mother's expression tempers emotion to the extent that it is separate and different from the primary experience, although crucially it is not recognized as the mother's experience, but as an organizer of a self-state. It is this 'inter-subjectivity' which is the bedrock of the intimate connection between attachment and self-regulation (Fig. 3.1).

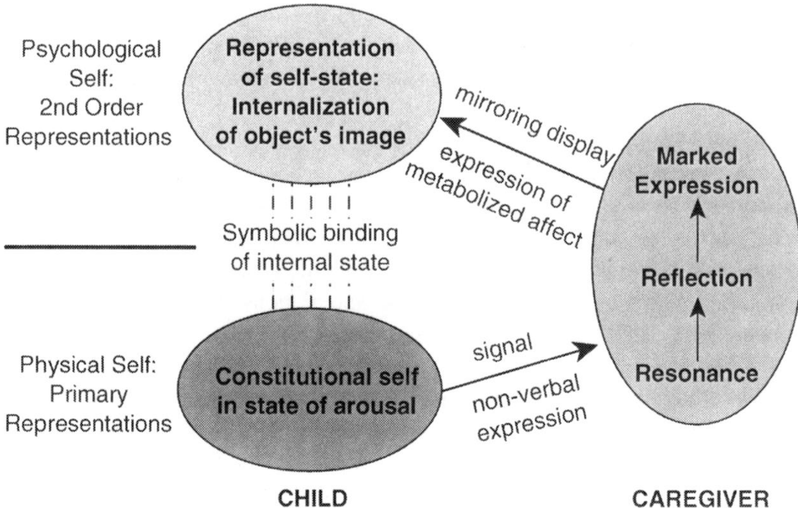

Fig. 3.1 Intersubjective space and the symbolization of emotion.

If the mother's mirroring is to effectively modulate her baby's emotions, and provide the beginnings of a symbolic system by means of which the capacity for self regulation can be further extended, it is important that as well as reflecting the emotion the child is feeling accurately (i.e. the mirroring is *congruent* with the child's emotional display), she signals in some way that what he is seeing is a reflection of *his own* feelings: otherwise it is possible that he will misattribute the feeling to his mother. Misattributing the expressed emotion would be especially problematic in cases where the mother is reflecting the infant's *negative* emotion states, say, his or her fear or anger. If the child thinks that the caregiver *has* the feelings she is displaying, his own negative emotion state, instead of being regulated in a downward direction, is likely to escalate, as the sight of a fearful or angry parent is clearly cause for alarm.

This attribution problem is solved by a specific perceptual feature of the parent's mirroring displays, which following Gergely and Watson we refer to as their '*markedness*'. Marking is typically achieved by producing *an exaggerated version* of the parent's realistic emotion expression, similarly to the marked 'as if' manner of emotion displays that are characteristically produced in pretend play. When the child is sensitive to markedness the child sees the mother's expression as mirroring him and thus not carrying its normal consequences. In this way the child moves away from interpreting reality 'as is' and imposes an alternative construction upon it. This constitutes a move away from the immediacy of physical reality. The marked display, nevertheless, is close enough to the parent's usual expression of that emotion for the infant to recognize its dispositional content. However, the markedness of the display inhibits the attribution of the perceived emotion to the parent: because it is contingent on the infant's behaviour, he therefore assumes that it applies to himself.

In infancy the contingent and congruent responding of the attachment figure is thus far more than the provision of reassurance about a protective presence. It is a principal means by which we acquire an understanding of our own internal states, which is an intermediate step in the acquisition of an understanding of others as psychological entities. In the first year, the infant only has primary awareness of being in a particular, internal, emotional state. Such awareness is non-causal or epiphenomenal in that it is not put to any functional use by the system. It is in the process of social biofeedback that these internal experiences are more closely attended to and evolve a functional role (a signal value) and a role in modulating or inhibiting action. Thus it is the primary attachment relationship that can ensure the move from primary awareness of internal states to a functional awareness. In functional awareness a concept corresponding to the feeling of anger (the *idea of anger* rather than *the experience of anger*) may be used to simulate and so to infer the other's corresponding mental state. It may also be used to serve a signal value to direct action. The robust establishment of these capacities may ensure that the individual can not only moderate his anger through self-regulation but can also use it to initiate actions that are likely to effectively deal with the cause. In the absence of functional awareness anger, once aroused, might be experienced as overwhelming and the individual will be at considerable disadvantage in the creation of effective strategies to address the cause of the dissatisfaction that generated this emotion. It should be noted that this is not the same as reflective awareness of emotion, where the individual can make a causal mind state become the object of attention before, and without it, causing action. Whereas functional awareness is intrinsically coupled with action, reflective awareness is separate from it. It has the capacity to move away from physical reality and may be felt to be not for real.

Many studies provide evidence consistent with the social biofeedback model. For example, a recent study of mothers singing to their infants in distress demonstrated that while securely attached mothers were able to combine maternal displays of incompatible emotions with maternal displays of congruent affect, avoidant mothers sang expressing incongruent emotions alone while mothers whose attachment classification was pre-occupied sang with sadness, mirroring the infant's affect (Milligan *et al.* 2003). Both the latter strategies would be considered in the Gergely–Watson model as non-optimal strategies for the achievement of affect regulation. Similarly, an unpublished study carried out in our laboratory showed that the rapid soothing of distressed six-month-olds could be predicted on the basis of ratings of emotional content of the mother's facial expression during the process of soothing; mothers of rapid responders showed somewhat more fear, somewhat less joy but most typically a range of other affects in addition to fear and sadness. Mothers of rapid responders were far more likely to manifest multiple affect states (complex affects). We interpreted these results as supporting Gergely and Watson's notion of the mother's face being a secondary representation of the infant's experience—the same and yet not the same. This is functional awareness with the capacity to modulate affect states.

We can assume that infants' discovery of their high degree of contingent control over their caregivers' reactions positively arouses them and gives them feelings of causal efficacy. They are also likely to experience the pleasurable changes in their affective states that the parent's affect-modulating soothing interactions bring about (and become associated with, see Gergely and Watson, 1996, 1999). Since such attuned interactions often involve affect-mirroring, infants may come to associate the control they have over their parent's mirroring displays with the ensuing positive change in their affect state, leading to an experience of the self as a self-regulating-agent (Gergely and Watson 1996, 1999). The establishment of second-order representations of emotions creates the basis for affect regulation and impulse control and provides an essential building block for the child's later development of the crucial capacity of mentalization. If the caregiver mirrors the baby's emotions inaccurately or neglects to perform this function at all, the baby's feelings will be unlabelled, confusing, and experienced as unsymbolized and therefore hard to regulate.

The caregiver who is able to give form and meaning to the young child's affective and intentional states, through facial and vocal mirroring and playful interactions, provides the child with representations that will form the very core of his developing sense of selfhood (see Fig. 3.2). For normal development the child needs to experience a mind that has his mind in mind and is able to reflect his feelings and intentions accurately, yet in a way which does not overwhelm him (for example when acknowledging negative affective states). This is the experience that a psychologically neglected child might never have, even if there can be no doubts about the provision of adequate physical care. The child who has not experienced the caregiver's integrative mirroring of his affective states cannot create representations of them, and may later struggle to differentiate reality from fantasy, and physical from psychic reality. This leaves the individual vulnerable to primitive modes of representing subjectivity and the agentive self which are not fully representational or reflective.

Psychic equivalence and the pretend mode

If, as we have argued, experiencing a thought as only a thought is a developmental achievement, what is psychic reality like before it is experienced as 'psychic'?

Attachment figure 'discovers' infant's mind (subjectivity)

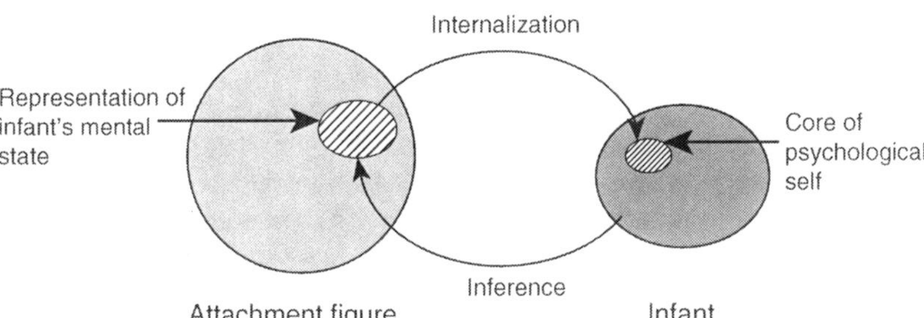

Infant internalizes caregiver's representation to form psychological self
Safe, playful interaction with the caregiver leads to the integration of primitive modes of experiencing internal reality → mentalization

Fig. 3.2 Birth of the psychological self.

We have suggested that early awareness of mental states takes place within two modes (Fonagy and Target 1996; Target and Fonagy 1996). One equates the internal with the external. What exists in the mind must exist in the external world, and what exists out there must invariably also exist in the mind. There cannot be differences in perspective about the external world because it is isomorphic with the internal. '*Psychic equivalence*', as a mode of experiencing the internal world, can cause great distress because the projection of fantasy to the outside world is felt to be compellingly real. A three-year-old boy asked his father to find him a Batman outfit on his trip abroad. The father had great difficulty, but eventually found a fancy dress shop and bought an expensive costume. Unfortunately, the costume was so realistic that the boy was frightened when he saw himself in the mirror, refused to wear it again and went back to using his mother's skirt as his Batman cloak.

The other mode, of '*pretend*' in relation to mental states is therefore essential. Here the child's mental state is decoupled from external or physical reality, but the internal state is thought to have no implications for the outside world. The child's inner experience is separated from the rest of the ego. The pretend mode is illustrated by a trivial incident where a child aged two and a half was playing with a garden chair on its side, pushing it around and evidently shooting at an imaginary enemy. However, when the child was asked, 'Is that a chair or is it a tank?' he immediately put the chair the right way up and walked away from the game. In the pretend mode there can be no connection between what is pretended and actual reality. In pretend mode the child can 'believe' that a chair is a tank, and yet not expect it to shoot real shells, and there have been experimental demonstrations that small children can keep alternative or changing beliefs in mind if they are doing a task in play rather than for real.[2] We believe Freud (1924) referred to vestiges of this developmental state when he described (in the paper on 'The loss of reality in neurosis and psychosis'): '... a domain which became separated from the real external world... kept free from the demands of the exigencies of life, like a kind of "reservation"; it is not accessible to the ego, but is only loosely attached to it' (p. 187). Ron Britton (1992) has also described 'an area of thinking protected from reality and preserved as an area of day-dream or masturbatory fantasy... a place where some people spend most of their lives' (p. 4). It is crucial to remember that for different reasons neither the pretend mode nor the psychic equivalence mode can create internal experiences that have the full quality of internal reality: psychic equivalence is too real while pretend is too unreal. In normal development the child integrates these two modes to arrive at *mentalization*, or reflective mode, in which thoughts and feelings can be experienced *as* representations. Inner and outer reality are seen as linked, but separate, and no longer have to be either equated or dissociated from each other.

In clinical work with borderline patients, words referring to internal states are most commonly used with the expectation on the part of the treater that these will have 'a real impact' on the patient. While the patient is in pretend mode, however, the words may be understood but can have no real implications for the individual to whom and about whom they are spoken. 'Therapy' can go on for weeks, months, sometimes even years, in the pretend mode of psychic reality, where internal states are discussed at length, sometimes with excessive detail and complexity yet no progress is made, and no real understanding is experienced. Indeed, along with the over-ready use of mental state terms, excessive complexity, the simultaneous presence of incompatible formulations or their ready alteration are all indicators of the therapy occurring in the pretend mode.

Mentalization

Mentalization, the capacity to think about mental states as separate from, yet potentially causing actions, is assumed by us to arise as part of an integration of the pretend and psychic equivalent modes of functioning. This happens optimally in the context of a playful parent–child relationship. In such a relationship feelings and thoughts, wishes and beliefs can be experienced by

---

[2]Gopnik and Slaughter (1991) created a 'pretend version' of the belief change task. They asked children to pretend that an empty glass had a chocolate drink in it, the glass was then 'pretend emptied' by the adult and the child was asked to pretend that the glass was now full of lemonade. Almost no 3-year-olds had any difficulty in remembering that the original imagined content was chocolate.

the child as significant and respected on the one hand, but on the other as not being of the same order as physical reality. Both the pretend mode and the psychic equivalent mode of functioning are modified by the interaction with the parent in what Winnicott (1971) incomparably termed, a transitional space. Mentalization as a concept has arguably been part of psychoanalytic thinking since its inception. It represents a major line of theorization in French psychoanalysis for at least the last forty years (Lecours and Bouchard 1997). In the French tradition the concept is limited to the transformation of drives and affects. A different tradition originates from Bion's theory of thinking (Bion 1957, 1962*b*). Andre Green (1975, 1977) came closest to successfully integrating Bion's concept with the Paris tradition of Pierre Marty (1991) and Luquet (1988).

Bion's theory of thinking identifies the origin of symbolic capacity in an analogous way to the Freudian notion that thinking arises out of frustration tolerance, perhaps better labelled impulse control or affect regulation. Bion considers that the progression to a mental event begins with sensory impressions. These have no psychic quality and are labelled 'beta elements'. They require 'alpha function' to be elaborated psychically. 'Alpha elements' are the building blocks of thoughts. Bion's concept of pre-conceptions, that is, inherited predispositions to patterns of thought, was initially controversial, but the literature on behaviour genetics has increasingly made it seem like a far less improbable assumption. It turns out that identical twins, even when reared apart, share patterns of thought at a quite sophisticated level, resulting in similar value systems and preferences (Plomin *et al.* 1997). The linking of alpha elements to create internal experience is similar to our conception of the mirroring of affect states and the creation of second-order representations. For Bion, thinking emerges when elements are linked to represent something that is not present (Bion 1962*a*, 1965). It is fascinating that Bion's notion of the origins of higher order thinking based on the idea of the 'not present', is basically identical to the current cognitive science notion of the conception of a false belief as the litmus test of the presence of mentalization (see below). Bion also, in agreement with the line of thinking advanced in this volume, emphasizes the intersubjective interactional processes that underpin the evolution of thought. In Bion's view the mother 'detoxifies' the infant's state of tension through her own reverie, which makes this tension thinkable for the baby through a process that he terms 'containment'. The emphasis on mentalization received an undoubted boost from progress in philosophy of mind and writings pertaining to 'the intentional stance' and 'the theory of mind' (Fonagy 1991; Fonagy and Target 1997, 2000; Fonagy *et al.* 2000). During the last decades philosophers (Dennett 1987; Fodor 1987, 1992; Bogdan 1997) and cognitive developmentalists (Astington *et al.* 1988; Wellman 1990; Perner 1991; Whiten 1991; Baron-Cohen *et al.* 1993; Hirschfeld and Gelman 1994; Baron-Cohen *et al.* 2000) have focused on the nature and developmental origins of our capacity to attribute causal mental states to others. Initially, it was Dennett (1987) who argued that applying such a mentalistic interpretational strategy, which he called the 'intentional stance', was a significant evolutionary adaptation that enabled us to predict others' behavior.

In opposition to the currently dominant cognitive developmental view, which holds that young children attribute intentional mental states (such as goals, emotions, desires, and beliefs) to others as the causes of their actions, from a psychodynamic perspective we argue that the capacity for mentalization is a developmental achievement greatly facilitated by secure attachment (Fonagy 1991, 1997). Evidence such as young children's performance on false belief tasks supports this argument. Wimmer and Perner (1983) were the first to demonstrate that three-year-olds who witness a person leaving an object in container A before leaving the room and who see the object being transferred to container B in that person's absence, make the (reality-based) error of predicting that she will search in container B (where the object actually is) rather than in container A (where she left the object) when she comes back. By the age of four or five, children do not commit this error any more: they tend to correctly predict that the person will look in container A, because they are able to attribute a false belief to him or her.

The acquisition of this capacity has come to be known as the development of a theory of mind. 'Theory of mind' is an interconnected set of beliefs and desires, attributed to explain a person's behavior. Baron-Cohen and Swettenham (1996) appropriately ask '...how on earth can young children master such abstract concepts as belief (and false belief) with such ease, and roughly at the same time the world over?' (p. 158). In current models of theory of mind development the child tends to be seen as an isolated processor of information, constructing a theory of mind using biological mechanisms which, where the child's endowment is less than optimal, have an expectable failure rate (see Carpendale and Lewis in press for a fresh but controversial alternative perspective). From the viewpoint of developmental psychopathology and its psychosocial treatment, this is indeed a barren picture, which ignores the central role of the child's emotional relationship with the parents in developing the child's ability to understand social interactions in psychological terms. The development of children's understanding of mental states is embedded within the social world of the family, with its network of complex and often intensely emotionally charged relationships, which are after all much of what early reflection needs to comprehend. Therefore it should not surprise us that the nature of family interactions, the quality of parental control (Dunn *et al.* 1991*b*), parental talk about emotions (Denham *et al.* 1994), and the depth of parental discussion involving affect (Dunn *et al.* 1991*a*) are all strongly associated with the acquisition of the intentional stance in observational studies. Perner *et al.* (1994) reported that pre-schoolers with siblings demonstrate false belief understanding at an earlier age than children without siblings.

Jenkins and Astington (1996) replicated this 'sibling effect', although they found it to be less pronounced in children with more advanced linguistic abilities. Lewis *et al.* (1996) also found that number of siblings and performance on false belief tests were associated, but overall they found a more consistent effect of older siblings and kin on the development of false belief understanding. Ruffman *et al.* (1998) found beneficial effects for older but not younger siblings in a series of experiments with a large number of participants. The sibling effect was not replicated, however, in two more recent studies involving working-class families (Cutting and Dunn 1999; Cole and Mitchell 2000). This suggests that it may be the nature of the relationships children experience rather than just the number of people in the household that influences development (Hughes *et al.* 1999). There is further evidence of correlations between social cognitive development and parenting style (Ruffman *et al.* 1998; Hughes *et al.* 1999; Vinden 2001), aspects of parent– child conversation (Sabbagh and Callanan 1998), attachment (Fonagy *et al.* 1997*a*, 1997*b*; Meins 1997; Meins *et al.* 1998; Symons and Clark 2000), mothers' education (Cutting and Dunn 1999), and socioeconomic circumstances (Holmes *et al.* 1996).

Furthermore, a number of studies have found correlations between language and social understanding (e.g. Happé 1995; Jenkins and Astington 1996; Cutting and Dunn 1999; de Villiers 2000). In longitudinal studies, forms of family talk about mental states have been found to be related to later success on false belief tests (e.g. Dunn *et al.* 1991*a*; Moore *et al.* 1994; Brown *et al.* 1996; Ruffman *et al.* 2002). In addition, mothers who think of their children in mentalistic terms ('mindmindedness'), and therefore presumably talk to their children about the psychological world, have children who are more advanced in understanding beliefs than are other children (Meins *et al.* 1998; Meins and Fernyhough 1999). Similar correlations between family interaction and the development of children's understanding of emotions have also been reported (e.g. Dunn *et al.* 1991*b*; Hooven *et al.* 1995; Kuebli *et al.* 1995; Steele *et al.* 1999). In a longitudinal study, Astington and Jenkins (1995) found that earlier language abilities predict later false belief performance but earlier false belief competence does not predict later language abilities, supporting the conclusion that language is important in social cognitive development.

Research with deaf children also provides evidence that social interaction is important for the development of a mentalistic understanding. Studies have shown that deaf children with hearing parents are delayed in the development of false belief understanding, whereas deaf children with deaf parents are not delayed (Peterson and Siegal 2000; Woolfe *et al.* 2002). This seems to be because deaf parents are native users of sign language and thus their children are exposed to normal conversation, but hearing parents are less fluent in sign language and therefore their children are not exposed to complex conversation about everyday events involving people's actions, beliefs, and emotions.

Conversation about the mental world may well be essential for the development of social understanding. The ability to give meaning to our own psychological experiences develops as a result of our discovery of the minds beyond others' actions.

For research purposes we have operationalized the ability to apply a mentalistic interpretational strategy as reflective function (Fonagy *et al.* 1998), as the plausible interpretation of one's own and others' behavior in terms of underlying mental states. This implies awareness that experiences give rise to certain beliefs and emotions, that particular beliefs and desires tend to result in certain kinds of behaviour, that there are transactional relationships between beliefs and emotions, and that particular developmental phases or relationships are associated with certain feelings and beliefs. We do not expect an individual to articulate this theoretically, but to demonstrate it in the way they interpret events within attachment relationships, when asked to do so. Individuals differ in the extent to which they are able to go beyond observable phenomena to give an account of their own or others' actions in terms of beliefs, desires, plans, and so on. This cognitive capacity is an important determinant of individual differences in self-organization as it is intimately involved with many defining features of selfhood such as self-consciousness, autonomy, freedom and responsibility (Cassam 1994; Bolton and Hill 1996). The intentional stance, in the broad sense considered here (i.e. including apparently irrational unconscious acts), creates the continuity of self-experience which is the underpinning of a coherent self-structure.

More recently, RF has been seen as linked to Bogdan's notion of interpretative capacity (Bogdan 1997, 2001). Interpersonal interpretative function (IIF) is considered to be the product of an overarching neural system which is involved in the processing of all new experiences and affects. This definition is more or less identical to Bion's basic model of thinking (see Bion 1962*a*, 1963, 1970), and involves a major shift from the original reflective function (RF) theory of mentalization which arose from a simple extension of Main's (Main and Hesse 2001) theory of metacognitive monitoring of relational experiences. In this new model, there is a strong tie with recent neuroscientific findings, such as Damasio's, (2003) and with Clarkin and Kernberg's psychopathological theory of affect-regulation (Clarkin and Lenzenweger 1996; Clarkin *et al.* 1999). The IIF consists of interpretive functions in the related domains of affect-regulation, attention, and reflective function.

The concept of the IIF brings together the basic elements of our developmental model. The primary emotional contact with the mother is via the process of 'parental affect mirroring', after Watson and Gergely as outlined above. This is crucial in the creation of second-order representations of basic constitutional experience of internal states, and provides the bases of the affect-regulation of the child. These second-order representations are at the crossroads of the psychic equivalence and pretend modes of functioning. This resembles Bion's dichotomy between the psychotic and the non-psychotic segments of the personality, which are based on the thinking or not-thinking of experiences (Bion 1957). The model now distinguishes two types of interpretative processes: those predominantly directed at interpreting the cognitions of self and other (IIF-c) and those that are directed at affect states (IIF-a). This dichotomy might help to explain why narcissistic PDs and psychopaths may have a high level of RF as measured on the AAI, while not being in touch with their own or others' emotions.

Reflective function and attachment

Reflective function is assessed and measured by scoring transcripts of the AAI according to guidelines laid out in the Reflective Function Manual (Fonagy *et al.* 1998). The characteristics of attachment narratives that raters look for as evidence of high RF include awareness of the nature of mental states (such as the opaqueness of mental states), explicit efforts to tease out the mental states underlying behaviour, recognition of the developmental aspects of mental states and showing awareness of mental states in relation to the interviewer. There was a strong relationship between scores on the RF scale and the strange situation behaviour of infants (Ainsworth *et al.* 1978) whose mothers and fathers had been assessed using the AAI before the birth of the child (Fonagy *et al.* 1991). In a subsequent study on the same sample, we found that RF was particularly predictive of secure attachments with mothers, in cases where mothers independently reported significant deprivation in childhood (Fonagy *et al.* 1994).

A growing body of evidence links mentalizing with attachment. The caregiver's awareness of the child's mental states appears to be a significant predictor of the likelihood of secure attachment. Recent evidence by Slade and her colleagues provided an important clue about the puzzle of intergenerational transmission of attachment security. They demonstrated that autonomous (secure) mothers on the AAI represented their relationship with their toddlers in a more coherent way, conveying more joy and pleasure in the relationship, than did dismissing and pre-occupied mothers (Slade *et al.* 1999). That the mother's representation of each child is the critical determinant of attachment status is consistent with the relatively low concordance in the attachment classification of siblings (van IJzendoorn *et al.* 2000). We believe that the parent's capacity to adopt the intentional stance towards a not-yet-intentional infant, to think about the infant in terms of thoughts, feelings, and desires in the infant's mind and in their own mind in relation to the infant and his/her mental state, is the key mediator of the transmission of attachment and accounts for classical observations concerning the influence of caregiver sensitivity (Fonagy *et al.* 1995*b*). Those with a strong capacity to reflect on their own and their caregiver's mental states in the context of the AAI were far more likely to have children securely attached to them—a finding which we have linked to the parent's capacity to foster the child's self-development (Fonagy *et al.* 1993). The association between parental reflective function and child security is strongest when there is adversity in the mother's history (Fonagy *et al.* 1994). We have suggested that the likelihood of intergenerational transfer of trauma and adversity is reduced by the mother's capacity to reflect on her own and others' thoughts and feelings related to her history. While it is clear that childhood maltreatment in the parent's own past is recognized as one important risk factor in the abuse of children (Widom 1989), this is not inevitably the outcome (Langeland and Dijkstra 1995). In one study, 10 mothers who had been able to break the cycle of abuse differed from 14 mothers who failed to do so in terms of their superior ability to talk about their past abuse in a coherent, meaningful, and integrated fashion that enabled them to reflect on their style of parenting their own children (Egeland and Susman-Stillman 1996). It is interesting to note in this context, that mothers of girls sexually abused by male abusers appear to have lower capacity to think of their child in mental state terms than mothers from similar demographic groups whose child was not maltreated (Normandin *et al.* 2002).

A series of studies by Arietta Slade and her group (Slade *et al.* 2001) have demonstrated that mothers with high RF on the AAI are also likely to have high RF on the Parent Development Interview (an interview that explores the parent's representation of her child) and to have infants securely attached to them. A further direct test of our hypothesis that mentalizing parenting engenders security of attachment in the infant was provided by Elizabeth Meins and colleagues (Meins *et al.* 2001). They analyzed the content of speech of mothers in interaction with their 6-month-old children and coded the number of comments the mother made on the infant's mental states (knowledge, desires, thought, interest), the infant's emotional engagement (e.g. assertions about the infant being bored), comments on the infant's mental processes ('are you thinking?') or comments about what the infant might think the mother thinks or attempts on the infant's part to manipulate the mother's mental state ('are you just teasing me?'). The comments were further coded as appropriate if an independent coder agreed that the mother was reading the child's mental state correctly, in line with the immediate history of the interaction, and was not cutting across the child's apparent intentions with assertions about putative mental states that were incongruous with the infant's current state of mind. The proportion of such 'appropriate mind-related comments' was highly significantly associated with attachment security in the child 6 months later and significantly contributed to the prediction even when traditional measures of maternal sensitivity were controlled for. In a further recent study Muzik and Rozenblum (2003) reported a study on a community sample of 100 mothers and their 7-month-old infants. Mothers' narratives were assessed via the Working Model of the Child (WMC) Interview (Zeanah and Benoit 1995).

Maternal behaviour was assessed via observations of mother–infant interaction during free play and structured teaching tasks. Scoring of these segments assessed (1) maternal behavioural sensitivity, and (2) maternal verbal sensitivity, or the number of mind-minded comments made by the mothers reflecting attributions of mental/emotional states to their infants (e.g. 'I think you are happy playing with the ball'). The study included three interactive segments: (1) in free play mothers and infants were left alone in a room with developmentally-appropriate toys and were told to spend time playing with their infant; (2) during the teaching task, mothers were given two challenging tasks to 'teach their infant' to put plastic balls into a clear plastic container, and then (3) to stack a series of block cubes. All three interactive episodes were three minutes long. Maternal behaviour was coded from videotape along several dimensions using a system developed by Miller *et al.* (2002). Behaviours assessed included maternal sensitivity, intrusiveness, rejection, positive affect, and anxiety. Reflective Function assessed in the working model of the child interview correlated 0.4 with mind-related comments made during the teaching tasks. Mothers with higher scores on the reflective capacity scale made more mind-minded comments, although these associations were only observed during the high challenge teaching tasks. Mentalizing comments and reflective capacity were both related to maternal behaviour during interaction, but unrelated to maternal affect. Balanced representations in the WMC interview are associated with more mind-minded statements during the teaching task. All in all, considerable evidence was found to confirm the hypothesis that the transgenerational transmission of secure attachment is normally achieved via the high reflective capacity of the mother in relation to past attachment relationships, that enhances her mentalization in relation to the infant both in terms of representations of the infant and mind-minded speech with the infant during demanding tasks.

More than mental state language, the coherence with which the child's mental state is perceived may be the critical variable. In a study by David Oppenheim, (Koren-Karie *et al.* 2002) mothers were asked to narrate a videotaped playful interaction that they had just had with their infant. Mothers who were reflective in their narratives, able to see various experiences through the child's eyes and gain new insights as they talked were far more likely to have securely attached infants than mothers who either had preset conceptions of the child which they appeared to impose or disengaged from trying to understand what was on the child's mind. Most pertinent was the observation that disorganized attachment classification was associated with mothers who were incoherent, switching between the above categories and not fitting well into any of them. Thus mentalizing and security of attachment in the caregiver appear to go together and are associated with a coherent working model of the child that is richly imbued with representations of internal states.

The above series of studies demonstrated that high levels of reflective function are associated with good outcomes in terms of secure attachment in the child. The interrelatedness of these two domains, mentalizing and attachment, are also underscored by observations of child development. As reviewed above (p. 73) there is a clear link between attachment security in infancy and precocious mentalization in early childhood. In a recent study of the relationship of attachment security in middle childhood and performance in the Happe advanced theory of mind tasks involving 78 children a correlation of $r=0.51$ was found between a four-point scale of attachment security and theory of mind performance (Target *et al.* in press). Our ability to give meaning to our own psychological experiences develops as a result of our discovery of the minds beyond others' actions. Security of attachment on the AAI in 131 moderately-at-risk adolescents (Allen *et al.* 1998) predicted low risk for conduct disorder (CD) and delinquency and was associated with peer competence, lower levels of internalizing behaviours, and low levels of deviant behaviour.

Co-operative relationship rooted in the coherence of the perception of the child's mental state may not be the only factor. The development of the key psychological capacities that underpin theory of mind may be grounded in the attachment relationship (Fonagy and Target 2002; Fonagy *et al.* 2002). It is quite probable that an important mediator of the association of secure attachment and theory of mind development lies in the regulation of physiological arousal. Secure attachment may be conducive to mentalizing because it facilitates an optimal level of arousal (Field 1985; Kraemer 1999; Panksepp *et al.* 1999). Similar arguments could be mounted in relation to effortful control. The capacity to inhibit a dominant response in place of a sub-dominant one is a key achievement of early development (Kochanska *et al.* 2000; Rothbart *et al.* 2000). It also appears to be powerfully predicted by security of attachment at one year (Kochanska *et al.* 2000; Kochanska 2001; Kreppner *et al.* 2001). Mentalizing involves setting aside immediate physical reality in favour of a less compelling reality of the other's internal state. Previous studies have linked the acquisition of effortful control to performance on the false belief tasks as they follow a common developmental timetable and share a common brain region and yield common types of pathology (Carlson and Moses 2001). Thus we would argue that children with a background of secure attachment are more rapid in their acquisition of mentalization in the context of social relationships because secure attachment has equipped them with the capacity appropriately to attend selectively to critical aspects of such interactions.

We suggest (1) that specific capacities (arousal regulation, effortful control) link the secure base that generates secure attachment with evolving symbolic function; (2) that the link of the secure base phenomenon to the development of mentalization will be increasingly understood to be causal rather than correlational in that the group of capacities that underpin adequate social understanding, what Bogdan (1997) called interpretation, are evolutionarily tied to it; in other words, that the evolutionary function of the attachment relationship in humans goes beyond the protection of the vulnerable infant; its evoluationary function is to provide an environment within which social understanding may be readily acquired; and therefore (3) that deficits in attachment create a vulnerability in the child to later environmental challenges because of deficits of interpretive capacity.

Neurological basis of mentalization

The contribution of secure attachment to mentalization can be understood on both neurobiological and psychosocial levels, and we believe that understanding the challenges to mentalizing in psychotherapy—for both therapist and patient—require this dual understanding. Schore (2001) has reviewed extensive evidence supporting his thesis that secure attachment is essential for optimal development of cerebral structures supporting mentalization. The right hemisphere is specialized for emotion and social cognition, and the right hemisphere is dominant in the first three years of life, providing an opportunity for attachment relationships to participate in the sculpting of the cerebral substrates of social-emotional behaviour and emotional self-regulation. As Schore put it, 'The attachment relationship thus directly shapes the maturation of the infant's right brain stress-coping systems' (p. 41). These systems mediate the capacity to regulate emotions in interpersonal relationships. He ascribes to the orbito-frontal cortex the implicit regulatory mechanisms associated with internal working models of attachment relationships. He notes further that the amygdala and orbito-frontal cortex, which conjointly contribute to emotional experience, remain highly plastic throughout life. Hence attachment relationships may continue to play a role in the development of cerebral regulation of emotions throughout the lifespan.

Although our grasp of the neurobiological basis of mentalization remains rudimentary, converging evidence from human and non-human primate studies with a wide range of methodologies (e.g. effects of brain lesions, neuroimaging, single-cell recording) implicate several brain areas in the processes of social engagement, social cognition, and mentalization (see Allen and Fonagy 2002). We can consider responsiveness to communicative facial expressions as prototypical of implicit mentalizing. Such responsiveness depends on highly processed visual information integrated in the temporal lobe (superior temporal sulcus) to provide identification of the individual and the individual's expressive cues (Bonda *et al.* 1996; Frith and Frith 1999, 2000; Emery and Perrett 2000); this identifying information is rapidly processed for emotional significance in the amygdala (Rolls 1999; Aggleton and Young 2000; Emery and Perrett 2000; Stone 2000). Mentalizing on-line in interpersonal interactions, however, requires executive control that includes flexibly and continually updating interpretations of emotional cues in conjunction with regulating one's own emotional states and expressions.

The orbitofrontal cortex plays a prominent role in this flexible responsiveness and self-regulation (Rolls 1999; Elliott *et al.* 2000) and, consistent with Schore's view, there is evidence for right hemisphere lateralization in this regard (Brownell *et al.* 2000).

Mentalizing depends substantially on optimal pre-frontal cortex functioning (Blair and Cipolotti 2000; Rowe *et al.* 2001; Stuss *et al.* 2001; Siegal and Varley 2002; Adolphs 2003). Medial and orbital pre-frontal cortices have been linked to the regulation of inter-personal relationships, social co-operativity, moral behaviour, and social aggression (Davidson *et al.* 2000; Greene and Haidt 2002; Kelley *et al.* 2002; Damasio 2003; Schore 2003). The optimal functioning of the pre-frontal cortex in turn depends on optimal arousal. Neurochemical regulation of the pre-frontal cortex is complementary to that of posterior cortex and sub-cortical structures[3] (Arnsten 1998; Arnsten *et al.* 1999*b*). Arnsten and Mayes (Arnsten 1998; Arnsten *et al.* 1999; Mayes 2000*b*) have argued that when arousal exceeds a certain threshold, it is as if a neurochemical switch is thrown. This switch shifts us out of the executive mode of flexible reflective responding into the fight-or-flight mode of action-centered responding. Those with insecure or disorganized attachment relationships are sensitized to intimate interpersonal encounters, experience higher arousal, and the relative level of arousal in the frontal or posterior part of the cortex readily shifts posteriorly.

Activation of the medial pre-frontal cortex (including the ventromedial pre-frontal cortex overlapping the orbitofrontal cortex) has been demonstrated in a series of neuroimaging studies in conjunction with a wide range of theory of mind inferences, in both visual and verbal domains (Fletcher *et al.* 1995; Goel *et al.* 1995; Happe *et al.* 1996; Gallagher *et al.* 2000; Klin *et al.* 2000). It appears likely that an extensive portion of the pre-frontal cortex (i.e. orbitofrontal extending into more dorsal medial cortex) is involved in mentalizing interactively in a way that requires implicitly representing the mental states of others. Of course, many experimental paradigms demonstrating medial prefrontal activation in theory of mind tasks require explicit responding (e.g. explicating the mental states of story characters). Yet explicit responses

---

[3]As level of cortical activation increases through mutually interactive norepinephrine alpha 2 and dopamine D1 systems, pre-frontal cortical function improves on capacities such as anticipation (shifting of attention), planning/organization and working memory. With excessive stimulation, norepinephrine alpha 1 and dopamine D1 inhibitory activity increases; the prefrontal cortex goes 'offline' and posterior cortical and sub-cortical functions (e.g. more automatic functions) take over. Increasing levels of norepinephrine and dopamine interact such that above the threshold, the balance shifts from pre-frontal executive functioning to amygdala-mediated memory encoding and posterior sub-cortical automatic responding (fight-flight-freeze).

often entail representational redescription of implicit representations such that medial pre-frontal cortex perforce plays a role in both implicit and explicit mentalizing regarding other persons.

Some evidence suggests that the anterior cingulate cortex plays a key role in mentalizing the self, at least in the domain of emotional states (Lane *et al.* 1997, 1998; Damasio 1999; Frith and Frith 1999). Lane has proposed more specifically that implicit self-representations (i.e. phenomenal self-awareness) can be localized to the dorsal anterior cingulate, whereas explicit self-representations (i.e. reflection) can be localized to the rostral anterior cingulate (Lane 2000). Moreover, intriguing findings regarding mirror neurons suggest that representations of self and others bearing on interpretation of intentional action promote mentalization by virtue of shared anatomical circuitry (Brothers 1997; Jeannerod 1997; Gallese 2000, 2001).

Other neural structures are undoubtedly involved in sustaining mentalizing as a psychological function and could account for its abnormalities in borderline patients. Hippocampal cortical structures are involved in autobiographical memory, which may provide material for mentalization. There is evidence for poor function or even atrophy in these brain areas in individuals with histories of severe maltreatment. This frequently includes individuals with BPD (Bremner *et al.* 1999*b*; Driessen *et al.* 2000; Teicher *et al.* 2002, 2003*a*).[4] An alternative source of material for mentalization are implicit memories that are procedures without content. These procedures are normally not accessible to reflection, but nevertheless are consciously influenced and maintain implicit mentalization, and are underpinned by neuroanatomical structures in the amygdala and thalamus (Herpertz *et al.* 2001). These structures are established in the first years of life and are less likely to be modified later.

Of these various structures involved in mentalizing, we would emphasize the prominent role of the pre-frontal cortex. The pre-frontal cortex plays a central role in executive functions, which include planning and temporal ordering of responses in the context of novelty and ambiguity. In Goldberg's (2001) view, social interactions place the highest demand for these executive capacities: 'imagine that you have to plan and sequentially organize your actions in co-ordination with a group of other individuals and institutions engaged in the

[4]The diminished left–right hemisphere integration and the smaller corpus callosum of patients with a history of childhood abuse is consistent with a model that assumes that individuals with BPD might have trouble shifting rapidly from a state that overvalues the logical left hemisphere to an alternative state which is highly negative, critical, and undoubtedly emotional, neurologically underpinned by the right hemisphere (Teicher *et al.* 2003*b*). The lack of integration of the two hemispheres may be brought into relief by the reduced effectiveness of mentalization, allowing a state to occur where the individual sees one person in an overly positive and another in an excessively negative light.

planning and sequential organization of their actions' (p. 107). Not surprisingly, he concludes, 'the pre-frontal cortex is the closest there is to the neural substrate of social being' (p. 111). Goldberg's view is consistent with extensive evidence-linking theory of mind to executive functions (Baron-Cohen 1999; Perner and Lang 2000). Although theory of mind and executive functions develop in tandem and share neurobiological substrates, they are distinct from one another, and the extent to which the development of theory of mind builds upon executive function or vice versa has yet to be determined.

But the critical link we wish to make between attachment and neurobiology is this: Mentalizing activity is contingent on an optimal level of arousal that sustains prefrontal functioning. As Schore (2001) argued, failure of attachment relationships can undermine the development of cortical structures needed to regulate affective arousal, and these are the same structures that are essential to the activity of mentalizing. Thus we have potentially interlocking vicious developmental circles in which attachment disturbance, affective hyperarousal, and failure of mentalization are all intertwined with catastrophic consequences.

The impact of an insecure base

Having established that a caregiving environment of mind-mindedness is a necessary condition for optimal development of the interpersonal interpretative function, we will argue that because of neglect (by which we do not mean only physical but also psychological neglect), individuals with BPD have an inadequate capacity to represent mental states—to recognize that their own and others' reactions are driven by thoughts, feelings, beliefs, and desires. This lack of reflective capacity results because they have not received the assistance they needed to integrate the two primitive modes of experiencing the internal world: pretend and psychic equivalence modes. The failure to mentalize creates a kind of psychic version of an auto-immune deficiency state that leaves these individuals extremely vulnerable to later sometimes quite brutal social environments. In such environments their 'psychic auto-immune deficiency' means there is an increased risk that at a certain moment they may cease to resist the brutalization, and start sustaining themselves through self-harm or social violence (e.g. Goodman and New 2000; Stone 2002).

The failure of mirroring

Previously we identified congruency and markedness as the qualities of the parent's mirroring of the child that are essential if the child is to develop the capacity for secondary representation of his/her affect states. If either of these qualities is absent, or if there is little or no attempt by the caregiver at interpretative interaction with the child, difficulties may result. Some mothers, because of their own emotional difficulties and conflicts, may find their infants' negative affect-expressions overwhelming, and may struggle to mirror their babies' emotions in a marked way. They are likely to react to their infant's negative emotions by reflecting them accurately, but in an unmarked, realistic manner. When this happens, the mirroring affect-display will be attributed to the parent as his or her real emotion, and it will not become anchored to the infant either. Consequently, the secondary representation of the baby's primary emotion-state will not be established, leading to a corresponding deficiency in self-perception and self-control of affect. Since the infant will attribute the mirrored affect to the parent, he will experience his or her own negative affect 'out there' as belonging to the other, rather than to himself. Instead of regulating the infant's negative affect, the perception of a corresponding realistic negative emotion in the parent will escalate the baby's negative state leading to traumatization rather than containment (Main and Hesse 1990). This constellation corresponds to the clinical characterization of *projective identification* as a pathological defensive mechanism characteristic of a borderline level of personality functioning (Klein 1946*b*; Segal 1964; Kernberg 1976; Sandler 1987*b*). The features of impoverished affect regulation, excessive focus on physical rather than psychic reality and over-sensitivity to the apparent emotional reaction of the other are clearly features that mark the mental functioning of certain individuals prone to violent acts and these might be traced back to these patterns of early mirroring. We hypothesize that sustained experience of accurate but unmarked parental mirroring in infancy might play an important causal role in establishing projective identification as the dominant form of emotional experience in personality development characteristic of individuals with BPD. On the other hand, if the caregiver's attempt at mirroring is *not congruent*, if it does not match the infant's primary experience, there will be a tendency towards the establishment of a narcissistic false-self-like structure where representations of internal states correspond to nothing real. In this latter case, second-order representations are created that have either no link or inappropriate links to constitutional self-states. Representations of internal states will be thought about but will not be adequately felt. This predisposes the individual to the pretend mode of experiencing internal reality. Labels for internal states will 'come cheap'. They will not carry the same weight of implication as a label to which congruent internal states are attached. This is in contrast with unmarked mirroring which predisposes to the persistence of a psychic equivalent mode of experiencing internal reality. In that case internal experience is made too real by the lack of mitigation which normally the marking of facial affect introduces.

Lack of playfulness

Playful parenting is prototypically responsible for the integration of the pretend and psychic equivalent modes of representing mental states. Parental playfulness and secure attachment have been linked for some time. For example, mothers whose narratives were classified as secure on the AAI and whose infants were later likely to be observed to be securely attached to them are rated as singing more 'playfully' to their infants in distress than dismissing or pre-occupied mothers whose infants are more likely to manifest avoidant or resistant attachments (Milligan *et al.* 2003). Evidence we have already reviewed above suggests that playful parenting attitudes characterize families where children acquire mentalizing capacities fastest (Dunn 1996; Dunn *et al.* 1999, 2000). Playful interplay between parent and child is least likely in families where there is child maltreatment (Emde *et al.* 1997). The child is forced to take any action on the part of the parent seriously as they have learned that frightening consequences may follow. The undermining of a playful attitude may be the most serious deprivation associated with child maltreatment. In a playful parent–child relationship feelings and thoughts, wishes and beliefs can be experienced by the child as significant and respected on the one hand, but on the other as not being of the same order as physical reality, allowing for modification of both the pretend mode and the psychic equivalent mode of functioning in a transitional space.

In individuals whose caregivers were unable to facilitate the development of the capacity for robust representations of internal states, the primitive modes of psychic reality, the pretend mode, and the mode of psychic equivalence, may be more likely to partially persist into adulthood. While extreme physical abuse or neglect of the kind that comes to the attention of child protection services will often undermine the acquisition of the capacity to mentalize through the mediation of the primary object (see below), much more subtle (what one might call 'middle-class') forms of psychological neglect are equally deleterious to the emergence of mentalization. Neglect associated with increasing financial and social pressures on the modern Western family is widely reviewed (at times in terms verging on moral panic) and will not be considered here. It is clear that single parent and dual employment households are increasing in proportion and that the amount of time parents (particularly fathers) spend with children is surprisingly low according to most surveys (e.g. NICHD Early Child Care Research Network 1996). The average father spends just 7.5 min per week in one-to-one contact with his child.

The caregiver's failure to provide a relationship in the context of which mentalization and the sense of self as a psychological entity can develop leads to the persistence of the more primitive modes of psychic reality. The persistence of the mode of psychic equivalence is a key aspect of the tendency of individuals with BPD to express and cope with thoughts and feelings through physical action, against their own bodies or in relation to other people. Violent individuals violate themselves as much as or more than they violate others (Gilligan 1997); examples from one of England's high security prisons include not just self-cutting and swallowing razor blades but gouging eyes out and inserting bedsprings into urethras. Not being able to feel 'themselves' (their self-states) from within, they are forced to experience the self through action (enactments) from without. Individuals with BPD may oscillate between this and the pretend mode of experiencing internal reality. Equally devoid of mentalization, in the pretend mode, the individual allows himself to imagine a mental world with the proviso that it must be completely separated off from physical reality. The heir of the pretend mode of psychic reality is dissociated thinking. In dissociated thinking, nothing can be linked to anything—the principle of the 'pretend mode', in which fantasy is cut off from the real world, is extended so that nothing has implications for anything else (Fonagy and Target 2000). The compulsive search for meaning is a common reaction to the sense of emptiness that the pretend mode generates. As we noted earlier, the borderline individual is at times hypersensitive to the emotional states of mental health professionals and family members, yet without achieving actual insight or intimacy. The reflective capacity is hijacked into the pretend mode of experience, in which psychological events, like relationships, are idealized but emptied of emotional depth.

Enfeebled affect representation and attentional control

The lack of a stable sense of a representational agentive self is of central importance to our understanding of BPD. The capacity for symbolic representation of one's own mental states is clearly an essential pre-requisite of a sense of identity. Those who lack it are not only deficient in self-love, they will lack an authentic, organic self-image built around internalized representations of mental states. The absence or weakness of a representational agentive self brings to the foreground a non-mentalizing self working on teleological principles, leaving the child, and later the adult, with an inadequate understanding of their own subjectivity and of the interpersonal situations they encounter on a daily basis, and consequently with sometimes intense affect which remains poorly labelled and quite confusing, and hence difficult to regulate. The capacity for attentional control, which enables the moderation of impulsivity, is also compromised. Posner and Rothbart have termed the ability to inhibit a dominant response to perform a subdominant response 'effortful control by attention' (Posner and Rothbart 2000). Early attachment, which allows the child to internalize the mother's ability to divert the child's attention from something immediate to something else (Fonagy and Target 2002), serves to equip children with this capacity. Longitudinal studies of self-regulation demonstrate that the capacity for effortful control is strongly related to a child's observed willingness to comply with maternal wishes (committed compliance) i.e. the degree to which they apparently willingly embrace the maternal agenda (Kochanska *et al.* 2001).

Inhibitory control may be essential to the capacity to mentalize. Inhibitory functioning is thought to contribute to individual differences and developmental changes in a wide array of cognitive abilities, including intelligence, memory and emotion regulation (Kochanska *et al.* 1996). Withholding an impulsive response is a pre-requisite for mentalizing, as this requires the foregrounding of a distal second-order non-visible stimulus (mental state) in preference to what immediately impinges on the child (physical reality). The successful performance of theory of mind tasks, for example, must involve the inhibition of the child's own prepotent knowledge of current reality to respond in terms of less salient representations of reality. Alan Leslie, one of the pioneers in the field, has come to consider theory of mind as a mechanism of selective attention. Mental state concepts simply allow the brain to attend selectively to corresponding mental state properties of agents thus permit learning about these properties' (Leslie 2000, p. 1245). Inhibitory control and mentalization share a developmental timetable and a common brain region, and it is likely that their joint absence yield a common psychopathology, such as BPD. The development of effortful control is powerfully influenced by attachment processes (see Fonagy and Target 2002). In a study of 3- and 4-year-old children, where inhibitory control and theory of mind was simultaneously assessed (Carlson and Moses 2001), the shared variance between inhibitory control and theory of mind was 44%. Inhibitory tasks requiring a novel response in the face of a prepotent but conflicting response (e.g. whispering the name of a figure that was well-known to the child) were most closely related to theory of mind performance in this study. In order to perform the theory of mind task, the child needs to be able to set aside their own salient knowledge to ascribe a new salient mental representation to another or to themselves.

Bowlby's (1980) formulation explicitly identified the role of the attachment system as the mechanism activated by the need to reduce fear-generated disequilibrium associated with internal or external stimuli. Thus, the major function of attachment is the control of distress, and attentional processes must play a key role if the attachment system is to achieve this objective (Harman *et al.* 1997). Michael Posner, amongst others, suggests that the interaction between infant and caregiver is likely to train the infant to control his distress through orienting the infant away from the source of distress by soothing and involving him in distracting activities. Self-regulation is taught (or more accurately modelled) by the caregiver's regulatory activity. It has been suggested that joint-attention with the caregiver serves a self-organizing function in early development (Mundy and Neal 2001). A study of infants who were disorganized in their attachment found that these infants also had difficulties with social attention coordination in interactions with their caregiver (Schölmerich *et al.* 1997). In a sample of 59 high risk infants prenatally exposed to cocaine, 28 had been coded as disorganized in their attachment in the strange situation (Claussen *et al.* 2002). Those with disorganized attachment at 12 months showed greatest dysfunctions of social attention coordination, not only with the caregiver but also with an experimenter (e.g. they initiated joint attention less often).

Evidence from late-adopted Romanian orphans with profound disorganizations of attachment suggests that quite severe attention problems are more common in this group than would be expected both in relation to other forms of disturbance and epidemiological considerations (Chugani *et al.* 2001; Kreppner *et al.* 2001). An interesting study of individuals vulnerable and non-vulnerable to depression linked the capacity for attentional control, mood disorder, and maternal caring (Ingram and Ritter 2000). The study demonstrated that induced negative mood could bring about errors in attentional monitoring of individuals who are vulnerable to depression (in terms of having had an episode of depression in the past) if they also had a history of low maternal caring. From the point of view of our model of borderline psychopathology, we argue that an enfeebled attentional control system is a likely consequence of attachment disorganization, perhaps linked with enfeebled affect representation, and serves to undermine the development of mentalization as well as its appropriate functioning in later development. It is probable that trauma further undermines attention regulation and is associated with chronic failures of inhibitory control (Allen 2001; Schore 2003).

There is extensive evidence for limitations in the capacity for effortful control in patients with BPD. In the classic task of effortful control, the colour naming (Stroop) test, BPD patients show more errors and delayed responding with emotional words relative to normal controls (Arntz *et al.* 2000). It is important to bear in mind that these, like all cognitive deficits of individuals with BPD, are limitations that manifest in emotionally troublesome domains of the patient's life. It is when an individual with BPD is confronted with the threat of abandonment, rejection, or abuse that they begin to use their cognitive systems in primitive ways. For example Korfine and Hooley (2000) used a directed forgetting paradigm when subjects are asked not to try to remember words which they are later asked to recall. Among other capacities this task assesses the extent to which patients are able to use effortful control to exclude things from their awareness. The findings indicated that BPD subjects had difficulties with this task (i.e. recalled words that they were asked not to) when the words related to specific borderline issues of abandonment, rejection, anger and rage, self-harm, or others being uncaring and unempathic.

Disorganization of attachment

The converse of the association of high levels of parental reflective function with good outcomes in terms of secure attachment in the child is naturally that low levels of reflective function generate insecure and perhaps disorganized attachment. The latter category of attachment in infancy is most likely to be associated with self-harming or aggressive and potentially violent behavior later in development. A good proportion of toddlers who go on to manifest conduct problems show disorganized attachment patterns in infancy (Lyons-Ruth 1996; Lyons-Ruth and Jacobovitz 1999). The nature and origin of this attachment pattern, characterized by fear of the caregiver and a lack of coherent attachment strategy (Main and Solomon 1986), is as yet poorly understood (Solomon and George 1999). Some evidence is available that links it with frightening or dissociated behaviour on the part of the caregiver (Schuengel *et al.* 1999; Lyons-Ruth *et al.* 1999*a*). Some attachment theorists have linked it with an approach-avoidance conflict in relation to the attachment figure on the part of the infant (Main and Hesse 1992), while others consider it reflective of a hostile-helpless state of mind in the caregiver (Lyons-Ruth *et al.* 1999*a*) or an indicator of inadequate self-organization (Fonagy and Target 1997; Fonagy 1999*b*). A series of studies by Arietta Slade and her group (Grienenberger *et al.* 2001; Slade *et al.* 2001) have demonstrated that high RF on the Parent Development Interview (the PDI is an interview that explores the parent's representation of her child) is associated with secure attachment. More relevant in the present context is the study by Grienenberger *et al.* (2001), which showed that mothers with low RF on the PDI are more likely to show intrusive, fearful, withdrawing and other behaviors that have been shown to be generative of disorganized attachment in the infant (Lyons-Ruth *et al.* 1999*b*). The suggestion here is that poor mentalization of the infant in the mother permits behaviours that undermine the healthy development of the infant's interpersonal interpretative function, which in turn undermines attachment processes, leading to the development of a disorganized self, parts of which are experienced as 'alien' or not really belonging to the self. In the absence of the capacity for mentalization, the coherence of this self can only be ensured by primitive psychological strategies such as projective identification. It is the impact of attachment disorganization upon an agentive self that might be most important for us in understanding BPD.

Establishment of the 'alien self'

An important complication arises if the processes that normally generate an agentive self fail. In early childhood, the failure to find another being behaving contingently with one's internal states and available for the intersubjective processes detailed above can create a desperation for meaning as the self seeks to find itself in the other. This desperation leads to a distortion of the intersubjective process and leads the individual to take in non-contingent reflections from the object. Unfortunately, as these images do not map onto anything within the child's own experience, they cannot function as totally effective experiences of the self. As Winnicott (1967) noted, inaccurate mirroring will lead to the internalization of representations of the parent's state rather than of a usable version of the child's own experience. This creates what we have termed an *alien experience within the self*: ideas or feelings are experienced as part of the self which do not seem to belong to the self (Fonagy *et al.* 1995*a*, 2000). The agentive self is not effectively established for the neglected child because the second-order representations of self states are distorted as they contain within them representations of the other.

These representations of the other internalized as part of the self probably originate in early infancy when the mother's reflective function at least partially but regularly failed the infant. The infant, trying to find herself in the mother's mind, may find the mother instead, as Winnicott (1967, p. 32) so evocatively put it. The image of the mother comes to colonise the self. Because the alien self is felt to be part of the self it disrupts a sense of coherence of self or identity, which can only be restored by constant and intense projection. Note that the projection is not motivated by conflict or guilt, but by the need to re-establish the continuity of self-experience (Fig. 3.3).

The residue of maternal non-responsiveness, this alien other, probably exists in seed form in all our self-representations, as we have all experienced neglect to a greater or lesser extent (Tronick and Gianino 1986). Normally, however, parts of the self-representation which are not rooted in the internalized mirroring of self-states are nevertheless integrated into a singular, coherent self-structure by the capacity for mentalization. The representational agentive self creates an illusion of coherence within our representations of ourselves by attributing agency, accurately or inaccurately assuming that mental states invariably exist to explain experience. Dramatic examples of this have been noted long ago in studies of individuals with neural lesions, such as individuals with surgical bisections of the corpus callosum, so called 'split-brain' patients

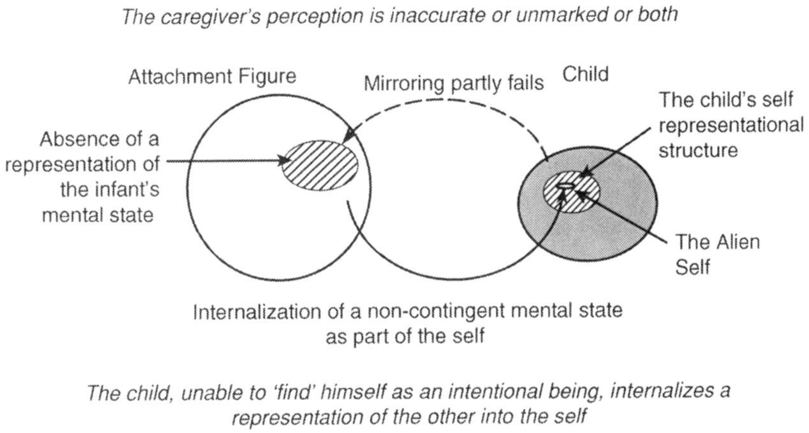

The caregiver's perception is inaccurate or unmarked or both

Attachment Figure
Mirroring partly fails
Child
The child's self representational structure
Absence of a representation of the infant's mental state
The Alien Self
Internalization of a non-contingent mental state as part of the self

The child, unable to 'find' himself as an intentional being, internalizes a representation of the other into the self

Fig. 3.3 Birth of the 'alien' self.

(Gazzaniga 1985). When presented with emotionally arousing pictures in the hemi-field without access to language, they would find improbable mentalized accounts for their heightened emotional state.

Controlling IWM

The normal process of attributing agency through putative mental states preconsciously works in the background of our minds to lend a coherence and psychological meaning to our life, our actions, and our sense of self. This may indeed be an important psychological function of the fully-fledged autobiographical agentive representational self. Individuals whose capacity for mentalization is not well-developed may need to use controlling and manipulative strategies to restore coherence to their sense of self. The 'alien' aspects of the self may be externalized into an attachment figure. Using processes often described in the clinical literature as projective identification, the attachment figure is manipulated into feeling the emotions that have been internalized as part of the self but are not entirely felt to be 'of the self'. These are not self-protective maneuvers in the sense of needing to shed feelings which the individual cannot acknowledge; rather, they protect the self from the experience of incongruence or incoherence that has the potential to generate far deeper anxieties (c.f. Kohut 1977; Kernberg 1982, 1983). The attachment figure thus performs a 'life-saving', or more accurately, a 'self-saving' function by ridding the self of the unbearable internal representations. Apparently coercive, manipulative behaviour reflects the individual's inability to contain the incoherence of his self-structure. Unfortunately, in performing this function, in becoming, for example, angry and punitive in response to unconscious provocation, the attachment figure is in the worst possible state to help restore the afflicted individual's mentalizing function, because she has lost touch with his mental world. Thus the controlling internal working model further undermines the child's possibilities to establish an agentive self-structure.

The mechanism described here may be a prototypical example of the psychoanalytic notion of pathological projective identification (Klein 1946*a*) or, more specifically, what Spillius (1994) has termed 'evocatory projective identification'. To state it simply: disorganized attachment is rooted in a disorganized self. Attachment research has demonstrated the sequelae of disorganized attachment in infancy to be extreme controlling and dominating behaviour in middle childhood (see Solomon and George 1999). The individual, when alone, feels unsafe and vulnerable because of the proximity of a torturing and destructive representation from which he cannot escape because it is experienced from within rather than from without the self. Unless his relationship permits externalization, he feels almost literally at risk of disappearance, psychological merging, and the dissolution of all relationship boundaries. Such need to externalize the alien part of the self may serve

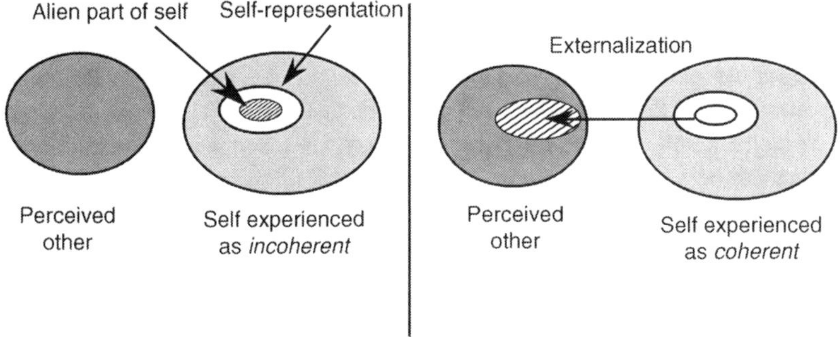

Fig. 3.4 Creating a coherent self-representation by controlling and manipulation: the controlling internal working model.

inadvertently to recreate relationships where the persecutor is 'generated' outside in the shape of relationships of emotional turmoil and significant negativity (Fig. 3.4).

The impact of attachment trauma

Attachment trauma is often, though not always, part of the history of individuals diagnosed with BPD (Cohen *et al.* 2001; Sansone *et al.* 2002) (see also Chapter 1). Although we know that different types of trauma play a significant role in the psychogenesis of PD (e.g. Johnson *et al.* 1999), we believe that it is the persistence of the mode of psychic equivalence, associated with early psychological neglect, that subsequently makes these individuals particularly vulnerable to such harsh social experiences. In cases where individuals with BPD are self-harming or violent, the brutalization of affectional bonds, in childhood or adolescence, and even in young adulthood, appears to be a necessary, but not a sufficient condition for self or other directed aggression. Weakness in the capacity for mentalization due to non-contingent mirroring and the absence of child-focused intersubjective interpersonal interactions undermines the links between internal states and actions and creates subsequent difficulties when the individual's resources to understand are challenged by the hostility and destructiveness of their social world. We suggest that the loose coupling of trauma and borderline states arises because early trauma (or more likely neglect) reduces the capacity to mentalize later traumatic experience. The case for early neglect or even abuse creating a significant vulnerability for the effect of later maltreatment is well-supported by epidemiological data. For example, a higher incidence of post-traumatic stress disorder (PTSD) in Vietnam veterans has been shown to be associated with a history of childhood physical abuse (Bremner *et al.* 1993*c*). Early trauma has also been shown to predispose adults to suffer PTSD following traumatic events in adulthood (Yehuda *et al.* 1995*b*). Thus, weak mentalization might amplify the impact of later trauma, but trauma also impacts on the capacity to mentalize, creating a severe self-reinforcing and highly destructive process.

Failure of mentalization

We believe that trauma commonly brings about a partial and temporary collapse of interpersonal interpretive function. We have both clinical and experimental evidence to support this view. The disorganizing effects of trauma on attention and stress regulation are well-known (Allen 2001). The capacity for mentalization is undermined in a significant proportion of individuals who have experienced trauma. Maltreated toddlers have difficulty in learning to use internal state words (Cicchetti and Beeghly 1987; Beeghly and Cicchetti 1994). Neglected children have greater difficulty in discriminating facial emotional expression and physically abused children show a response bias towards angry expression and show greater variance in their interpretation of facial affect (Pollak *et al.* 2000). A study of sexually abused Canadian girls demonstrated that children with sexual abuse histories had lower RF scores on the childhood attachment interviews (CAI) in relation to self than demographically matched controls (Normandin *et al.* 2002). In the same study, dissociation was shown to be closely related to the low RF of abused children. Whereas 75% of those with low RF on the CAI scored high in dissociation, only 20% of those with high RF could be said to be dissociating. Young adults who have been maltreated experience greater difficulty with the reading the mind in the eyes test (a relatively simple measure of implicit mentalization that involves identifying photographs with one of four mental states) (Fonagy *et al.* 2001). In a further investigation we found that while 'objective' (Court or SRS record) based assessment of maltreatment related to explicit mentalization as measured by RF on the AAI, implicit measures predicted subjective reports of abuse ('How badly did you feel abused?') (Fonagy *et al.* 2003).

We have suggested that a key to an understanding of severe PD is the inhibition of mentalization, perhaps prototypically in response to trauma. We have argued that patients with BPD will defensively avoid thinking about the mental states of self and others, as these experiences have led them to experiences of unbearable pain in the course of maltreatment (Fonagy 1991). Especially in individuals in whom the capacity for mentalization is already weak, trauma may bring about a complete collapse. The collapse of mentalization in the face of trauma entails a partial loss of awareness of the relationship between internal and external reality (Fonagy and Target 2000). Where the ability to mentalize is lost, the modes of experiencing psychic reality that antedate the achievement of mentalization in normal development re-emerge. The mode of 'psychic equivalence' is apparent when the traumatized individual starts fearing his own mind, not wanting to think. Flashbacks are terrifying as they are memories experienced in the mode of psychic equivalence. The alternative to this mode of functioning, the heir of the pretend mode of psychic reality, is dissociation in the wake of trauma. The most characteristic feature of traumatization is the oscillation between these two modes of experiencing internal reality.

There is considerable evidence that is consistent with the claim that individuals with a history of abuse who are also limited in their capacity to think about mental states in themselves and others in the AAI are highly likely to have a diagnosis of BPD (Fonagy *et al.* 1996). This finding has been replicated by other researchers with other traumatized samples. For example, in the Kortenberg-Leuven Process-Outcome Study of in-patient treatment of PD (Vermote *et al.* 2003), a significant negative correlation was reported between RF measured on the Object Relations Inventory (Blatt *et al.* 1996) and SKID-II diagnosis of BPD and an even stronger correlation with clinical observation of self-harm.

A number of other findings are consistent with the central claim that severe PD is marked by a failure of mentalization in the face of emotional arousal. (1) There is something like 'an interpersonal perception deficit' in BPD patients leading such patients to be poor in judgments of personality and interpersonal situations. For example, in one study patients were asked to view film clips with emotional themes centered on abandonment, rejection, and abuse and requested to write down their spontaneous reactions to the six film personalities (Arntz and Veen 2001). The findings suggested that severe PD was associated with poorly differentiated evaluations with a low number of trait dimensions and lower complexity of evaluations of people. (2) Patients with severe PD have unexpected difficulties in recognizing affects and manifest symptoms akin to alexithymia. For example, in one study individuals with ASPD were contrasted with a normal control group and were found to have highly significant elevations on the Toronto Alexithymia Scale that was not associated with general psychiatric disturbance (Sayar *et al.* 2001). (3) Maltreatment in childhood and adolescence leads to profound deficits in interpersonal relatedness that may be interpreted as consequent upon a failure of mentalization. This literature was in part reviewed in Chapter 1. For example, it will be recalled that emotion regulation skills of maltreated children have been shown to be less adaptive than non-maltreated controls (Shields *et al.* 1994; Shields and Cicchetti 1997) and that sexually maltreated 6–12-year-old girls demonstrate lower levels of emotion understanding for both anger and sadness as compared to their non-maltreated peers (Rogosch *et al.* 1995; Shipman *et al.* 2000). (4) In a study of a variety of verbal indicators of mentalization, PD diagnosis was found to be best predicted by a combination of poor mentalization of one's own negative affects, low RF as measured in the AAI, and poverty of high level defenses (Bouchard *et al.* submitted). (5) Early maltreatment is likely to have its long-term impact upon the capacity to form romantic interpersonal relationships via impairment of attachment specific mentalization. Consistent with this, in a follow-up study of pre-schoolers referred for maltreatment to the Menninger Hospital pre-school (Fonagy *et al.* 2003) the best-fitting statistical model of the relationship of early adversity, adult RF, and adult personality functioning showed that attachment-related mentalization may be the mechanism through which early childhood adversity impairs functioning in adult romantic relationships. Adolescent neglect (probably associated with sexual abuse) had only a small direct adverse effect on romantic relationships, which was not linked to mentalization once early adversity was controlled for.

Changes to the arousal 'switch'

Although psychological trauma is a functional route to impaired mentalizing, neurobiological approaches underscore how trauma may compromise the development of cerebral structures that support mentalizing. As noted earlier, Schore (2001) reviewed extensive evidence that secure attachment relationships are essential to the normal development of the pre-frontal cortex and thus to affect regulation. Hence early maltreatment, which is associated with extremely compromised (disorganized) attachment (Barnett *et al.* 1999; Lyons-Ruth and Jacobovitz 1999; Lyons-Ruth *et al.* 1999*a,b*), is most likely to undermine the development of cortical structures key to mentalization. In our review of the literature on neurocognitive impact of trauma we found significant evidence for the involvement of frontal structures that are also involved in the regulation of attention and arousal. The anterior cingulate cortex, a region of the medial prefrontal cortex, is part of an executive attention system that is activated during decision-making and novel or dangerous situations (Posner and Petersen 1990). Above, we have considered the central role of attention and affect regulation to the achievement of mentalization. Thus there seems to be considerable evidence (reviewed in Chapter 1) to suggest that trauma, including neglect, (together with constitutional vulnerability), may have part of its impact on psychological functioning via its impact on brain processes that are crucial to the achievement of this aspect of symbolic thought.

Not only may trauma undermine the development of cerebral structures crucial to mentalization, but the re-experiencing of trauma (i.e., in post-traumatic flashbacks) may be associated with alterations in cerebral functioning consistent with impaired mentalization as Mollon (2002) described. Arnsten (1998; Arnsten *et al.* 1999) and Mayes (2000*b*; 2002) have linked extreme stress to altered dynamics in arousal regulation in a way that is highly pertinent to trauma.

They describe how increasing levels of norepinephrine and dopamine interact with each other and differentially activate receptor sub-types so as to shift the balance between pre-frontal executive control and posterior sub-cortical automatic control over attention and behaviour. Mild to moderate levels of arousal are associated with optimal pre-frontal functioning and thus to employment of flexible mental representations and response strategies conducive to complex problem solving. On the other hand, extreme levels of arousal trigger a neurochemical switch that shifts the individual into posterior cortical–subcortical dominance such that vigilance, the fight-or-flight response, and amygdala-mediated memory encoding predominate. In effect, high levels of excitatory stimulation (at alpha-1 adrenergic and D1 dopaminergic receptors) takes the pre-frontal cortex off-line. This switch in attentional and behavioural control is adaptive in the context of danger that requires rapid automatic responding. Yet Mayes (2000*b*) points out that early stressful and traumatic experiences may permanently impair the dynamic balance of arousal regulation, altering the threshold for this switch process. Hence sensitized individuals may be prone to impaired pre-frontal functioning in the face of stress, with automatic posterior sub-cortical responding taking control of attention and behaviour, undermining flexible mental representations and coping. In line with this suggestion is the observation that *N*-acetyl-aspartate (NAA), a marker of neural integrity, is lowered in the anterior cingulated region of the medial pre-frontal cortex of maltreated children and adolescents (De Bellis *et al.* 2000).

These proposals regarding impaired arousal regulation and shifting the balance of pre-frontal-posterior cortical functioning are consistent with neuroimaging studies employing symptom provocation in persons with PTSD. As we have seen in Chapter 1, such induced post-traumatic states are associated with diminished medial pre-frontal and anterior cingulate activity (Rauch *et al.* 1996; Bremner *et al.* 1999*a*,*b*; Lanius *et al.* 2001; Shin *et al.* 2001). A similar observation was reported in a PET study comparing sexually abused women who had PTSD with women with a similar history who did not. The PTSD sufferers were found to have lower levels of anterior cingulate blood flow during traumatic imagery (Shin *et al.* 1999). This suggests that some BPD symptoms may be connected to an impairment of medial pre-frontal cortical functioning (Zubieta *et al.* 1999). Van der Kolk and colleagues viewed findings showing deactivation in Broca's area in post-traumatic states as indicative of 'speechless terror' and concluded that, in such states, 'the brain is "having" its experience. The person may feel, see, or hear the sensory elements of the traumatic experience, but he or she may be physiologically prevented from translating this experience into communicable language' (p. 131). Thus dysfunctional arousal may play a part in the re-emergence of the subjective state we have described as psychic equivalence.

We propose a synergy between psychological defenses, neurobiological development, and shifts in brain activity during post-traumatic states such that mentalizing activity comes to be compromised. The shift in the balance of cortical control locks the traumatized person either into the psychic equivalence mode, associated with an inability to employ alternate representations of the situation (i.e. functioning at the level of primary rather than secondary representations), much less the ability to explicate the state of mind (meta-representation), or into the pretend mode, associated with states of dissociative detachment.

Psychic equivalence, shame, and the teleological stance

The weakness of the capacity for mentalization and the re-emergence of more primitive modes of experiencing psychic reality make individuals with a history of psychological neglect exceptionally vulnerable to brutalization in attachment contexts. The attacks cannot be attenuated by mentalization of the painful subjective experience engendered. Unmentalized shame is not an 'as if' experience. Whereas an individual with a robust capacity for mentalization might be able to see what lies behind the attack, its meaning, and not mistake it for the possibility of a real destruction of the self, a person in whom this capacity is weak or absent will experience the subjective experience of humiliation evoked by helplessness as tantamount to the destruction of the self. It would not be an exaggeration to label this emotion 'ego-destructive shame'. The coherence of the self, identity itself, is under attack. Ultimately, brutalization, if sufficiently severe, will generate ego-destructive shame even in those with exceptional capacities for mentalization. The humiliation can be so intense that all things felt to be internal (subjectivity) become experiences to be resisted. In describing their experience of brutalization, maltreated prisoners frequently report finding the very act of thinking unbearable. Explicit phrases such as: 'I stopped thinking' or 'I went numb', 'I could not bear to think' are quite common antecedents to the point where victim turns into victimizer.

Impulsivity in BPD may be seen as representations of intentional actions generated by the 'teleological stance' (see p. 61). The principle of rational action still guides impulsive acts but as a function of available evidence about the '*pragmatic*' aspects of a goal object, about the specific situational constraints on action, and about the dispositional constraints characteristic of the actor. Thus, prior intention is often not attributed to the other and the consequences of the action are not predicted, commonly leading to sizable interpersonal conflicts and other social disasters. Only visible (concrete) goals of action are accepted as valid. (Real physical contact is necessary to generate an experience of being loved. Inferring it from others' actions or what they say is insufficient, empty, lacking in meaning.)

Why should the brutalization of affectional bonds be associated with such an intense and destructive sense of self-disgust verging on self-hatred?

The shame concerns being treated as a physical object in the very context where special personal recognition is expected. Unbearable shame is generated through the incongruity of having one's humanity negated, exactly when one is legitimately expecting to be cherished. Violence or the threat of violence to the body is literally soul-destroying because it is the ultimate way of communicating the absence of love by the person inflicting the violence, from whom understanding is expected. As Freud (1914) taught us, the self is sustained by the love of the object so it can become self-love; the sign of a self starved of love is shame, just as cold is the indication of an absence of heat (Gilligan 1997). And just like cold, shame, while painful as an acute experience, when intense and severe is experienced as a feeling of numbness or deadness.

Failure of mentalization and the exposure of the 'alien self'

As we saw earlier, when in infancy mirroring fails, when the parent's perception is inaccurate or unmarked, or both, the child internalizes a non-contingent mental state as part of a representation within the psychological self. These internalizations sit within the self without being connected to it by a set of meanings. It is this incoherence within the self-structure that we refer to as an 'alien self' (Fonagy and Target 2000). As we have said, such incoherencies in self-structure are not only features of profoundly neglected children, and the coherence of the self, as many have noted, is somewhat illusory. This illusion is normally maintained by the continuous narrative commentary on behaviour that mentalization provides, which fills in the gaps and makes us feel that our experiences are meaningful. In the absence of a robust mentalizing capacity, with disorganized patterns of attachment, the disorganization of the self-structure is clearly revealed.

But when trauma inhibits mentalization, the self is suddenly experienced as incoherent. There are parts within that feel like the self yet also feel substantively different, sometimes even persecutory. The persecutory nature of the alien part of the self arises as a sequel to maltreatment in childhood, adolescence, or even adulthood. Anna Freud described the process by which the child aims to gain control over powerful hostile, external forces through the process of identification with the aggressor (Freud 1936). If the cohesion of the self structure has been weakened by limited mentalization and the discontinuity within the self represented by the alien part of the self is well-established, the 'identification' with the maltreater is most likely to occur with the help of this alien part of the self-structure. In slight disagreement with Anna Freud, we do not look at this process as an identification, as that would imply (following Sandler's (1987*a*) clarification of the concept) a change in the shape of the self in the direction of achieving more significant similarities to that of the abusive figure. It is more like a kind of 'colonization' of the alien part of the self by the child's or adolescent's image of the mental state of the abuser.

The aim of the strategy is to have a sense of control over the uncontrollable. This is ultimately a highly maladaptive solution, as the persecution from the maltreating person is now experienced from within. A part of the self-structure is felt to wish to destroy the rest of the self. This may be one aspect of the massive impact that maltreatment can have upon the self-esteem of those subject to abuse (e.g. Mullen *et al.* 1996). They feel evil because they have internalized evil into the part of the self that is most readily decoupled from the self but nevertheless is felt as part of the self. A way of coping with the intolerable pain which this self-persecutory self within the self represents, is externalization into the physically proximal other. The part of the self that is so painful is forced outside and another physical being is manipulated and cajoled until they behave in a way that leads the patient to experience that they no longer own the persecutory alien part of the self (see Figure 3.5). The only way the individual can deal with this is by constantly externalizing these alien parts of the self-structure into the other, so that he can feel whole. At the simplest level, the world then becomes terrifying because the persecutory parts are experienced as outside. At a more complex level, it is felt essential that the alien experiences are owned by another mind, so that another mind is in control of these parts of the self. This might be part of the explanation why, strikingly, persons with BPD frequently finds themselves in interpersonal situations where they are maltreated or abused by their partner.

While accepting that the relationship between childhood maltreatment and BPD is complex, the statistics on the sequelae of childhood sexual abuse seem quite relevant to this point. It is known that victims of childhood abuse who are revictimized are most likely to suffer from severe mental health problems including (as we have seen frequently) BPD. According to one study, 49% of

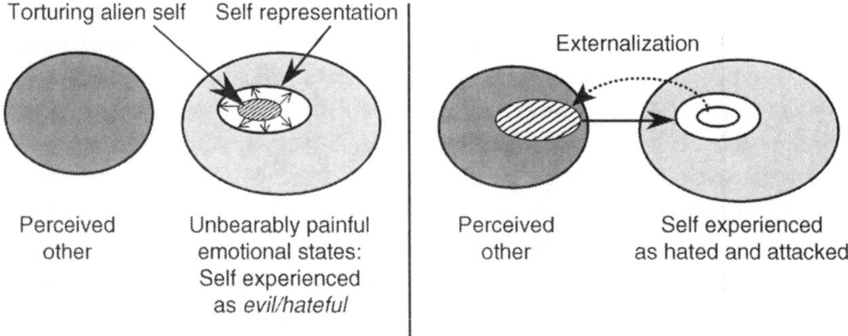

Fig. 3.5 Self-destructiveness and externalization following trauma: Coercive, controlling behaviour is used to reduce the experience of unbearably painful emotional state of attack from within—externalization becomes a matter of life and death.

abused women compared to 18% of women without the experience of sexual abuse had been battered by their partners (Briere and Runtz 1987). In a large study with a sample representative of San Francisco (Russell 1986), between 38% and 48% of women abused (depending on the severity of abuse) had physically abusive husbands compared to 10–17% of non-abused women. This should in no sense be taken to mean that the men involved in the battering are any less culpable. Individuals with experiences of maltreatment appear to be drawn to individuals who are likely to maltreat them, we would argue, in order to increase the opportunity of externalizing intolerable mental states concerning themselves. As might be expected on the basis of this, many sexual assaults experienced by college-aged survivors of sexual abuse occur at the hands of a known individual (Gidycz *et al.* 1995). Indeed, one survey demonstrated that 81% of the adult sexual assaults experienced by revictimized women were perpetrated by male acquaintance of the survivor (Cloitre *et al.* 1997).

Interpersonal relating and the transference

The other is essential not just to create the illusion of coherence. This restores the individual's equilibrium. But the other is also there to be destroyed. In this sense attacks on the other are a gesture of hope, a wish for a new beginning, a desperate attempt to restore a relationship, even if in reality they may have a tragic end. This is why borderline patients require rather than enjoy relationships. Relationships are necessary to stabilise the self-structure but are also the source of greatest vulnerability because in the absence of the other, when the relationships break down, or if the other shows independence, the alien self returns to wreak havoc (persecute from within) and to destabilize the self-structure. Vulnerability is greatest in the context of attachment relationships. Past trauma leaves an impoverished internal working model from the point of view of clear and coherent representations of mental states in self and other. This representational system is activated by the attachment relationship with the consequence that the mental states of the other are no longer clearly seen. The physical other is desperately needed to free the self from its inwardly directed violence, but only as long as it acts as the vehicle for the patient's self state. While this happens, dependence on the other is total. Substitution is inconceivable, no matter how destructive or hopeless the relationship might seem from the outside.

Our approach owes much to that of Otto Kernberg, John Clarkin, Frank Yeomans and their group (Clarkin *et al.* 1996, 1998, 1999; Kernberg 1992; Kernberg *et al.* 2002*b*). In many respects, the model of the mind that underpins our approach is the one brilliantly advanced by Kernberg over the last decades (Kernberg 1975, 1976, 1980, 1984*a*). However, there are also important differences and nowhere are these differences more apparent than in our approach to the transference. In the transference-focused psychotherapy (TFP) model, as outlined in Chapter 4, patients are seen as re-establishing dyadic relations with their therapists that reflect rudimentary representations of self–other relationships of the past (so called 'part-object relationships'). Thus, TFP considers the externalization of these self-object-affect triads to be at the heart of therapeutic interventions. We do not differ from the TFP therapist in emphasizing the externalization process, but we are far less concerned with the apparent relationship which is thus established between patient and therapist. In our model, the role-relationships established by the patient through the transference relationship are considered preliminary to the externalization of the parts of the self the patient wishes to disown. In order to achieve a state of affairs where the alien part of the self is experienced as outside rather than within, the patient needs to create a 'relationship' with the therapist through which this externalization may be achieved. The patient subtly and unconsciously manipulates the therapist to experience particular intense feelings, sometimes quite specific thoughts. These originally belong to the patient but following a period of coercive interactions are reassuringly seen by him to be outside, in the therapist's mind. Once the externalization is achieved, the patient has no interest in the relationship with the therapist and may in fact wish to repudiate it totally. At these moments the therapist may feel abandoned. Some instances of boundary violations may be related to the therapist's difficulty in coping with the implicit rejection which the patient's wish to distance themselves from a disowned part of their mind entails. Focussing the patient's attention on the relationship can be felt by them as undermining of their attempts at separating from the disowned part of themselves and can consequently be counterproductive, leading the patient to prematurely terminate the treatment. The focus of the TFP therapist is on the dyad that is established through the externalization.

Self-harm

We are now also in a position to gain some understanding of the acts of violence committed by certain sufferers of BPD against others or themselves. For such individuals, self-harm may entail a fantasy of eradicating the alien part of the self unconsciously imagined to be part of their body. Self-mutilators report a range of conscious motivations, including self-punishment, tension reduction, improvement in mood, and distraction from intolerable affects (Favazza 1992; Herpertz 1995). Following the act, the individual mostly reports feeling better and relieved (Favazza 1992; Herpertz 1995; Kemperman *et al.* 1997). We suggest that in the absence of a person who may act as a vehicle for the alien part of the self, a person with BPD achieves self-coherence through the externalization of this part of the self into a part of their body. Attempts at self-harm are acts carried out in a mode of psychic equivalence when a part of the body is considered isomorphic with the alien part of the self, at the same time as creating a respite from intolerable affects. Attempts at self-mutilation are more common when the patient is in isolation, or critically, following the loss of an 'other' who up to that point could fulfil the task of being a vehicle for the persecuting alien part of the self.

Suicide

Clinical and epidemiological studies have demonstrated that between 55% and 85% of those who self-mutilate also attempt suicide (Stanley *et al.* 1992; Dulit *et al.* 1994) and BPD carries a suicide risk of around 5–10% (Stone *et al.* 1987; Fyer *et al.* 1988). Most consider attempted suicide to be on a continuum of lethality with other types of deliberate self-harm (e.g. Linehan 1986). Our model of suicide attempts indeed understands them as at the extreme of attempts at self-mutilation often consequent on experience of loss of the other. In such states feelings of despair, hopelessness, and depression predominate. The loss of the other as vehicle for the alien parts of the self, the disruption of the process of externalization signals the destruction of the constitutional or real part of the self. Hence the sense of despair is not from the loss of the object who normally would not have been a genuine attachment figure in the first place but the anticipated loss of self cohesion. The act of suicide is at least in part an act in the psychic equivalence mode aimed at destroying the alien part of the self (hence the continuum with self-harm). When BPD patients attempt suicide their subjective experience is decoupled from reality (in the pretend mode of subjectivity) and in a sense they believe they will survive (or their true self will survive) the attempt but their alien self will be destroyed forever. Consistent with our view is evidence that suicide attempters with BPD features perceive their suicidal attempts as less lethal, with a greater likelihood of rescue and with less certainty of death (Stanley *et al.* 2001). In fact in some patients suicide is felt as "a secure base", a reunion with a state that can reduce existential fear.

Impulsive acts of violence

The same models of pathology that account for self-harming behaviour are generally held to be applicable to certain categories of acts of interpersonal violence (Meloy 1992, 2001; Dutton 1995; Fonagy *et al.* 1997*c*; Gilligan 1997, Fonagy 1999*a*). As with BPD, we see interpersonal violence of an explosive or affective type (Vitiello and Stoff 1997) which is often associated with ASPD. It may help at this stage to summarize the model we have described (see Figure 3.6). We see internally or externally directed impulsive acts of violence as arising from a vulnerability consequent on (1) poor contingency caregiver responsiveness, and related to this (2) a weakness of secondary representation of psychological states which in turn brings with it (3) a persistence of dual mode of psychic reality. With (4) acts of brutalization in the context of attachment relationships that frequently include exposure to domestic violence not just direct victimization, two further structural changes occur: (5) the identification with the aggressor leads to the colonization of the alien

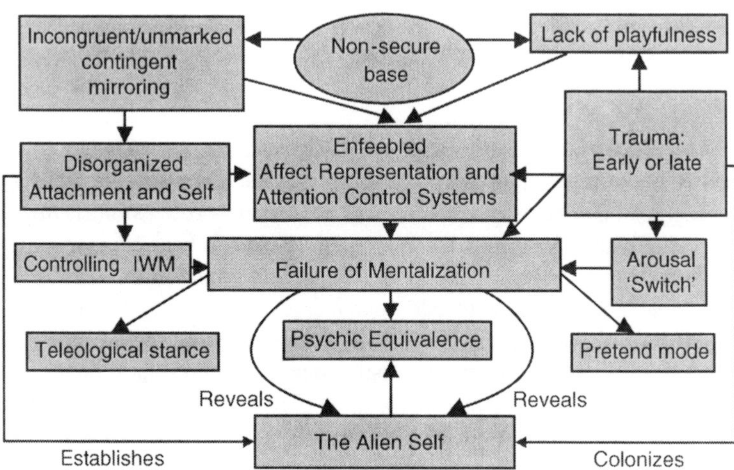

Fig. 3.6 Attachment model of trauma-related psychopathology.

part of the self by the maltreating figure and (6) vulnerability to a malevolent mind brings with it the defensive inhibition of mentalizing capacity. (7) The act of violence itself is usually the consequence of a failure of the externalization of the alien self. It is when the 'other' refuses to be a vehicle for intolerable self states, he or she refuses to be 'cowed' or humiliated, that the vulnerable mind of such an individual turns to interpersonal destruction. (8) An important trigger for this is the experience of 'ego-destructive shame'. The lack of a coherent sense of agentive self has created a massive vulnerability in such individuals to humiliation which is felt as the other refuses to accept a role of complete passivity and through manifesting agency presents unbearable humiliation to the violent mind. (9) The challenge is unbearable in the mode of psychic equivalence, where shame is experienced not just as an idea or feeling but as having the actual power to destroy the self. The destruction of the other through violence is an expression of the hoped for destruction of the alien self; it is an act of hope or liberation and is often associated with elation and only later with regret. The absence of mentalization at these moments is of course of further assistance.

(10) Not being able to see the other as an intentional being, the lack of empathy or identification with his or her pain or suffering clears away what is probably an evolutionary obstacle to violence against conspecifics. In itself, lack of empathy is insufficient; it is a necessary but not a sufficient condition for violence. As we have seen, there are many more that lack empathy than are interpersonally violent. The act of violence may represent the perverted restoration of a rudimentary mentalizing function. Whether impulsive or calculated, the act of violence is rarely one of blind rage. Rather, it is a desperate

attempt to protect the fragile self against the onslaught of shame, often quite innocently triggered by an other (the act may often seem disproportionate to the provocation). The experience of humiliation, which the individual tries to contain within the alien part of the self, comes to represent an existential threat and is therefore abruptly externalized. Once outside, and perceived as part of the representation of the victim in the perpetrator's mind, it is seen as possible to destroy once and for all. In this sense violence is a gesture of hope, a wish for a new beginning, even if in reality it is usually just a tragic end.

Clinical illustration[5]

Henrietta, with a history of abuse and a suspended sentence for manslaughter, presented for treatment in her late twenties with anxiety-related problems. The early years of her treatment were punctuated by episodes of self-harming, suicidal manipulations, or intense emotional outbursts as well as dissociation.

Henrietta's mother, probably herself a 'survivor' of abuse, had had a prolonged post-natal depression after the birth of her second child when Henrietta was two. She withdrew almost completely from both Henrietta and Henrietta's father, and eventually left the family. Her father sought solace from at first cuddling, then rubbing against and finally vaginally and then anally penetrating his daughter. I suspect this happened when she was about seven and went on for at least four years. Henrietta recalls initially welcoming his attention (even encouraging it) and gradually, when 'the pain' started, going blank and this helped him get inside her. She describes imagining herself as one of her lifeless dolls. This strategy of inhibiting her mentalizing in response to the brutalization of attachment is critical. It was impossible for Henrietta to understand how her father could contemplate hurting her as part of what grew out of an act of affection. The disavowal of mental states was an adaptation, distancing her from a mind with truly malevolent ideas about the fragile child. As she turned away from mental states in him, and herself, she was forced to fall back on the non-reflective organization within the self—the alien other.

As we have seen, the alien self is internalized in place of, yet also as part of, the self. Henrietta, neglected and unrecognized as a small child, internalized an image of absence or vacuousness as the representation of her state of distress. Not surprisingly, it was this state which was re-activated in moments of her brutalization, since this too was an experience of feeling unrecognized. Reflectiveness temporarily abandoned, the self–other boundary destroyed, the abusing father's cruelty was internalized into the alien self-representation. Thus, the alien part of the self became torturing as well as vacuous. Her experience of abuse by a teacher at boarding school, after the age of eleven, simply reinforced this deeply pathological self-organization. Finding others to

[5]A more extended version of this case history was first presented in P. Fonagy and M. Target (2000). Playing with reality III: The persistence of dual psychic reality in borderline patients. *International Journal of Psychoanalysis*, **81**(5): 853–74.

be a vehicle for this torturing part of Henrietta's self-representation became a matter of life and death. Her experience of self-coherence depended on finding someone willing to torture her. Her teacher was perhaps the first. A line of severely sado-masochistic relationships testified to the fact that he was certainly not the last. Over many sessions her tragic story unfolded. She regularly had allowed herself to be sexually maltreated by her boyfriend. Normally, she somehow felt 'cleansed' by the experience, particularly by his sense of shame about his own actions. But on the last occasion, she saw contempt in his eyes. This, she could not tolerate. 'I think that is why I had to kill him' she said. 'I couldn't bear him thinking I was disgusting'. She screamed and shouted at him. He ridiculed and disparaged her. She picked up the knife and as he moved towards her, still mocking and sneering, she stabbed him. And with this action she hoped to have killed the threat to her self-representation, her self-hatred, and humiliation.

Henrietta resorted to violence to destroy a mental state, which was hers and yet not hers at the same time. The impact of her boyfriend's affect could not be reinterpreted through the mediation of mentalization. Because of her primitive experience of psychic reality, it actually threatened the destruction of her 'self'. She wished to disown the humiliation she felt, but felt no control over it. A murderous act was the only solution. The act of violence performed a dual function. First was the unconscious hope that through its dramatic destruction the torturing alien self would be gone forever. Perceiving the terror in the eyes of her victim, she felt strangely reassured. But the terror she created also helped her to recreate and re-experience the alien self within the object. Henrietta's frenzied and prolonged sadistic act was crucially not lacking in empathy. It seemed essential that she saw her victim's reaction and, within that, something which she would otherwise have to experience as part of herself. His struggle, bleeding, and suffering, were vital features of this experience. Her rage was not at all 'blind'. There were subtle and specific links between the emotional states she found intolerable, and the emotions she attributed to her victim during her attack.

In a sense, given the reality of her shame in the mode of psychic equivalence, we may say that Henrietta killed in self-defence. Violence is a defence against the destructive actuality that humiliation and ego-destructive shame experienced in the mode of psychic equivalence generate. At the moment of murder she felt alive, coherent, and real, out of reach of the deadly rejections, insults and taunts, momentarily once again feeling vital self-respect.

Remembering trauma

That memory is by no means mechanical was clear to Freud as early as 1899 (Freud 1899). Freud recognized what gestalt psychologists of the next generation came to see as the active nature of memory, that is, that *remembering is reconstruction*. Freud, however, held to a belief which was popular at the time, that all experience was laid down in the brain and thus in principle accessible given sufficiently deep analysis. Present-day psychoanalysts and psychotherapists often appear to share this 'mechanical' or 'archival' view of memory as an exhaustive store of all experience (e.g. Blum 2003). While many of Freud's views of memory can be seen to resonate with recent developments in cognitive neuroscience (Pugh 2002). There are also differences. In Freud's day, memories were conceived of as concrete physical structures, laid down in the mind/brain. We now know that the brain does not really 'store memories' (Goldman Rakic *et al.* 2000; Mayes 2000*a*; Schacter *et al.* 2000; Baddeley 2002). It stores traces of information that are later used to create memories. As a consequence it rarely, if ever, expresses a completely veridical picture of past experienced reality. A complex neural network involving many different parts of the brain, acts to encode, store, and retrieve the information, which can be used to create memories. Different memory systems crucially depend on different brain structures (explicit memories appear to depend on the hippocampus and related cortical areas, memories for emotional events on the amygdala). But no one-to-one correspondence exists between memory type and anatomical location. Also, the memory systems interact. But we have to accept that what we know about the psychological and neuropsychological basis of memory is for the most part incompatible with the view that unearthing an apparently forgotten experience may somehow be intrinsically therapeutic. Constructing a putative past experience that makes sense of a current way of being, of feeling, and thinking, is naturally and invariably helpful and perhaps more helpful for being veridical rather than self-serving. None of this implies that it is the remembering rather than the thoughts and feelings consequent upon the memory construction that lead to greater inner peace and a better capacity to work, love, and play.

Whilst an individual's memory, particularly of how they were looked after by parents, correlates quite strongly with adult outcomes, particularly psychological disorders, the agreement between the child's perception of their experience and the perspectives of others is quite poor (e.g. Gerlsma *et al.* 1990; Parker *et al.* 1992). Thus, in retrospective accounts of childhood, we are likely to be tapping representations of the past that are irretrievably distorted by fantasy and defence, that may have been more important in determining psychological development than the objective attributes of the parents (Sandler and Rosenblatt 1962). Retrieval of information from storage is analogous to perception and is biased by the same 'top-down' processes that have been shown to affect perception (Kosslyn 1994). For example, expectations of what is to be recalled influences memory in just the same way that expectations about what will be perceived have been shown to influence what is seen, heard, and so forth. In other words, memory in some respects appropriately seems like perception but this implies that it is at least as vulnerable to illusion and distortion as is perception. The imagery of memory is perceptual, but the vividness represents the neural structures common to perception and memory and not a confirmation of access to direct, actual experience.

All that we know about memory cautions us about the possibility of taking personal recollections too seriously. Subjective confidence in the accuracy of recall appears to be a poor guide. Nevertheless, the gist of experience recalled is far more likely to be accurate than inaccurate (Christianson 1992; Heuer and Reisberg 1992; Riccio *et al.* 1994). Early memories of traumatic events, for example, are quite likely to be broadly accurate (Usher and Neisser 1993). The fact that episodic memory does not develop until age five clearly need not mean that children do not encode and store many experiences that they are unable to recall.

Whilst in general childhood memories, even when recalled in adulthood, may be accurate (Brewin *et al.* 1993), this does not mean that systematic working through of such experiences is helpful in the treatment of patients with BPD. The reason for this is precisely because these individuals are quite likely to have experienced trauma in their development. Trauma interferes with autobiographical memory. We have known this for some decades, particularly from studies of combat veterans suffering from PTSD (Fisher 1945; Sargant 1967; Kazniak *et al.* 1988; Christianson and Nilsson 1989; Bremner *et al.* 1992). In particular early trauma may disrupt the normal functioning of the memory system (Teicher *et al.* 1994). Repeated experiences of maltreatment have been shown to generate hippocampal damage (Bremner *et al.* 1993*b*) and the hippocampus is critically important in the integration of experiences in memory. In the absence of such an integrative function, patients are likely to be left with unintegrated images and emotions that they are unable to combine with their life narrative or self-schema. Thus, whilst it is highly unlikely that psychogenic amnesia is a particularly relevant model for understanding the impact of early trauma on individuals with BPD, the impact of traumata on the developing nervous system may indeed point to limitations in the memory capacity of individuals who present with BPD. It has been suggested that patients with frontal lesions or lesions of the limbic system commonly manifest profound memory dysfunction. They have been observed to confabulate memories and to concoct stories to make sense of the visual and auditory memories that they retrieve. The frontal lobes appear to play a key role in the attribution of a source to the individual's memories. Illusions of memory may be due to the failure of an attributional process that monitors how a memory image has been generated. Illusions of memory are likely to occur when an individual is trying hard to remember. Monitoring the source of the memory image is momentarily relaxed, and prior information such as knowledge, expectations, and beliefs creates an unusually vivid set of ideas or images. Psychotherapy may be a context in which source monitoring is compromised by the intensity of the emotions generated. The focus by a therapist on recreating and reviving memories will inevitably introduce a further bias. This is a possibility rather than a demonstrated fact. However, the therapist must be aware that the cognitive monitoring functions normally available to individuals to prevent confusion between fantasy and memory may be specifically compromised by the therapeutic process itself.

Some, and we are not amongst these, might argue that using reconstruction to identify a child within the patient, traumatized by (say) rejection at the time of her sibling being born, serves to collude with the patient's need to avoid the massive depressive anxiety associated with her hatred of her own child and the multifarious roots of her self-hatred. In that sense, these clinicians might argue that reconstruction is invariably somewhat collusive with the patient's defences, to the extent that it serves to displace primitive and intense guilt from the present into the past while also making others (rather than the patient) culpable. We think that reconstruction does indeed carry such a risk. But so does any effective psychotherapeutic intervention. Any psychotherapeutic technique must take into account the patient's defences (address the conflict from the point of view of the ego) and ensure that it is (broadly) acceptable to the patient in the way it presents what we recognize is inherently difficult to contemplate. We believe that reconstruction is probably essential to the therapeutic process because: (1) it provides a means to bring the patient's mind into contact with what it has previously found intolerable; (2) it provides a place where threat to the ego and therapeutic goal are reasonably balanced; (3) it generates a coherent self-narrative assuming a historical continuity of self which may itself be of therapeutic value (Schafer 1980; Spence 1994; Holmes 1998).

While reconstruction of how things actually were in childhood may significantly contribute to therapeutic action, this does not however mean that the outcome of reconstruction, the remembering of a hypothetical autobiographical event, has anything whatever to do with "cure". It is the process of re-working current experiences in the context of other, in this case childhood, perspectives, that we believe to be curative. The crucial component is the provision of a perspective or a frame for interpreting subjectivity that is beyond that which the patient has ready conscious access to apart from the analytic encounter. But the 'other perspective' need not be that of the patient's childhood, it could be the analyst's current experience, or the way the patient is experienced by others close to him (as in the group therapy described in this volume for example). Given the historical, theoretical, and even geographical specificity of psychotherapeutic focus on particular historical reconstructions (taking up primal scene memories, sibling rivalry, birth trauma, toilet training, sexual abuse, separation trauma, etc.) it is most unlikely that any specific type of reconstruction per se is essential; the creation of a narrative is quite probably helpful. The deep exploration of subjectivity from alternative perspectives is almost definitely essential. The questioning of current ways of being and thinking, inevitably implied by any act of reconstruction, is no doubt therapeutic.

Not all forms of interpretation of current experience as reminiscence carry equal risks. The interpretation of current physical symptoms as body memories

(Dewald 1989; Kramer 1990) depicting childhood traumatic events, particularly sexual experience at an early age (Frederickson 1992) may be especially unwarranted. The same physical symptoms can emerge in the absence of child sexual abuse (CSA). The bodily symptoms may be a consequence of strongly held beliefs rather than actual experiences, in just the same way as dramatic bodily change can be caused by current beliefs (Early and Lifschutz 1974; Roediger *et al.* 1993). The interpretation of unusual gestures or odd behaviours as evidence of CSA might be relatively common, but probably is also ill-advised. Many consider behavioural re-enactions to be the most common response to childhood trauma, particularly covering the period of infancy (Dewald 1989; Terr 1991, 1994); the notion of procedural memory provides a good psychological basis for this view (see Clyman 1991), but the link to trauma is by no means compelling (Hartmann 1984). In fact, much of early experience is probably encoded in terms of procedures. Thus, there is no reason to believe that traumatic experiences are specifically more likely to be encoded in this way, nor is it clear why re-enactments would be of accurate memories rather than fantasies.

The interpretation of manifest dream content as memory is similarly probably unwise. Despite Freud's skepticism (Freud 1900), some therapists appear to interpret the manifest content of dreams literally, as accurate reflections of early memory (Schuker 1979; Williams 1987; Bernstein *et al.* 1990). There is no physiological evidence to support this view (Horne, 1988), and it is more likely that dreams depicting CSA reflect the content of therapy sessions (Nielsen and Powell 1992) than that they verify hypotheses about early traumatic experiences.

The inadvertent enhancement of the patient's confidence in vague recollections, and the treatment of them as clear memories, may serve to immunize the patient against appropriate doubt (Olio 1989; Blume 1990; Courtois 1992). Treating natural doubt as an indication of resistance of defensiveness may also enhance patients' confidence in the accuracy of their memories, which may well alter their unconscious strategies and lead them to produce further, fully-fledged memories of ill-treatment (Haaken and Schlaps 1991; Yapko 1993). Therapists sometimes also make inappropriate 'expert' statements about the kind of mental representations that they expect to see in patients with a history of abuse. Yet most therapists' experience in this area is quite limited. It does not permit them to speak of CSA in general, and their exposure to individuals who have not suffered psychiatric disorder despite having experienced CSA is, in all probability, minimal. It is almost impossible for them to know which aspects of the patient's representations are causally linked with the CSA experience and which follow from family pathology or from other factors in the etiology of psychiatric disorder. We mention these problems as the rationale behind our caution in exploring our patients' past histories and our almost exclusive focus on the patients' current psychological experience.

Conclusion

This chapter has presented a developmental model of BPD. It is focused around the development of the social affiliative system which we consider to be driving many higher-order social cognitive functions that underpin interpersonal interaction, specifically in an attachment context. We considered four of these in detail: affect representation and, related to this, affect regulation; attentional control, also with strong links to the regulation of affect; the dual arousal system involved in maintaining an appropriate balance between mental functions undertaken by the anterior and posterior portions of the brain; and finally mentalization, a system for interpersonal understanding within the attachment context. To psychoanalytic readers the focus on attachment and a range of neurocognitive mechanisms may sound insufficiently dynamic to be considered in the context of a psychoanalytic theory of borderline pathology. However, we would maintain that our model is dynamic insofar as we consider the above capacities to evolve in the context of the primary caregiving relationships experienced by the child and vulnerable to extremes of environmental deficiency as exemplified by severe neglect, psychological or physical abuse, childhood molestation, or other forms of maltreatment. We suggest that when in place the capacities above normally control or obscure the potential for a more primitive form of subjectivity. This form of subjectivity is dominated by modes of representation of internal states and the relationship of internal and external that are normally observable in the mental functioning of young children. These processes, in combination with a profound disorganization of self-structure, explain many facets of borderline personality functioning. We do not attribute a central role to the trauma, although we expect that in individuals made vulnerable by early inadequate mirroring and disorganized attachment to highly stressful psychosocial experiences in an attachment context, trauma will play a key role in both shaping the pathology and directly triggering it by undermining the capacity for mentalization. We see mentalization as having the power to protect individuals who have been subjected to the same kinds of psychosocial experience but appear to have suffered little or no adverse effects. It makes conceptual sense, therefore, that promoting mentalization should be a focus for therapeutic intervention if we are to bring the primitive modes of mental functioning of borderline individuals under better regulation and control.

4 Current models of treatment for borderline personality disorder

We will now contrast our own theoretical approach with that of others in an attempt to highlight the similarities and differences. A number of approaches to therapy with borderline personality disorder (BPD) have so far been manualized, including psychoanalytic psychotherapy (Kernberg *et al.* 1989), dialectical behaviour therapy (DBT) (Linehan 1987), object relations/interpersonal approaches (Dawson 1988; Marziali *et al.* 1989) and cognitive-analytic therapy (Ryle 1997). Non-manualized approaches have also been described and even subjected to outcome research (Stevenson and Meares 1992) although in Chapter 2 we saw not only how sparse outcome evaluation has been in the field of personality disorder (PD) but also how little comparative outcome research has been done. In part, this is because it is hampered by a lack of specificity in psychological approaches to therapy (Roth and Fonagy 1996) and some have argued that the considerable overlap between psychotherapies compromises the possibility of reaching conclusions concerning relative effectiveness (Goldfried 1995) even if they are manualized. Nevertheless, there are differences between therapies which are apparent and in this chapter we review some of the distinctions between our own approach and other current therapies although some of the differences may seem, occasionally, more theoretical than practical. Establishing variance between therapies is particularly problematic in the case of long-term approaches, which includes all of the above methods, since practitioners make complex choices taking into account both behavioural and dynamic factors when making interventions. So, even when we and others define the important strategies and tactics of treatment, skilled practitioners may end up doing very similar things under the guise of differently-named interventions.

Whenever we talk about the approach described in this book, people are struck by some of the similarities to the therapies that they themselves practice. This is not surprising since all psychotherapeutic approaches to the treatment of BPD construct a similar framework around treatment within which therapeutic interventions take place. All effective therapies for BPD are well-structured, devote considerable effort to enhancing compliance, have a clear focus, and encourage a powerful attachment relationship between therapist and patient, enabling the therapist to adopt a relatively active rather than a passive stance. Some are deliberately well-integrated with other services available to the patient whilst others are avowedly separate. In our treatment programme, psychiatric care is integrated within treatment and not separated off elsewhere to ensure that prescribing and other aspects of psychiatric and social care are fully informed by transference and countertransference processes. Medication is prescribed by members of the treatment team and is considered in the context of transference and countertransference issues arising within individual and group psychotherapy (see p. 195).

Whilst there is overlap between therapies in the framework of treatment, a number of features of the framework of our treatment approach are distinct from other major approaches. For example, mentalization-based treatment (MBT) is a relatively long-term therapy whilst others are short (e.g. CAT is recommended for 24 sessions); some therapies have contracts whilst others do not; some allow contact with the therapist outside sessions whilst others actively discourage it. These variations in the framework and theory of approaches are summarized in Fig. 4.1. Differences are found both within theory and in the translation of those principles into practice, especially in the shape and content of clinical interventions. To this extent theoretical differences are not simply nuances of intellectual distinction but determine how therapy is actually practised. In the next section, we abbreviate our treatment to MBT.

Transference-focused psychotherapy (TFP)

Transference-focused psychotherapy (TFP) is a unique psychodynamic approach in having a coherent theoretical frame of reference as well as a well-manualized set of technical procedures that includes measures of adherence (Yeomans *et al.* 1992; Clarkin *et al.* 1999; Kernberg *et al.* 2002*a*). It is rooted in Otto Kernberg's (1967) theory of borderline personality organization (BPO), which defines BPO as characterized by (a) identity diffusion, (b) primitive defences, (c) generally intact but variable reality testing and (d) characteristic object relations. Identity diffusion, a term which originates in the work of Erik Erikson (1959), is seen as rooted in the disparate, disconnected (split) self-representations which fail to cohere into an organized concept of the self. Thus identity diffusion is a reflection of a failure of developmentally expectable integration of aspects of the self. Primitive defences (splitting, idealization/devaluation, projective identification) are residues of early developmental phases, and what Melanie Klein (1937) has described as the paranoid-schizoid position. While BPO has in common with psychotic personality organization (PPO) both primitive defences and identity diffusion, the quality of reality testing distinguishes BPO from PPO. Unlike PPO, individuals with BPO are able to differentiate self

	MBT	TFP	CAT	DBT	TC
Framework Frequency Length Setting	 2–5 x week 18-months OPD/Partial Hospital	 2 x week 1year OPD	 1x week 6 months OPD	 2 x week 1year In-patient/OPD	 5 x week 1–2years In-patient
Key Constructs	Self-structure Psychic equivalence Pretend Mode Teleological Stance Mentalization	Object relationships Identity diffusion Aggression	Reciprocal roles Self states	Affect dysregulation Invalidating environment Dialectical failure	Communality Permissiveness Democracy Social analysis
Modalities	Individual Group analytic Expressive	Individual	Individual	Individual Social skills group Homework	Groups
Core Techniques	Interpretation Transference Mentalizing Affect and meaning Integrated psychiatric care	Interpretation Transference	Reformulation Interpretation	Problem solving Validation Skills training Affect control Mindfulness	Sharing Social understanding

Fig. 4.1 Comparison of treatments.

from non-self, internal from external reality, and have empathy with social criteria of reality. It should be noted that this distinction between BPO and PPO may not be as clear-cut as originally suggested by Kernberg. Psychotic symptoms have been increasingly commonly noted in individuals with a formal diagnosis of BPD (Gunderson 1984).

Individuals with BPO are seen as manifesting poor impulse control and anxiety tolerance because of a general, non-specific weakness of the ego. Primitive defences will also interfere with current object relations and the limited capacity to sublimate will interfere with the capacity to engage in productive work. The dominance of part-object as opposed to whole-object relations and, associated with this, the failure of full structuralization, leaves the individual with BPO with potentially severe superego pathology (antisocial tendencies) and, more commonly, deep disturbances of sexual functioning (both inhibition of sexuality and chaotic sexuality). Kernberg's model is sophisticated in terms of putative etiology of BPD and considers both genetic and neurophysiological vulnerabilities. The assumed final common pathway is via abnormal affectivity, particularly high levels of aggression. It is assumed that the integration of good and bad object representations is undermined by uncontrollably high levels of aggression, projected on to the object who is then experienced by the infant as an overwhelming and terrifying threat. The 'depressive position', perceiving the good and bad object as one and the same, and recognizing one's role in the distortion, is never reached. It is assumed that under peak affect states, the infant internalizes representations of the self in relation to the other. Further, it is assumed that these initially coalesce into those with positive and those with negative affect. If the child is environmentally or constitutionally predisposed to give greater weight to negative than positive experience, the negative experiences will be isolated and split off and an originally normal developmental split will not be resolved. For example, a relationship representation bringing together a maltreated figure (self) with an object representation of a harsh authority figure accompanied by fear may exist side by side with a representation of the object as an ideal, giving figure and the self as childish and dependent. The affect associated with the self–object relationship representation is love. Temperamental factors may also play a part in disrupting object relations, particularly in the realm of achieving appropriate capacities for self-regulation. Etiological factors outside of the individual include pathology of early attachment relationships, trauma inside and outside the attachment relationship, and family pathology. Individuals with pervasive aggression, antisocial features, severely restricted object relations and poor sublimation because of low intelligence and shifting lifestyle, are regarded as more likely to respond poorly to therapeutic intervention.

The therapeutic approach of TFP is based on the assumption of a mental world populated by object relations dyads. In the split world of BPO, representations of positive interactions between the self and the object are kept apart from representations of negative interaction. The aim of therapy is to move towards normal organization where the individual is conscious of the complexity of self and object and accepts that good and bad parts exist in both. However, traditionally in therapy, the poorly integrated self–object representations of the patient are externalized so the therapist may be seen as a harsh authority figure one moment and an idealized, giving figure the next. Further, considerable oscillation may characterize the relationship with the therapist moving from the self to the object pole of a dyadic representation or the representations themselves changing from benign to negative.

The first stage of the therapy may be marked by considerable chaos in the sessions where fragmented and partial self and object representations activated in rapid succession may make therapists feel bombarded with chaotic and contradictory object relations. The therapist's task is to tolerate the confusion, accept the uncertainty, and refrain from overactivity. In the second step, dominant object relations are defined. In a further step, the protagonists of the dominant object relations are named while the therapist attends to the patient's reactions. These steps constitute the primary strategy or long-term objective of TFP. Other strategies include the observation and interpretation of role reversal in the active dyads, the observation and interpretation of linkages between object relation dyads that defend against each other and thus maintain internal conflict and fragmentation, and finally the elaboration of the patient's capacity to experience a relationship differently in the transference and review the patient's other significant relationships in the light of this exchange.

Transference-focused psychotherapy helpfully distinguishes long-term objectives above (strategies) from tactics and techniques. Tactics are tasks the therapist is asked to undertake in the context of each individual session, while techniques are consistent, habitual ways of addressing what happens from moment to moment. Techniques include clarifying, confronting, interpreting, analyzing the transference, managing technical neutrality, and utilizing awareness of the countertransference. The TFP manual defines each of these techniques carefully. For example, clarification is requesting clarification and explicitly not the offering of clarification. The manual thus guards against the therapist experiencing himself as an omniscient other. Using clarification, the patient's distortions may be elaborated, particularly those experienced in the context of the transference. Confrontation is also an honest enquiry rather than a hostile challenge. Upon identifying contradiction in the patient's communication, the therapist invites the patient to reflect on this apparent inconsistency. Underlying this technique is the assumption that the contradiction represents separate aspects of the self split off from one another and the confrontation can prepare the way to integration. This kind of contradiction can manifest as a discrepancy between different channels of patients' communication. A verbal account of affection may be delivered in an angry, hostile manner, or alternatively contradiction may manifest in a rapidly changing perception of the therapist in the eyes of the patient. Interpretations are conceived of as existing at different levels. The first level of interpretation concerns interpreting acting out, or interpreting primitive defences mounted to avoid awareness of internal experience. A second level of interpretation is aimed at addressing the currently active object relations dyad and/or reversals of this dyad. A third level of interpretation addresses the dyad that is defended against and attempts to address the putative motivation for this defence.

Tactics of TFP, the tasks the therapist needs to have in mind in each session with the patient, include contract setting, maintaining the treatment frame, selecting a focus for intervention, attending to the general priorities of the treatment, appreciating and interpreting the positive and negative transference and primitive defences, and regulating the intensity of affective involvement. The contract between therapist and patient defines the responsibilities of each and, as far as this is possible, protects the therapist's ability to think clearly and reflect. The contract is seen as providing a safe place where the dynamics of the patient's internal world may unfold. It sets the stage so that deviations from the contract may be interpreted at later stages of the therapy. It provides an organizing frame that permits therapy to become a point of reference in the patient's life. The contract will typically contain references about attendance, fees, and free disclosure of thoughts and feelings as part of the patient's responsibilities. The therapist's responsibilities include scheduling, attempting to understand, and clarifying the limits of involvement. Contracting is achieved after a process of dialogue that may itself be therapeutic, where threats to the patient's treatment are identified and elaborated. The most obvious threats are suicidal and self-destructive behaviour, but lying and censoring information, abusing drugs, or excessively intruding into the therapist's life may all be significant threats. The recommended path around suicidality may at first glance seem quite 'draconian' in TFP. If the patient does not feel that the urge to kill himself/herself can be controlled and if he/she is unwilling to go to the emergency room to have this evaluated, then the therapist will arrange an ER visit but then will end the therapy. If the patient is hospitalized, therapy is suspended until the patient is discharged. If the patient refuses hospitalization even though it is recommended, the therapist calls an end to the treatment. If the patient takes suicidal action in the course of therapy, and calls the therapist, the therapist does what is needed at that moment but then ends the therapy.

The choice of what material to address in any one session is guided by four principles. First, interventions should concern issues where there is most affect. Second, material to be addressed should go from the defence towards the impulse, that is, from identifying a defensively activated object relations dyad and as a second stage identifying the impulsive object relations dyad that it shields from consciousness. Third, closely related to the above, object relations dyads should be seen as most likely alternating with each other in an impulse–defence interaction, thus the self may be depicted as meek and victimized to defend against an image of the self as powerful and controlling. Finally and crucially, TFP identifies a hierarchy of thematic priorities which directs the therapist initially to address obstacles to transference exploration e.g. suicide threats, contract breaches, acting out inside or outside the session. Second in the hierarchy are overt transference manifestations (verbal references to the therapist, non-verbal references to the therapist or inferred references to the therapist such as seeing the patient's discussion of other figures as being displaced commentaries on the therapist). Third in the hierarchy is non-transferential affect-laden material. The treatment manual comprehensively addresses complications of TFP, including erotization of the transference relationship, hatred of the therapist in the transference, threats to drop out of treatment, paranoid reactions to the therapist, the enactment of traumatic experiences in the therapy, etc.

Under optimal circumstances, therapy results in greater integration of object relations dyads and brings about structural change (the forming of psychic structures of id, ego, superego from object relations dyads). Indications of such change include greater ability on the part of the patient to accept the interpretation of primitive defences, increased capacity to contain and tolerate the awareness of hatred, the capacity to consider fantasies and confront the pathological or grandiose self. Progress is indicated by the patient's comments indicating reflection on and exploration of the therapist's intervention. Change is seen to occur as the patient moves towards a greater integration of the self-concept simultaneously with greater integration of concepts of others.

Affective experience will become enriched and modulated and previously dissociated or split-off affect states come to be integrated into a more coherent, better-structured organization. A further mechanism is identified as the increased capacity for empathy in relation to self and others and the concurrent development of in-depth relationships.

Evaluation

Undoubtedly, TFP is the most coherent, comprehensive, and best specified psychoanalytic psychotherapy in existence for any patient group. It has a range of admirable features: (1) It is firmly rooted in psychodynamic theory and closely linked to the most widely practiced method of psychodynamic intervention that will surely facilitate training in TFP and the generalization of TFP training to other patient groups. (2) The operationalization of TFP is highly sophisticated, far more so than the manualization of most other psychotherapeutic treatments including DBT, CAT, and CBT. For example, the integration with pharmacological therapies is clearly defined with a specific set of algorithms in treating cognitive perceptual symptoms, affect dysregulation symptoms and behavioural dyscontrol symptoms of BPD (Soloff 1998). There are specific modules of TFP designed to address particular complicating features of the disorder such as depression or suicidality. As a therapeutic package, TFP is realistic in terms of both intensity and duration, making widespread cost-effective implementation a real possibility. Finally it is accessible to empirical testing and therefore potentially compatible with the demands of evidence-based practice.

There are some important differences between this formulation of borderline pathology and the model advanced in this volume. Many of these differences are subtle and only some have practical implications. TFP views the emergence of the agentive self differently from MBT. It errs on the side of early attribution of agentive thinking, and this may translate to the attribution of intentionality to the patient in contexts where MBT might not. Secondly, at the core of TFP is the understanding that externalizations in the transference are externalizations of mental representations of self–other relations internalized at moments of peak affect. Within MBT many such externalizations would not be seen as primarily relational, but rather, as externalizations of parts of the unmentalized self, particularly the core self or the alien self. An important technical implication of this is that MBT would not expect the patient to understand much of the discourse that the therapist might verbalize in relational terms. The self and the therapist are experienced as perceived (unquestioning psychic equivalence), and this is sometimes strikingly without relationship implications. Third, and related to this, projective identification in TFP is seen as protecting the ego from destruction by aggression. Within MBT its principal role is ensuring the coherence of the self-organization. Fourth, affect dysregulation is attributed to constitutional anomalies, temperamental differences, the absence of effortful control in TFP, but is seen in MBT as a consequence of symbolic failure, particularly associated with incongruent mirroring.

There are technical differences in clinical approach between TFP and MBT. Some of these are most likely to be the function of differences in setting of the two treatments. TFP is an out-patient therapy whilst MBT was initially developed for a partial hospital setting. Adaptation of MBT to an out-patient setting is likely to blur the treatments further. TFP is offered on a fee for service basis or the fee is covered by insurance companies to a greater lesser extent controlled by Health Maintenance Organizations (HMOs). MBT is offered as part of a comprehensive health and social care service (the NHS) that prides itself on being unequivocally free at the point of delivery. Perhaps most importantly under this heading, TFP is delivered by experienced psychoanalytic therapists; therapy in the MBT context is offered by nurses, psychologists, and social workers who are supervised by psychoanalysts. The differences in setting may be associated with differences in the theoretical origins of these approaches. TFP represents a most creative integration of drive theory and object relations theory. MBT is also an integration, but most specifically an integration of cognitive and psychoanalytic developmental theory and attachment theory.

Notwithstanding these differences, there are many common aspects to the systems. Both focus on affect and affect-related cognitions, emphasize countertransference awareness, and ask the therapist to consider relationship representations and parallels between relationship patterns. Both approaches turn away from classical psychoanalytic therapy by de-emphasizing deep unconscious concerns in favour of conscious or near conscious content. They share the therapeutic aim of achieving representational coherence and integration and conceptualize their mode of action as working with endogenously-activated representational systems.

There are some apparent incompatibilities that on closer scrutiny turn out to be shared aspects of these approaches. For example, TFP emphasizes neutrality whilst MBT accepts 'reflective enactment'. In MBT the therapists' occasional enactment is seen as a necessary concomitant of therapeutic alliance. In MBT it is assumed that the therapist is an essential vehicle for the alien part of the patient's self, and that this permits the therapist to perceive and reflect on the patient's constitutional self (that which is left behind following the externalization). For the patient to tolerate the relationship, the therapist needs to become that which the patient needs her to be. But both approaches recognize that beyond enactment the therapist, in order to be helpful, must be able to preserve a 'neutral' part of their mind that is able accurately to mirror, to reflect the patient's internal state *following* successful projective identification.

Mentalization-based treatment does not involve contracting with the patient. For TFP this is an important stage in the initial phases of negotiation. Is psychodynamic psychotherapy possible for individuals with BPD without an explicitly negotiated contract? Quite possibly not. MBT recommends defining the rules of treatment (see Chapter 5); for example violence in the treatment context will trigger police involvement and a time out from the treatment. Drug and alcohol use, as judged by two independent treaters, will result in temporary exclusion from the program. The definition of roles of mental health professionals involved in patient care is a key part of MBT's equivalent to aspects of the TFP contract. However, there are differences too. The one-team approach is an important part of MBT and would not admit of some aspects of the TFP role definition of the therapist which imply a splitting of responsibilities.

There are further commonalities in the structure. Both treatments reject "commune-ism", democracy, and egalitarian principles, but also authoritarianism, controlling attitudes, and mindless enforcement of views. The authoritative framework in both TFP and MBT counteracts the reactive, fragmented, and unreliable aspects of "treatment as usual", that usually presents a fragmented version of the patient for mirroring. Both approaches recognize that patients in these treatments perceive and exploit inconsistency, and therefore the treatment protocol has to minimize inter and intraprofessional disputes. TFP is MBT's closest ally among the psychological therapies.

Dialectical behaviour therapy

Developed by Marsha Linehan (1987), dialectical behaviour therapy (DBT) has engendered considerable interest around the Americas, Europe, and elsewhere because it was the first psychotherapy shown in a randomized controlled clinical trial to have effects on symptoms of BPD (see p. 47). DBT, a broad-based behavioural treatment, is founded on a dialectical and biosocial theory of BPD that determines the form and content of the interventions.

It is not possible to do justice to the complexity of the dialectical formulation of BPD but three aspects of the theory—dialectics, affect dysregulation, and mindfulness—will be summarized here since they offer alternative theoretical formulations that contrast with our own approach and lead to different styles of treatment intervention in practice.

Dialectics

Dialectics form the core of the strategies in DBT and determine the therapist's attitude and stance towards the patient. In the context of behavioural treatment, dialectics imply that analysis of small components or individual parts of a system is of limited value and the part needs to be viewed in relation to the whole. In this way DBT differs from standard behavioural treatment, which focuses on breaking down the whole into components and eschews examination of the complete picture. The DBT therapist using dialectic understanding may tackle a specific problem from a skill-based perspective but relate it to areas of the patient's life; he may take the attitude that learning new skills may on its own not be enough; he may recognize that well-used skills may need to be lost as others are learned. In addition, dialectic suggests that individual reality comprises opposing forces, a thesis and antithesis, which are not static; any synthesis may release another set of opposing forces but the borderline patient is stuck within polarities without synthesis, the most fundamental of which is accepting himself as he is and recognizing a need for change. Thus reality is viewed as being in a state of continuous flux and intervention in DBT is less about structure and content than change and process. Within this system of opposites, getting what is desired may be as problematic as being denied; learning new skills that lead to improvement may invalidate personal integrity which has been maintained by grievance. These are dialectics.

Not surprisingly, these dialectical aspects of DBT overlap considerably with psychoanalytic ideas about BPD. For example dialectics has much in common with conflict and object relational models of psychopathology. Rey (1979) summarizes borderline patients as being stuck between oedipal and pre-oedipal, between psychosis and neurosis, between male and female, between paranoid-schizoid and depressive positions, between fear of the object and need for the object, between inner and outer, between body and mind. Others view the core of the problem as being conflict about need for closeness accompanied by fear of abandonment by the object on the one hand and rejection, retreat, and withdrawal from intimacy, on the other hand. These internal fluctuations and the extreme internal splits described from a psychoanalytic perspective are characterized in DBT as dialectical failures. For DBT, the continuation of conflict is a dialectical failure because there is opposition between firmly rooted but contradictory positions, wishes, and desires which have not been transcended through synthesis—the conflict has not been worked through.

The dialectical approach is a philosophical position or a world view whereas our position is developmental and informed by attachment research. As has been said, the absence of mentalizing capacity and of accurate second-order representations of internal states (feelings, beliefs, wishes, ideas) in BPD leads in our view to failure in establishing an agentive sense of self. Emotional fluctuations, opposing beliefs, proneness to action, all arise from an inability to experience a sense of self as agentive, especially within the context of monitoring and interpreting correctly the relevant mind-state cues that are available in intimate attachment relationships. The borderline patient needs to rely on rigid structures and schematic beliefs in order to protect and maintain an illusory stable self.

Despite this difference of understanding of psychological process, it is the dialectic component of DBT that inevitably leads to a focus in DBT on the relationship between the patient and therapist which is, of course central to all psychoanalytically-orientated treatments. To this extent DBT is more similar to dynamic therapies than other behavioural treatments. Linehan states that 'the therapeutic relationship is central to effective treatment with suicidal and borderline individuals' (Linehan 1993*b*, p. 1) and that DBT, in some aspects, is 'more similar to the psychodynamic emphasis on transference behaviours than it is to any aspect of standard cognitive behavioural therapies' (Linehan, 1993*a*, p. 21). Indeed in some respects transference and countertransference may be considered as a clinical manifestation of an internal 'dialectic' and points to the fundamental deficit in self-other differentiation.

In both DBT and MBT, and probably in all therapies, a positive therapeutic alliance is fostered and the relationship is a vehicle through which strategies are implemented, but in MBT there is an additional role for the relationship in that it is the core of therapy. The relationship between patient and therapist is used to understand the behaviours, feelings, desires, and beliefs of the patient and to effect change. Transference and countertransference, teased out within the therapeutic interaction, are considered essential elements of therapy (see p. 207) and are harnessed to bring about change. This is not to suggest that in MBT the therapist takes a passive stance, commenting on what the patient brings to the relationship and reflecting back in the way that analytic therapies are often characterized (or caricatured) but that the therapist actively mentalizes about the patient within the context of the relationship and tries to establish the meaning of behaviours and feelings experienced within the here-and-now of the relationship. Understanding of transference and countertransference are used for this purpose. Further, there is no place for prescient relational statements from the therapist about the patient because both have the task of considering each other's mind states. Mistakes in understanding on the part of the therapist are acknowledged and seen as the best understanding that the therapist had at the time, which in the light of further consideration, are recognized as incorrect. Of course it is not therapeutic to simply capitulate when challenged by a patient but equally it is not conducive to a therapeutic alliance to deny mistakes. This balance in the therapist between an open and closed 'mind' within the mentalizing process shares aspects in common with the acceptance and change stance of the DBT therapist.

Emotional dysregulation

A further aspect of DBT is the emphasis on emotional dysregulation which is seen as the outcome of biological disposition, environmental context, and the transaction between the two during development. To some extent this interactional, developmental view is shared by all psychotherapeutic approaches but DBT gives a crucial developmental role to the invalidating environment in which erratic and inappropriate responses are given during childhood by insensitive and thoughtless caregivers—a child who expresses anger may be dismissed, one who says she did her best is told that she did not. Persistent divergence between inner experience and outer responses, the invalidating environment, not only leads to emotional dysregulation by failing to teach the child the skills to modulate arousal and tolerate strong feelings but also results in an uncertainty in later life about the validity of inner experience and the accuracy of one's interpretation of events. The emphasis on affective hyper-responsiveness is not fully supported by empirical data. Studies have shown that borderline patients do not show electrodermal hyporesponsiveness which would predispose them to stimulus-seeking and disinhibited, impulsive behaviour (Herpertz *et al.* 2001*a*) and self-report data and physiological data suggest that the intensity of affective response in BPD is no different from controls (Herpertz *et al.* 1999). Whilst agreeing that borderline patients have significant problems with emotions, we take an alternative view about the core of the emotional difficulty. It is not that the child fails to develop the skills to modulate emotions but that she cannot easily identify emotions and distinguish whose they are or give meaning to them. The deficit is not one of regulation but it is the inaccessibility of the *experience* of feeling regulated. The borderline patient both misunderstands and misattributes them and finds them perplexing.

According to our model, adaptive affect–reflective interactions between mother and child result in expressed affect being identified and decoupled from the parent. The parent first has to ensure that the emotion is accurately perceived and reflected (categorically congruent) and second that the feeling is recognized as either hers or the baby's through marking the emotion (perceptual marking). Invalidation is but one example of failure of categorization and/or inappropriate perceptual marking rather than the underlying cause of the difficulty so the emphasis on invalidation in DBT as a causal phenomenon is too narrow and exclusive. The selective lack of either markedness or category congruence produces deviant mirroring styles that, if dominant in the infant's experience, are likely to lead to characteristic pathological consequences of emotional identification and expression. A secondary representation of emotional states, which acts as a buffer between feelings and actions, does not develop and so the patient has no psychological process through which to modulate or soothe feelings. This is discussed in detail on pp. 64, 83.

Mentalization and mindfulness

Mindfulness is a core skill of DBT. In essence the skills of mindfulness are intrapsychic, psychological, and behavioural versions of meditation, in particular those associated with Zen spiritual practices. These include 'what' skills (such as observing, describing, participating) and 'how' skills which consist of taking a non-judgemental stance, focusing on one thing in the moment, and being effective. These skills are used to balance states of mind within the individual of which there are three—'reasonable mind', 'emotional mind', and 'wise mind'. In a reasonable mind state an individual is able to think rationally and logically whilst in an emotional mind state the individual's mind is dominated by a current feeling; reason and logic are problematic. The 'wise' mind, an integration of reasonable and emotional mind, allows the individual to add intuition to emotional experience and logical thought, bringing about a greater synthesis and stability and it is 'Wise mind' which may be nearest to mentalization but, again, it is seen as a skill in DBT rather than a complex developmental psychological process. This imaginative adaption of Zen principles is unusual in CBT but anticipated other approaches (Teasdale *et al.* 2000). There have also been efforts to link psychoanalytic and Zen perspectives (Twemlow 2001*a*, *b*).

In relation to MBT it is worth pointing out that mentalization is not seen by us as a skill which is learned but a high-level mental function that mostly takes place outside consciousness and it is this developmental approach to its evolution which informs our therapy. It develops through a presentation to an individual of a view of their internal world which is stable, coherent, and can be clearly perceived by them and may be adopted as the reflective part of their self (the self-image of the patient's mind). It is intimately related to the development of both the purposeful and the representational aspects of the self: both the 'I' and 'Me' and therefore involves not just a self-reflective element but also an interpersonal component. In combination, these provide the individual with a capacity to distinguish inner from outer reality, intrapersonal mental and emotional processes from interpersonal communications, and what is self from what is not. These functions are not part of mindfulness. The development of mentalization critically depends upon interaction with more mature minds, which are both benign and reflective in their turn; hence our requirement for therapists themselves to show a capacity to take a mentalizing position (see p. 203) as a basic therapeutic stance and for the programme to be arranged in a way that encourages self-reflection within an interpersonal milieu.

The development of a capacity to modulate affect states, which is one purpose of mindfulness skills, is closely related to mentalization. Affect regulation is a prelude to mentalization and yet we also believe that once mentalization occurs, the nature of affect regulation is transformed. It is no longer simply modulated. 'Mentalized affectivity' allows the individual to discover the subjective meanings of his own affect states and this recognition of meaning as a fundamental aspect of mentalization distinguishes it from mindfulness. Mentalized affectivity represents the experiential understanding of one's feelings in a way that extends beyond intellectual awareness. It requires not only an internal recognition but also an appreciation that feeling has an interpersonal context and full understanding necessitates a grasp of one's own mind as represented within the mind of another. Not surprisingly such a complex mental function, not part of mindfulness, becomes subject to resistances and defences. We can misunderstand what we feel and what others think of us or think that we feel one thing while truly feeling another emotion. So, in this respect one task of therapy is not to teach mentalization but to identify how defensive processes interfere with its functions.

Practice

The differences outlined above may seem to the reader to be merely theoretical but in fact they have consequences for practice even though the format of the two treatments is similar. Both DBT and MBT provide a package of treatment in group and individual sessions with regular meetings between therapists and skilled supervision to ensure co-ordination of treatment. But the underlying reasons for the combination of group and individual therapy differ. The individual treatment in DBT is for attention to dialectics and motivational issues whilst the group is for skills training. In MBT the individual therapy allows detailed exploration of the self-structure within a dyadic relationship, a concentration in a secure environment of transference and countertransference process, the development of a secondary representation, and actively encourages mentalization about group treatment. Conflict between intimacy and distance can be explored within the here-and-now of the relationship. The individual therapist asks the patient to think about their emotional actions and reactions within the group during the individual sessions. To facilitate this, the group and individual sessions are linked together through regular meetings of the therapy team. In the group sessions there is a focus on consideration of other 'minds' and emphasis on appropriate expression of affect through an understanding of personal motivations and those of others. Patients are asked actively by the therapist to consider their understanding of the reasons for others' behaviour as well as questioning their own. The emphasis is on interpersonal process and how this reflects underlying internal processes and there is no specific focus on acquisition of skills. In short DBT offers skills training in groups whilst MBT offers group therapy to understand oneself in relation to others.

Supervision or consultation to the therapist is an integral part of both MBT and DBT to ensure that therapists are 'on-model' and keep within the frame. In DBT maintaining the therapeutic relationship is done through 'cheer leading'. If this means giving support, helping the therapist retain optimism when feeling hopeless, moving the therapist from bewilderment to understanding, then 'cheer leading' is a part of all supervision. But there are other purposes. In DBT the role of supervision is described within a dialectical principle—just as the therapist applies DBT to the patient so the supervisor applies DBT to the therapist to act as a dialectical balance—if the therapist moves too close to the patient, the consultant/supervisor remains at a distance; or the consultant may move back to encourage the therapist to become closer to the patient. In MBT transference and countertransference aspects of the patient–therapist relationship are considered and the relationship between consultant and therapist may be used to understand the current psychological processes within treatment but supervision is not therapy. Through the process of transference and countertransference, the borderline patient may 'push' the therapist too far into or away from the relationship. Even experienced therapists can end up behaving and feeling in ways that interfere with effective treatment and such occurrences are related to aspects of both the patient and therapist. No assumption is made in MBT that all events, problems, and emotional crises arise solely from the patient. This is particularly important to emphasize since the prevailing mythology is that psychoanalytically-based therapies consider the patient to be responsible for everything that happens. In fact we consider problems that arise in therapy as representing a dynamic within the relationship that needs exploring in the context of other relationships and this can include the supervisory relationship. In keeping with the principle of mentalization the most important aspect of therapy is the activity of teasing out what belongs to whom. Countertransference experience may, in fact, represent unresolved aspects of the personality of the therapist. Borderline patients often unconsciously pick up our weak spots.

Overall these differences reflect the different stance and attitude of the therapists and, to some extent, are part of a dialectic between problem-solving strategies, skills, and learned behaviour on the one hand and relationships, transference, and meaning on the other. Impulses, desires, feelings, and beliefs are firmly placed within a relationship frame within MBT and their meaning comes from an exploration of the interaction with the therapist and others. Crises are dealt with through attempts to understand the underlying motivations that are compelling an individual to cut or overdose or threaten others and not from a point of view of skills coaching. This is done within the group and individual sessions. Out-of-hours contact between team and patient does not occur since it is a time when the responsibility for actions lies with the patient including a decision to access the emergency psychiatric services. In the day unit programme, the weekends are the most problematic for patients and the link between a sense of abandonment and destructive actions is continually explored within the groups. During office hours patients may telephone a member of the team if in crisis and may be seen briefly if it is felt that this meeting will reduce fear and anxiety, stabilize the self, and minimize risk.

Reinforcers and aversive contingencies are not used in MBT but are present in DBT. In MBT no draconian contracts linked to discharge are placed on patients. BPD is a condition that is characterized by fear of rejection and abandonment. Seriously chaotic patients find it difficult to attend consistently, and emotional expression tends to be through action. These factors suggest that confronting behaviour with behaviour is likely at times to be traumatic rather than therapeutic, and the very problems that are the focus of treatment can become the same ones that result in discharge. All aspects of behaviour and attitude are discussed within the programme rather than being subject to contract. In DBT patients are discharged from treatment if they fail to attend for four consecutive weeks of skills training. In our view this sort of contract should only be made with patients who are functioning reasonably well, and even then it is of dubious value if used as an aid to reduce serious suicidal behaviour (Kroll 2000). Those that show chaotic lifestyles with unstable social circumstances and antisocial traits simply see contract 'rules' as a further example of the authoritarian and coercive regimes that they have experienced either in their early lives or later, for example, when in prison. Whilst our attitude to contracts may sound permissive and akin to letting patients do whatever they please, we emphasize the importance of attendance on a regular basis and have an active programme of engagement in therapy in which we contact patients who fail to attend. On one occasion we were reported for harassment for contacting a patient too much and trying to help him attend! In our research the drop-out rate was only 12%. This was much lower than expected and probably resulted from our careful attention to underlying reasons for patient non-attendance which were addressed in the individual session, the group sessions, and occasionally by home visit. Failure to attend is seen as interfering with everyone's therapy—a group is not a group unless all members turn up and are active within it. A patient begins to understand that his behaviour has consequences for others in the same way as theirs does for him. He is asked to consider the effect his non-attendance may have had on the others to encourage the process of 'mentalization'.

Overall the differences between DBT and our approach are best seen as lying, respectively, within the contrasts of behaviour and meaning, of support and expression, of rationality and emotion, of learning and identification, and of change through acquisition of skills and change through transference work. Yet it is inevitable that these stark contrasts are not absolute and that within DBT there is identification, within MBT there is support and so on. The borderline patient needs a flexible, thinking but consistent therapist, whether it is to assist them with learning mindfulness skills or with developing mentalization, and those characteristics are not the exclusive property of any one therapy but more a function of the therapist himself.

Cognitive behavioural therapy

Cognitive behavioural formulations of BPD are already as diverse as those of psychoanalysis, even though it is only over the past decade that cognitive therapists have turned their attention to PDs. Given the plurality of both approaches, it is difficult to do justice to the similarities and differences although this has been reviewed elsewhere (Bateman 2000).

A clinically-based approach has been proposed by a number of workers who have developed detailed conceptualizations and treatment strategies for each of the PDs. Initially these formulations built on the general view of psychopathology taken by cognitive therapy in which biased thinking patterns are considered as the core of a patient's problem and modification of these is necessary if the patient is to improve. Standard cognitive therapy focuses a great deal of attention on automatic thoughts and assumptions or beliefs. Automatic thoughts are akin to an internal running commentary which is evoked under particular circumstances, for example when writing a chapter for a book the anxious individual may continually say to himself 'I am never going to get this done and the editors will think that I am lazy'. Assumptions function at a deeper level of cognition and are tacit rules that give rise to automatic thoughts. But it was soon apparent that this formulation was overly simplistic and inadequate and a reformulated model has been proposed to take into account the complex psychological processes and behaviours found in BPD. In a revised model, Beck and associates (Alford 1997) define personality in terms of patterns of social, motivational, and cognitive-affective processes, thereby moving away from a primary emphasis on cognitions. However, personality is thought to be determined by 'idiosyncratic structures' known as schemas, whose cognitive content gives meaning to the person. But the term schemas has been used in various ways, on the one hand being considered as structures of cognition that filter and guide the processing of information, and on the other hand being viewed as the building blocks of latent, core beliefs. The latter is the commonest use of the term and implies basic rules that individuals apply to organize their perceptions of the world, self, and future, and to adapt to the challenges of life.

The concept of the schema is the cornerstone of cognitive formulations of BPD. Patients with BPD show characteristic assumptions and dichotomous thinking. Basic assumptions in the borderline commonly include 'the world is a dangerous place', 'people cannot be trusted', 'I am inherently unacceptable'. Dichotomous thinking is the tendency to evaluate experiences in terms of mutually exclusive categories such as good and bad, love and hate. Extreme evaluations such as these require extreme reactions and emotions, leading to abrupt changes in mood and immoderate behaviour. The assumptions, dichotomous thinking, and weak sense of identity are considered to form a mutually reinforcing and self-perpetuating system that governs relationships. Schemas that were adaptive during childhood persist even after they have become seriously dysfunctional. They are maintained in the face of contradictory evidence because of distortion, discounting, and seeing the evidence as an exception to the rule and extinction of the maladaptive systems does not take place as a result of negative reinforcement. In fact new experiences are filtered by the dysfunctional schemas in such a way that new experiences support existing dysfunctional beliefs and behaviour patterns. Young (1999) has argued vociferously for a 'fourth level of cognition' to be added to Beck's cognitive model, namely Early Maladaptive Schemas (EMS). These are stable and enduring patterns of thinking and perception that begin early in life and are continually elaborated. EMS are unconditional beliefs linked together to form a core of an individual's self-image. Challenge threatens the core identity, which is defended with alacrity, guile, and yet desperation since activation of the schemas may evoke aversive emotions. The EMS gives rise to 'schema coping behaviour', which is the best adaptation to living that the borderline has found. These schemas are different conceptually from some of those discussed by Beck, which are not unconditional beliefs about the self. Beck refers to core beliefs and conditional beliefs, both of which are labelled schemas. Core beliefs are more like EMS but conditional beliefs require an additional context to become active—'if he gets close to me he will find out how awful I am and then reject me'.

Safran and Segal (1990) have integrated schemas within an interpersonal context, arguing that the impact of an individual's beliefs and schemas is not purely cognitive but interacts with interpersonal behaviour which in turn has a reciprocal effect on beliefs. Thus the person is seen as being in a state of dynamic balance to the extent of provoking responses from others that perpetuate underlying assumptions. The borderline patient holds poorly integrated views of relationships with early caregivers and has extreme and unrealistic expectations that determine both behaviour and emotional response. This is exacerbated by problems of identity and a fragile identity leads to a lack of clear and consistent goals and results in poorly co-ordinated actions, badly controlled impulses, and unsustained achievement. Relationships become an attempt to establish a stable identity through dependency, assertiveness, and control. From this viewpoint, cognitive therapy is more than just changing assumptions. It becomes much more complex, lasts longer, and requires new techniques. The therapist cannot rely on modifying beliefs through review of evidence that contradicts maladaptive or negative conclusions. Borderlines cannot be argued out of their beliefs especially when they are dissonant with their affects. This has been recognized in CBT and attempts are made not only to challenge maladaptive beliefs but also to help the patient to identify, support, and develop alternative schemas.

Despite all the theoretical formulations there is limited information about clinical application of cognitive behavioural therapy for BPD although Davidson (2000) has published a treatment guide. The schema focused and interpersonal cognitive models, show the greatest overlap with psychoanalytically-based models, sharing a focus on exploration of the childhood origins of current problems and using the therapy relationship to develop an understanding of the individual's relationships. One difference often cited is the neutrality of the analytic therapist compared with the active, directive approach of the cognitive therapist. But it will become clear to readers of this manual that whilst the therapists in our treatment programme endeavour to remain neutral, eschewing judgment and moralization, they are not passive or inactive. On the contrary it is important for the therapist to 'keep talking' during crises and not to sit silently. One area that is distinctly different is that schema therapists now provide 'limited re-parenting', attempting to meet partially the unmet emotional needs of the patient in order to 'heal' schemas (Young 1999). This is in marked contradistinction to analytic approaches in which the 'real relationship' (see p. 216) is considered to be on a path towards boundary violation, antitherapeutic, and a probable manifestation of countertransference enactment.

Cognitive analytic therapy (CAT)

Cognitive analytic therapy (CAT), developed by Ryle (1990), shares elements of both cognitive and psychoanalytical therapies but is commonly promoted as an integrative and 'stand-alone' therapy with a distinctive theory and practice rather than as an off-shoot of either. It was initially developed as a short-term, structured treatment useful for treatment of neurotic disorders, and has been adapted for the treatment of BPD (Ryle 1997).

Reciprocal roles

It is well-known that borderline patients display widely diverse states of mind and induce powerful mental states in therapists. In order to conceptualize this clinical finding, Ryle developed a theory of reciprocal roles in which there is a role for the self, a role for the other, and a paradigm for their relationship. The quality of the reciprocal roles varies and may range from the benign, albeit perhaps pathological, for example caregiver/care receiver, to the harsh, such as bully/victim, abuser/abused. Reciprocal roles act as templates; when a patient takes one role there is a commensurate push for the therapist to take-up the congruent pole. Both patient and therapist may, of course, be unaware of this and the reciprocal roles may be appropriate, but more often the repertoire of the borderline patient is harsher and uncompromising and so the therapist begins to reciprocate in non-therapeutic ways.

Three levels of abnormality of the internalized reciprocal role structure are described. The first is the relative scarcity of roles that borderline patients have in their repertoire which is in contrast to the large number that other people can deploy. This relates to our own suggestion that borderline patients, when faced with complex interpersonal situations, default to repetitive and schematic representations of relationships. The second level of difficulty is the problem of switching gracefully and appropriately between roles. Borderline patients may switch suddenly leaving the reciprocator rather bewildered, uncertain, and unclear why things have changed. Finally there is incapacity to self-reflect and to exert self-control within the reciprocal roles.

It will not surprise the reader that we are, to some extent, in agreement with this sort of formulation which is clearly developed within a psychoanalytic frame. Ryle suggests that the concept of reciprocal roles is a less-mystifying version of projective identification and countertransference but in fact it is less specific rather than less mystifying and has more in common with the dynamic formulation of role responsiveness put forward by Sandler (1976), that of evocative projective identification suggested by Spillius (1994), or even that of complementary and concordant countertransferences suggested by Racker (1968). But the main problem with regard to the CAT formulation of reciprocal roles is that there appears to be little concern for the underlying reasons in borderline patients for the limited repertoire of roles, the difficulty in switching between them smoothly and appropriately, and the paucity of self-reflection. This lack of interest in latent meaning may account for the abandonment of interpretation of any kind as an intervention in CAT.

We have already discussed our views about why the borderline patient experiences problems in self-reflection and the relationship this has with an unstable sense of self, which in turn leads to affects remaining unlabelled and confused (see p. 64ff). During development, the absence of a stable reflective self creates a gap within the self-structure which is filled by internalizing a version of the other's state rather than by a metabolized or an appropriately reflected version of the child's state. This creates an alien self (see p. 89) which once internalized undermines self-cohesion and leads to confusion between inner and outer, between thoughts and feelings, between self and other. Feelings that are experienced within do not seem to belong to the self. Stability can only be maintained if the alien self is forcibly projected and it is this that leads to the distorted and limited reciprocal roles described in CAT. Interventions are likely to be ineffective unless the underlying purpose of the sudden switches and the reasons for the rigidity of roles, namely the stabilization of the self and the need to establish a basic continuity of self-experience, is understood by the therapist. In addition, there must be recognition that enacting such roles is at a considerable personal cost for both patient and partner. The enforced nature of the roles is resented by partners who may refuse to enact the assigned role. This not only leads to potential abandonment but also to a return of the alien self which further destabilizes the self-structure. This process is sometimes re-enacted within psychiatric services when patients are summarily discharged from treatment at their moment of desperation, for example when demanding hospital admission.

The fact that MBT looks at the underlying developmental reasons for the enforcement of reciprocal roles and the reasons for their common abnormalities has significant implications for practice.

Reformulation and interpretation

From our point of view, it is inadequate just to plot roles out in sequential diagrammatic reformulations even if these are agreed with the patient. The diagrammatic representation of roles possibly acts as an aid to non-collusion but the suggestion that this method places the CAT therapist in a less powerful and authoritarian role than the analytic therapist is only accurate if a false characterization of the contemporary understanding of unconscious process and its application in therapy is promulgated. Borderline patients are desperate for meaning and as a result are willing to take in reflections from others even if they do not map well onto anything within their own experience. Rather than clarifying feelings and processes this can lead to further development of the alien self as reflections and reformulations are desperately, but dissonantly, mapped onto their experiences. There is a risk that they may internalize representations of the therapist's view, rather than a usable version of their own experience as reflected by the therapist. This danger applies as much to the diagrammatic identification of roles as it does to interpretation of unconscious process. Both types of interventions can be applied with various degrees of competence and either can be an 'opaque, authoritarian, and potentially disabling form of discourse' (Ryle 1997 p. 106).

Ryle states that interpretation is not used in CAT because this 'invests the "unconscious" with mysteries to which he or she (the analyst) holds the key'. Yet in giving a reformulation a CAT therapist may fall into the very trap that CAT seeks to avoid by not using interpretation, namely of becoming prescient, all-knowing, and powerful. Interpretations are used in MBT. Their primary purpose is to increase the level of mentalization within therapy and to provide an alternative perspective. It is implicit and explicit during treatment that at times the therapist understands more than the patient and yet at other moments the reverse is true. However, interpretation is not enforced in some dictatorial way but offered as the start of trying to make sense of what otherwise may be an apparently meaningless event or feeling. It becomes a way in which a therapist can demonstrate that they are thinking in their own mind about the patient's mind and inevitably it can be given with varying degrees of competence and sensitivity.

Ryle claims that diagrammatic reformulations speed up the process of therapy and he asserts that a relatively brief intervention of CAT is effective over the longer-term. But, as yet, there is no evidence that this is the case (Margison 2000) (see p. 46). Overall the evidence is against such a conclusion. Most short-term therapies have limited results in treatment of BPD, and there are no studies linking the intervention of diagrammatic reformulation itself with outcome. Nonetheless a reformulation may help concentrate the therapist's mind and reduce the likelihood of perverse enactments. In MBT a dynamic formulation is completed by the individual therapist at the beginning of therapy as a method of demonstrating that coherent thought is possible about apparently non-understandable experience and to demonstrate that our minds, as a team of therapists, and our understanding, are different from that of the patient. The written formulation is given to the patient after completion and is revised by the patient and therapist during treatment. It is a working hypothesis rather than a visionary, divinatory statement and is developed and modified over time. Importantly it contains predictions of some problems that are likely to be encountered in treatment and to that extent has a far-sighted, foreknowing aspect embedded within it. For example, if a patient has had many short-lived relationships and has left them all in the context of violent, abusive acrimony, a dynamic formulation will consider this in terms of the individual's development and identify any features within treatment that may lead to such an outcome in therapy—forewarned is forearmed and the therapists must plan with the patient how such an outcome is to be avoided.

In summary, CAT shares a number of features with MBT and, even though Ryle is sharply critical of psychoanalysis and some of the theoretical ideas associated with mentalization, his focus on self-states and relationships leads to some commonality between treatments. This overlap of CAT and psychoanalytic approaches is reviewed by Denman who argues that CAT offers a base from which to develop a meta-theory for integration of psychotherapy (Denman 2002) in the treatment of BPD. This remains to be seen.

Psychodynamic-interpersonal

Russell Meares and his co-workers have made considerable efforts to develop a coherent and identifiable treatment approach based on Kohut's self-psychology, Winnicott's developmental approach, and the work of Robert Hobson. They have provided data on its effectiveness (Stevenson and Meares 1992, 1999). Treatment is based on the notion that BPD arises in the context of a disruption in the development of the self. Whilst this conception is, to some extent, in line with our own view about maintaining a focus on the self and its development, their underlying theoretical stance is different. Their principal assumptions are that a certain kind of associative, affect laden mental activity (not conceptualized as mentalization) develops through reverie, that symbolic play is necessary for the generation of the self and that this psychological process is disrupted through repeated 'impingements' of the social environment such as sexual and physical abuse. According to mainstream self-psychology, there is a persistent split of an archaic grandiose and idealizing self-configuration in BPD, which leads to fluctuating and highly conflicting and contradictory self-states as well as corresponding intense and contradictory selfobject needs. The term selfobject refers to the self-regulatory function of other people (or animals or valued objects). Lacking adequate regulatory functions of the self, the BPD patient is all the more dependent on others. The hallmark of BPD, the intense and unstable relationships to other people, is the behavioural manifestation of these intense self-object yearnings. An available other is desperately needed in order to feel worthy and vital. The BPD tragedy is that the tolerance for the inevitable self-object failures is limited, leading to affective storms and frequent rejection of the very source of vitality on which they depend. This paradox, e.g. the pervasive dependency and the rejection of the other, may be perceived as unbearable and may result in confusion and self-destructive acts.

Hobson (1985) worked within a similar frame and sought to design a therapy that had a greater interpersonal and collaborative focus than traditional psychoanalytic therapy which he saw as a one-sided and asymmetrical relationship.

He drew on psychodynamic principles but added some humanistic and interpersonal elements. Originally a conversational model because the aim was to develop a 'mutual feeling language' and a relationship of 'aloneness-togetherness', it has become known as psychodynamic-interpersonal therapy (PI) following its use in research trials for depression (Shapiro and Firth-Cozens 1987; Barkham *et al.* 1996), somatization and self-harm (Guthrie *et al.* 1991, 1999*b*, 2001), perhaps because the name states more clearly its fundamental assumptions.

The model has been conceptualized as consisting of seven different, but integrated, components. These are summarized by Guthrie (1999*a*). Although many of these form part of the non-specific aspects of therapy, together they form a discrete and definable therapy that is relatively easy to learn and is understandable to patients. The seven components are: exploratory rationale, shared understanding, staying with feelings, focus on difficult feelings, gaining insight, sequencing interventions, and making changes.

Psychodynamic interpersonal therapy is organized as a 12-month therapy for BPD and is offered in a modified form with careful attention given to the therapeutic alliance. The overall aim of therapy is maturational and more specifically to enable the patient to represent a personal reality in terms of an emotionally meaningful inner life. In order to achieve this, the first task is to establish an enabling atmosphere in which generative mental activity can develop. A key technique is empathy with the patient's plight, but it is accepted that this will fail or be experienced as failing. The failures are used as a key to understanding the underlying mental processes that inhibit development. Indications of failure include negative affect, linear thinking, focus on the outer world, and a change in the self-state (grandiosity, contempt). Transference phenomena are used to explore the detail of the empathic failures. It is important that therapy is sequenced carefully but that the therapist works flexibly. Initial sessions establish the interpersonal links of the patient's symptoms and identify the main problem areas by exploring carefully the relationships of the patient, agreeing a focus, and establishing a symptom history. Intermediate sessions may explicitly use transference to explore hidden feelings, stay with feelings, and link change in symptoms with interpersonal events. This is followed by final sessions in which ending may be linked to earlier losses, negative feelings are scrutinized, gains are explicated, and ways in which the patient can continue working on himself afterwards are discussed.

Guthrie (2001) has used the model to treat patients who self-harm, some of whom are likely to have been borderline patients, and demonstrated its effectiveness in a randomized controlled trial in reducing the behaviour. Her modifications may be useful when a borderline patient is in crisis. The therapist's first task is to explore the circumstances that precipitated the self-harm episode. Emphasis is placed upon exploring the patient's feelings, and bringing those feelings into the 'here and now'; i.e. bringing them alive in the session.

The problems that have precipitated the self-harm are explored and a rationale, linking feelings, problems and relationships is developed. Shared understanding is important in the process of PI and is formed through therapist and patient clarifying what the patient is really experiencing and feeling. In order to do this, a language of mutuality is developed; the therapist consciously uses terms such as 'I' and 'We'. The therapist expresses a more active involvement than is often recommended in psychoanalytic therapy, but many of the interventions are similar with the use of metaphor and interpretation. Interpretations are construed as tentative hypotheses and offered with less conviction than interpretations in classical psychoanalytic therapy. The aim is to produce a meaningful dialogue between patient and therapist in which suggestions can be worked with, but modified and owned by the patient. This emphasis on interpretation as a hypothesis to be worked in, the focus on formation of a therapeutic alliance, the use of interpersonal events to understand underlying emotions, the importance of empathy and mutuality, is in line with our own approach but the use of metaphor as a key component of therapy distinguishes PI from MBT.

Metaphor concentrates and enriches emotional understanding through the use of representation and symbolization and may be an effective aspect of psychotherapy, particularly in the treatment of patients with neurotic disorders. However, as we have already discussed, borderline patients demonstrate an enfeeblement of secondary representation of primary emotional states leading to a deficit in symbolic binding of affective states which is necessary to give meaning and context to feelings. The result is over-arousal, bewilderment about emotions, and affective volatility. In addition, the persistence of psychic equivalence, in which internal and external correspond, results in emotions being experienced as 'out there' and 'happening'. This makes the use of metaphor in therapy problematic. It confuses the patient who cannot distinguish reality from representation and may heighten emotion rather than bind it. It is for these reasons that simple 'here and now' interpretation is used in MBT and use of metaphor or focus on conflict is rarely applied, at least at the beginning of therapy. If psychological progress occurs, the use of more complex interpretation involving expression through metaphor may be used towards the end of treatment.

Therapeutic communities (TC)

Although there is no unified treatment approach within therapeutic communities, their defining characteristic involves 'communalism in sharing tasks, responsibilities and rewards; permissiveness to act in accord with one's feelings without accustomed social inhibitions; democratic decision making; reality confrontation of the subject with what they are doing in the here-and-now; as well as social analysis or Main's culture of enquiry' (Norton 1992). There is an attempt to minimize the 'power relationship' between patient and therapist. All these features create a social structure and milieu which are harnessed to promote psychological change. We have reviewed some outcomes data relevant to this approach in Chapter 2. In MBT there is no communalism of tasks, democratic decision making, or permissiveness to act without consideration of cultural social inhibitions, and there is no blurring of patient and staff roles leading to the criticism from therapeutic communities that, as in other therapies, there is a power relationship. In fact there is clarity of roles and responsibilities without denial of difference. This is an important distinction. In MBT the difference between patient and staff is clear within delivery of treatment. We have already mentioned that a central feature of borderline patients is that whenever they develop a relationship of personal importance, for example engaging in therapy, their interpersonal representational system becomes unstable. The representation of their own internal states and those of others becomes fluid and so they are unable accurately to recognize what they are feeling and thinking in relation to the other or to know what the other is feeling or thinking in relation to them. The relative absence of clarity of roles and responsibilities in a therapeutic community can create panic rapidly in some borderline patients leading to confusion and terror as their grasp on reality becomes tenuous. This results either in a retreat from therapy which may account for the greater drop-out rate from therapeutic communities than from other more structured treatments or in a shift into a more grandiose state in which the patient dominates the community and holds power of admission and discharge of other patients. Neither response is likely to be therapeutic to the individual or to others.

Despite the distinction between the therapeutic community approach and MBT, there is little doubt that the creation of a positive therapeutic milieu is essential in the treatment of PD. There is no place for authoritarian, custodial, and controlling attitudes but every place for interest, thoughtfulness, concern, and attempt to understand. Of course MBT takes place within a therapeutic milieu in the day hospital format but it does not rely on the milieu as the agent of change in the way that therapeutic communities do. In the out-patient version, the milieu is defined by the responsiveness of the staff and the atmosphere created within the service in the same way that it is with all out-patient services.

Other North American approaches

There is little doubt that the inclusion of Axis II in the DSM-III stimulated research into PD and increased its recognition in clinical practice. A number of practitioners were quick to take on the mantle of research into PD and developed considerable expertise in treatment. Although it is invidious to pick out a few and we run the risk of offence, they include John Gunderson, Glen Gabbard, Paul Pilkonis in the USA and Heather Monroe-Blum, Elsa Marziali, and John Livesley in Canada. Many others, namely, John Oldham, Paul Soloff, Andrew Skodal, M. Tracie Shea, and Thomas McGlashan have contributed equally to our present state of knowledge.

John Gunderson is one of the most prolific writers on borderline disorders and developed the Diagnostic Interview for Borderlines (DIB) (Gunderson *et al.* 1981), which was a landmark in reliable diagnosis of the disorder. His lifelong experience of treating patients has now been distilled in a seminal book in which he places his own perspective on different approaches to treatment (Gunderson 2001). Whilst he himself does not have a 'named' therapy for borderline patients, his approach integrates psychodynamic techniques and psychiatric care in the same way that we do and, over the years, we have drawn on some of his suggestions. His recommendations are rarely model-driven but rather based on severity of symptoms and psychological dysfunction, less influenced by preconception than individual consideration, and above all thoughtful rather than reactive.

From a theoretical point of view, Gunderson suggests that intolerance of aloneness is a core deficit of borderline patients and should be used as an essential criterion, necessary though not sufficient, for diagnosis (Gunderson 1996). This contrasts with the importance that we place on identity disturbance as a core phenomenon. However, Gunderson links the intolerance of aloneness to problems of attachment, suggesting that anxious/ambivalent and disorganized patterns of attachment are present in borderline patients, exemplified by clinging behaviours, separation anxiety, reluctance to become attached etc., because of failure to develop object constancy during childhood. In this regard, many of his ideas are compatible with those of Paul Pilkonis (Pilkonis *et al.* 1997), whose empirical and clinical work has focused on identifying abnormal attachment styles in PDs. In empirical investigations Pilkonis and colleagues have demonstrated that the degree of insecurity of attachment predicted outcome in a follow-along study of almost 150 personality-disordered patients (Meyer *et al.* 2001).

This attachment-based formulation has a number of consequences for therapy of which the most important is addressing the borderline patient's intolerance of loneliness. Gunderson suggests that the primary way to do this is by regulating therapist contact. There is no universally agreed number of times for a therapist to see a patient but once a week will be insufficient for the more unstable patients. Their acute sense of loneliness and abandonment destabilizes them and more frequent contact with a treatment team or therapist is required. We conceive of this as a failure of patients to keep a mindful therapist in their mind, resulting in loss of internal stability and an experience of abandonment, rather than as a simple repetition of an anxious/ambivalent attachment pattern. Gunderson considers therapist accessibility as a transitional phenomenon to help the patient bridge mental gaps and recommends use of a number of other transitional options when the therapist is absent.

These include another therapist substituting for the primary therapist, tape-recording sessions, giving directives, or even offering items from the therapist's office. Self-initiated options include increasing contacts with friends and relatives, distracting oneself, and more social networking. In general we do not become so directive in treatment and would not give a patient an object from the unit. Nonetheless, when an individual therapist is planning to be away from the unit, the team discuss the vulnerability of the patient and decide if an alternative session with another therapist should be offered to bridge the gap. This is then discussed with the patient who has freedom to decide.

Overall Gunderson's approach is pragmatic and its strength lies within its flexibility and humanity. Not surprisingly, he has generated a committed group with a number of co-workers at McLean Hospital who themselves have been productive, working within a special clinic for treating borderline patients. Amongst them Mary Zanarini has established a body of work which has furthered our understanding of BPD and continues to do so. Working in collaboration with Gunderson and others she revised the DIB to differentiate better between BPD and other PDs and has undertaken a large study of the longitudinal course of BPD (Zanarini *et al.* 2003). It seems likely that the McLean group will continue to take a lead in research and treatment of BPD.

Another major figure in the field who has originated a 'pragmatic psychotherapeutic approach' is Glen Gabbard. In a highly innovative model practice that is probably rooted in the Menninger Clinic's deeply humanistic approach to this group of patients, where Glen Gabbard was Medical Director for a time, he has evolved an approach to individual therapy which has transference and countertransference issues at the core of therapy (Gabbard *et al.* 1994; Gabbard 1995, 2000*a*; Horwitz *et al.* 1996). Gabbard's approach focuses on the impact on the therapist of the borderline patient's fluctuating stance between idealization and devaluation. He has identified, perhaps more clearly than any other author writing on this topic, the risks associated with therapeutic engagement with this group of patients, risks which are most acute in the context of individual psychotherapy, whether in an out-patient or an in-patient context. His writings are particularly helpful to therapists as they struggle with issues of self-esteem under the impact of repeated barrages of demeaning devaluations, as well as the seductiveness of idealization and the risk of boundary violations (Gabbard and Lester 1995). In an important book on the nature of love and hate in the analytic setting, he takes a strong and coherent position in relation to the pressure towards self-disclosure that is increasingly sanctioned by the intersubjectivist interpersonalist tradition (Gabbard 1996). His concept of 'disidentification with the aggressor' (see p. 186), where the analyst is drawn into a fantasy that a transcendent love, cleansed of hate, will heal the patient, is a good illustration of the pragmatic approach which Gabbard takes in psychodynamic therapy with these patients. Whilst having transference and countertransference clearly in his sights, these do not become an exclusive focus for Gabbard, and he is able to retain a balance between supportive and expressive therapeutic approaches, and considers the appropriate strategy to be determined by the particular defensive configuration presented by an individual patient. At the heart of Gabbard's approach is the emphasis on maintaining 'therapeutic space', space which is threatened to be eroded by relentless transference hatred that is unresponsive to interpretation (Gabbard 1991). He recommends long periods of containment as opposed to confrontation or active interpretation, in contradistinction to Kernberg, which will permit both therapist and patient sufficient time to integrate intensely negative feelings mixed with more positive affects. The aim is to regain the capacity to process analytical experiences in a reflective analytic space. In his more recent writings (Gabbard 2001, 2000*c*), Gabbard has been able to incorporate and creatively build on a number of the concepts we have reviewed in this volume. In particular he has been able to bridge a conceptual gap between Thomas Ogden's and the present ideas (Bram and Gabbard 2001).

Munroe-Blum and Marziali have taken a completely different approach and proposed ways in which group treatment, interpersonal group psychotherapy (IPG) can achieve positive outcomes in BPD based on the group as a vehicle for providing social role models and involving multiple interpersonal interactions giving a range of feedback. Rather than using active therapeutic techniques such as interpretation, the emphasis is on engaging the patients in determining the process of their treatment and empathy. Their thesis is that the activity of the therapists provides the patients with the means to damage their therapy and to make themselves worse as they try to access help. Instead of 'doing' something the therapist 'sits there' and encourages the patient to define his problem and to formulate it in social terms. The patient then sets the agenda and group sessions are offered in an unstructured and informal manner with discussion ranging from everyday problems to recent world events. This is called 'no-therapy therapy' by some which is a misnomer because it is in fact therapy but with a different aim. Responsibility for the therapy is placed with the patient and not the therapist and when the therapist feels forced to take responsibility, say when a patient is suicidal, this is done with expressed reluctance and acceptance that the therapist will make errors unless given direction by the patient. This approach is reminiscent of paradoxical responsiveness or even dialectical balance and may well prevent the borderline patient forcing therapists into specific roles and then attacking them for taking that role—if the therapist becomes the helper he will be attacked for not helping so it is better to 'sit back' and be directed by the patient on how to help. This approach is of considerable interest to the extent that it is in marked contrast to most other therapies and has been the subject of empirical investigation. The approach is manualized which forms an excellent basis on which to develop research. Monroe-Blum and Marziali (1995) randomly assigned 38 borderline patients to thirty $1^1/_2$ hour session of IPG and 41 to weekly individual psychodynamic therapy. Both groups showed similar improvement at 1 year which was sustained on follow-up a year later. There was a high rate of non-completion of treatment but the results suggest that the treatment deserves more interest than it has received.

Other European approaches

The increased harmonization of national regulations in the European Union appears to have done little to unify treatment approaches to PD across Europe. Some countries, for example Germany and, perhaps to a lesser extent, Holland continue to focus on in-patient treatment whilst others, for example Spain and Italy, take an uncompromising out-patient approach. Scandinavian countries are in-between and were some of the first to emphasize the importance of day-hospitals (Karterud *et al.* 1992; Karterud 1998). This is a tradition that has continued with a network of day-hospitals in Norway (Karterud 1998) and units in Copenhagen, Aarhus, and Aalborg in Denmark all developing treatment facilities for PD. In England there has been pressure to move from in-patient services to day-hospital and out-patient treatment, a shift primarily determined by financial pressure rather than a clear evidence-base. Whilst the context of treatment is shifting towards out-patient care, there continues to be debate about the best model and all countries have their proponents of different approaches. DBT has been developed in some hospitals and clinics in Germany (Bohus *et al.* 2002), Holland (Verheul *et al.* 2003), England and other countries whilst dynamic approaches continue to be the main focus in other centres. Peter Tyrer in the UK has suggested a new form of treatment known as Nidotherapy (Tyrer 2002*a*) in which the environment is shaped around the patient rather than the patient having to change to fit the external world, but further work is needed on this concept to evolve and widely implement this approach.

The Cassel and Henderson Hospitals in the UK continue to offer therapeutic community treatment for a select group of patients with PD, many of whom are borderline. Over the past 5 years there has been replication of the Henderson hospital and two further in-patient units have opened. The Cassel is an in-patient psychotherapy hospital with a long-standing tradition for the psychosocial treatment of patients with PD within the severe spectrum (Main 1989; Chiesa and Fonagy 2000). The treatment programme consists of a combination of individual psychoanalytically-oriented psychotherapy and an intensive sociotherapeutic programme based on the principles of psychosocial nursing (Griffiths and Leach 1998). The Adult Unit has traditionally functioned as a tertiary service with a national catchment area. About 55% of the patients receive in-patient treatment for an expected 1 year while other patients are admitted to the hospital's therapeutic milieu for an expected set period of 6 months, at the end of which they are discharged to out-patient treatment. The results of this treatment are discussed on p. 49. Patients are expected to become active participants in the life of the hospital throughout their stay, by sharing work, domestic and social activities, and taking on responsibilities for aspects of their ongoing existence in the community. The work of the day is structured around group activities (work groups, unit meetings, community meetings, catering meetings etc.), which allows the expression, channelling and working through of the patient's personality difficulties. The Henderson Hospital takes a similar approach but there are no individual sessions and the organization of admission, treatment, and discharge follows therapeutic community principles more specifically, and patients are not allowed to take medication following admission. Other notable practice sites following therapeutic community principles include Winterbourne House in Reading (Haigh 1999) and Francis Dixon Lodge in Leicester (Davies *et al.* 1998).

A less specialist but no less important approach has been the development in North Devon of a PD service organized within the general psychiatric services by Jeremy Holmes. The service was set up as it became apparent that patients suffering from PDs were (a) among the most troublesome to general psychiatric services, disproportionately to their numbers (b) not well-served by general psychiatric services which often reinforce rather than redress the difficulties which this client group present. The aims of the service are to reduce the burden which personality-disordered patients impose on community mental health workers, to reduce length of in-patient stay, to reduce the incidence of risky behaviours including deliberate self-harm and substance abuse, to stabilize often chaotic and/or stuck clinical situations, to engender hope that there can be improvement, and where relevant, to improve the parenting skills of PD sufferers and thus to reduce the impact of their difficulties on their children. A few of the general principles which inform the service are the provision of continuity of care over months and years with a stable therapeutic team in order to redress the breaks in care that are frequently characteristic of these patients' history; a 'holding in mind' of the patient and his/her difficulties between sessions and over time; and an offer of a range of treatment options and possibilities—including individual and group psychoanalytic therapy, DBT, CAT, and supportive psychotherapy—in order to counteract stereotyped responses. The emphasis in therapeutic work on 'affect consciousness' in order to help patients understand how their actions and perceptions are often dominated by unmodulated feelings rather than more considered appraisal; and the containment of anxiety both at the level of the service itself, so that the anxiety such patients create can be tolerated by the various teams they come in contact with, and also within the patient him/herself, are all components that we would argue increase the development of mentalization.

Overall the future for treatment of PD in Europe looks positive and the International Society for the Study of Personality Disorder (ISSPD) has an active European section.

Mentalization: The common theme in psychotherapeutic approaches to borderline personality disorder

So far we have considered a number of approaches to the treatment of BPD. As we have seen, whilst the focus of each approach is unique, the approaches share many features. This is perhaps inevitable since all aim to address a common set of problems, the challenges of offering a psychosocial therapy to a group of individuals characterized by the remarkable turbulence of their interpersonal relationships. It is not surprising, then, that the establishment of reasonable relationship processes in the therapeutic context is in the foreground of most approaches. While it is relatively easy to discuss this topic under the heading of non-specific factors in psychological therapy, and there can be no doubt that the provision of warmth, acceptance, and a supportive environment contributes to the effectiveness of all forms of psychotherapy, we believe that it is desirable and possible to be far more precise about the specific aspects of relationship processes that are therapeutic for individuals with BPD. It is the guiding construct of our therapeutic approach that psychotherapy with borderline patients should focus on the capacity for mentalization, by which we mean the implicit or explicit perception or interpretation of the actions of others or oneself as intentional, that is, mediated by mental states or mental processes. We believe that an important common factor in the psychotherapeutic approaches described in this chapter is the shared potential to recreate an interactional matrix of attachment in which mentalization develops and sometimes flourishes. The therapist or therapeutic milieu mentalizes the patient in a way that fosters the patient's mentalizing, which is a key facet of the relationship. As we have stated above, the crux of the value of psychotherapy with BPD is the experience of other human minds having the patient's mind in mind. It should be clear from this that, unlike a number of the approaches considered above (Kernberg, Ryle, Meares etc.) we consider *the process* of interpretation to be at the heart of the therapy, rather than *the content* of the interpretations or the non-specific supportive aspects of therapy. *The explicit content of interpreting or educating is merely the vehicle for the implicit process that has therapeutic value.*

We recognize that this is not by any means a novel approach. Concepts such as insight, empathy, the observing ego, and even introspection have been around throughout the 'psychotherapeutic century' (Allen and Fonagy 2002). The concept of mentalization, in our view, crystallizes the biological and relational processes that underpin the phenomena that these venerable clinical concepts denote. It is important to remind ourselves that mentalization is not the same as introspection. Mentalization can be both implicit and explicit. Implicit mentalization is a non-conscious, unreflective, procedural function. As Simon Baron-Cohen put it, 'We mind-read all the time, effortlessly, automatically, and mostly unconsciously.' (Baron-Cohen 1995) Explicit mentalization is only likely to happen when we hit an interactive snag (Allen 2003). Explicit mentalization, particularly when it is of a higher order, can be the apparent substance of psychological therapy, for example Person A can reflect upon his awareness of what Person B thinks about Person A's feelings or thoughts. Elsewhere we have pointed out that such explicit mentalization (metacognition) can only be considered genuine and productive when the link between these cognitions and emotional experience are strong. We have referred to this as mentalized affectivity (Fonagy *et al.* 2002). Others have approached this metaphorically in talking about 'making a feeling felt' (Siegel 1999, p. 149). In fact the dissociation between implicit and explicit mentalization in the course of development may be a defining criterion of psychological disturbance.

So what are the strong arguments in favour of mentalization as a key aspect of effective psychotherapeutic process? Firstly, the foundation of any therapeutic work must by definition be implicit mentalization. Without social engagement there can be no psychological therapy, and without mentalization there can be no social engagement. Secondly, since the work of John Bowlby (1988) it has generally been agreed that psychotherapy invariably activates the attachment system and as a component generates secure base experience. In our view this is important because the attachment context of psychotherapy is essential to establishing the virtuous cycle of synergy between the recovery of mentalization and secure base experience. The experience of being understood generates an experience of security which in turn facilitates 'mental exploration', the exploration of the mind of the other to find oneself therein. Thirdly, the therapist of all patients, but particularly those whose experience of their mental world is diffused and confusing, will continually construct and reconstruct in their own mind an image of the patient's mind. They label feelings, they explain cognitions, they spell out implicit beliefs. Importantly they engage in this mirroring process, highlighting the marked character of their verbal or non-verbal mirroring display. Their training and experience (e.g. striving towards therapeutic neutrality) further hones their capacity to show that their reaction is related to the patient's state of mind rather than their own. It is this often rapid non-conscious implicit process that enables the patient with BPD to apprehend what he feels. Fourthly, mentalizing in psychological therapies is prototypically a process of shared, joint attention, where the interests of patient and therapist intersect in the mental state of the patient. The shared attentional processes entailed by all psychological therapies in our view serve to strengthen the interpersonal integrative function (Fonagy 2003). It is not simply what is focused on that we consider therapeutic from this point of view, but the fact that patient and therapist can jointly focus on a shared content of subjectivity. Fifthly, the explicit content of the therapist's intervention will be mentalistic regardless of orientation, whether the therapist is principally concerned with transference reactions, automatic negative thoughts, reciprocal roles, or linear thinking. These approaches all entail explicit mentalization in so far as they succeed in enhancing coherent representations of desires and beliefs. That this is the case is supported by the common experience that such efforts at explicit mentalization will not be successful unless the therapist succeeds in drawing the patient in as an active collaborator in any explication. One may view psychotherapy for borderline individuals as an integrative process where implicit and explicit mentalization are brought together in an act of 'representational redescription', the term Annette Karmiloff-Smith (1992) used to refer to the process by which 'implicit information in the mind subsequently becomes explicit knowledge to the mind'. (p. 18). Sixthly, the dyadic nature of therapy inherently fosters the patient's capacity to generate multiple perspectives. For example, the interpretation of the transference may be seen as presenting an alternative perspective on the patient's subjective experience. We view this as optimally freeing the patient from being restricted to the reality of 'one view', experiencing the internal world in a mode of psychic equivalence. This process also becomes accessible through engagement in group psychotherapy. In either setting, mental states are perforce represented at the secondary level and are therefore more likely to be recognized as such, as mental representations. It should be remembered that this will only be helpful if implicit and explicit mentalization have not been dissociated and feelings are genuinely felt rather than just talked about.

In sum, it is our belief that the relatively safe (secure base) attachment relationship with the therapist provides a relational context in which it is safe to explore the mind of the other in order to find one's own mind represented within it. While it is quite likely that this is an adaptation of a mechanism provided to us probably by evolution to 'recalibrate' our experience of our own subjectivity through social interaction, it is a unique experience for individuals with BPD, because their pathology serves to distort the subjective experience of the other to a point where they have little hope of finding their constitutional self therein. The maladaptive interpersonal processes, whether we label these projective identification or pathological reciprocal roles, in most ordinary social contexts only enable these patients to find in their social partner parts of themselves that they desperately needed to discard in the first place, be that terror, contempt, excitement, or pain. The engagement in a psychotherapeutic context, either individually or in groups, thus does far more than provide nurturance, warmth, or acceptance. The therapist, in holding on to their view of the patient, and overcoming the patient's need to externalize and distort the therapist's subjectivity, simultaneously fosters mentalizing and secure attachment experience. Feeling recognized creates a secure base feeling that in turn promotes the patient's freedom to explore herself or himself in the mind of the therapist. Increased sense of security in the attachment relationship with the therapist as well as other attachment relationships, possibly fostered by the therapeutic process, reinforces a secure internal working model and through this, as Bowlby pointed out, a coherent sense of the self. Simultaneously, the patient is increasingly able to allocate mental space to the process of scrutinizing the feelings and thoughts of others, perhaps bringing about improvements in fundamental competence of the patient's mind interpreting functions, which in turn may generate a far more benign interpersonal environment. A limitation of therapy lies in the therapist's capacity to mentalize, constricted by his own attachment history, his current interpersonal circumstances and his constitutional capacities. It is the threat to the mentalizing capacities of the therapist that borderline patients represent that Glen Gabbard (see above) has so helpfully drawn our attention to. Our capacity to mentalize freely is readily compromised by the patient's teleological stance and their insistent use of psychic equivalence and pretend modes of representing subjectivity. These, and the experience of our minds being taken over by the alien parts of the patient's self, may dramatically curtail our value to these patients when we feel unsafe, threatened, depressed, or just empty of mind in their presence.

Conclusion

Placing mentalization as central to therapy with borderline patients may unify numerous effective approaches to the treatment of this challenging group of patients. While providing a common understanding of why a range of disparate approaches all 'work', the implication of this formulation is not that all approaches are equally effective and the best approach is a judicious combination of existing techniques. In the following chapters, we will elaborate the technical implications of focusing therapeutic work on the patient's capacity to mentalize. It should be clear from the above that therapists will need (a) to identify and work with the patient's limited capacities; (b) to represent internal states in themselves and in their patient; (c) to focus on these internal states; and (d) to sustain this in the face of constant challenges by the patient over a significant period of time. In order to achieve this level of focus, mentalizing techniques will need to be (a) offered in the context of an attachment relationship; (b) consistently applied over time; (c) used to reinforce the therapist's capacity to retain mental closeness with the patient. The manner in which we have organized treatment ensures a felicitous context for therapists and patients to focus their work in these ways and to concentrate on mentalization techniques. In the next two chapters we outline our approach. But we are aware that our method is not the only way in which good outcomes can be achieved and we make no claim that our organizing principles are necessarily the best way to arrange treatment. In fact we hope that rather than being followed slavishly, our description will encourage others to develop more efficient approaches.

5 Treatment organization

Introduction

In the previous chapter we suggested that a focus on mentalization is central to effective therapy with borderline patients. But techniques to improve mentalization need to be given within a carefully organized framework of treatment if interventions promoting change are to be delivered within an optimal context. This chapter describes the way in which we organize treatment to ensure that techniques of therapy have the best chance of being effective. But the Halliwick model is not the only way that treatment can be arranged, although it has been honed from our experience over many years, and we therefore outline other potential models here. The different models are not mutually exclusive and, to some extent, can be run in parallel with patients of greatest severity being treated using a team approach and those of less severity being managed and treated using a divided-functions model.

Service models

The most complicated challenge arising in the treatment of borderline patients is the question of how to deal with their tendency to externalize unbearable self-states, and the strong countertransference responses which this can produce. This has led to the development of models that recommend splitting the transference by creating alternative foci for the patient's feelings. This has become known as 'split treatment' and customarily refers to the separation of psychiatric treatment involving medication, hospital admission, medico-legal issues, and emergency procedures in the event of suicidal or homicidal impulses from a psychotherapeutic programme (Meyer 1999*a*,*b*). This is a two-person (Gabbard 2000*b*) or divided-functions model (Bateman and Tyrer 2003) since it usually involves a psychotherapist and a psychiatrist and has the advantage that different mental health professionals work together, bringing different perspectives to bear on the patient's problems and diluting the transferences. Each practitioner works autonomously but with some reference to the other. Therapy is not contaminated by discussions of medication or formal assessments of risk and the therapist, medical or non-medical, is free to explore the patient's problems. But the two-person model is a recipe for dangerous splitting with one professional being idealized and the other denigrated. Further, the patient may idealize or denigrate the different aspects of treatment, for example, at one time idealizing a biological approach and medication and decrying the psychological treatment; and at another, doing quite the reverse. Enactments may then occur between the professionals themselves and interfere with the coherence of treatment. For the severe personality-disordered patient we recommend a **one-team model**, which allows but contains splits and minimizes the risk that they are dangerously enacted.

One-team model

In a fully integrated team, there is no need for split treatment and less danger of ambiguity of clinical responsibility. The responsibility for the assessment of risk of suicide, violence, impulsive behaviour, prescribing, for example, lies with the team. Under these circumstances it is incumbent on the team to work together to combine all aspects of treatment into a coherent whole. Our programme is designed with this in mind and includes mental health professionals with different skills, including a psychiatrist, nurses, psychologists, and occupational therapists.

The one-team model contains within it a subsidiary two-or-more person model, thereby allowing many of the advantages of the two-person model without the disadvantages. The transferences are split between members of the same team rather than between independent practitioners, with the group and individual therapists being central to this dynamic model. Rules of confidentiality ensure that the team discuss the patient's actions and reactions and so repair split transferences, integrating them within the team before beginning to integrate them with the patient. Powerful countertransference feelings can also be contained and understood, thereby preventing the all-too-common situation of an independent professional being pushed into inappropriate enactments.

The programme itself is a combination of group and individual therapy, enabling the patient to use a model of split therapy whilst having to integrate both aspects over time. The treatment team value group and individual therapy equally, recognizing the need for both to address different aspects of the personality-disordered patient's problems. Borderline patients tend to idealize one aspect of treatment and denigrate the other and we have found that most patients prefer the individual sessions and find group interactions painful and frightening. Working with the patient's anxiety about group therapy is therefore a primary task of individual therapy early in treatment. The therapist helps the patient think about himself in the group from the vantage point of the individual session, attempting to understand the patient's underlying fears.

Thinking about themselves in another situation from within a significant relationship helps borderline patients place adequate distance between aspects of themselves—the 'me' in the group is considered by the 'me' in the individual session. Early in treatment this makes it safe for the patients to consider their own actions and reactions without being overwhelmed by emotion, and encourages mentalization.

Treatment context

The context in which the one-team model is applied varies both within and between countries. Some countries continue to offer prolonged in-patient treatment for selected patients whilst others have systematically closed specialist in-patient provision for personality disorder (PD). In England and other countries of Europe, for example Holland, therapeutic communities and in-patient units for PD remain, and in Germany it is possible for patients to admit themselves to specialist in-patient units for a period of stabilization. In contrast, in the USA nearly all long-term in-patient treatment for PD has been abandoned in the face of managed care. This trend is now discernible throughout most psychiatric services in Europe and elsewhere, with an increasing focus on day-hospital and out-patient provision as costs become the driving force behind all health care provision. Norway in particular has a well-developed network of day-hospitals involved in treatment of PD that has resulted in many influential papers (Karterud *et al.* 1998, 2003).

Despite the rampant closure of in-patient units, the evidence is not yet available to determine who should be treated in what context (Chiesa *et al.* 2002*a*) and whether some patients are treated more safely and effectively as in-patients. On the positive side, many governments are recognizing the importance of PD to the individual, the community, and society and insisting on some level of service provision. It can no longer be used as 'a diagnosis of exclusion' (DoH 2003) within psychiatric services and there have been a number of valiant attempts to issue treatment guidelines.

Treatment guidelines

The publication of the Clinical Practice Guidelines for the Treatment of Patients with Borderline Personality Disorder (BPD) by the American Psychiatric Association (American Psychiatric Association 2001) was a milestone in the annals of psychiatric treatment. Never before had such an influential organization concentrated on such a contentious topic and issued recommendations for treatment. Not surprisingly, the guidance met with a mixed reaction although most people recognized it had many positive features, including recognition of the multi-dimensional aspect of borderline pathology, a refreshingly non-partisan approach about models of treatment, and an attempt to distil clinical opinion in an unbiased way. On the negative side, the guidance is seen as premature, drawing on a limited-evidence base, being written in a way too favourable to dynamic psychiatry, and relying too much on a large raft of expert opinion (McGlashan 2002; Paris 2002; Sanderson *et al.* 2002; Tyrer 2002*b*). Nevertheless, they are likely to exert considerable influence on future treatment and research into BPD.

Recommendations in the American guidance include careful initial assessment in which safety issues are given priority, development of a clear and explicit psychotherapeutic treatment framework, organization of psychiatric management, use of pharmacotherapy in an adjunctive role, and consideration of multiple versus single clinician treatment. Our programme fulfils all these criteria and we have chosen to integrate psychiatric management and pharmacotherapy (see p. 195) using a team approach rather than opting for treatment by a single clinician or using a split treatment with multiple clinicians acting independently.

The National Institute for Mental Health in England has issued policy implementation guidance for the development of services for people with PD (DoH 2003), which is expected to have some influence on psychiatric services although financial restrictions may limit its execution within clinical settings. The document recommends the development of specialist multi-disciplinary PD teams to target those with significant distress or difficulty who present with complex problems and the formation of specialist day-patient services in areas with high concentrations of morbidity. This document is of further interest because it contains within it a section outlining the views of service-users who continue to feel stigmatized by the term PD—'a very sticky label' and 'the patients psychiatrists dislike' (Lewis and Appleby 1988). As early as 1988, Tyrer and Ferguson (1988) likened PD to body odour, 'indubitably affected by constitution and environment, a source of distress to both sufferer and society, yet imbued with ideas of degeneracy and inferiority so that its possession is also a personal criticism'. This attitude continues within psychiatric services, with users feeling blamed for their condition and staff acting in a belittling or patronizing manner. A negative reaction at the initial assessment makes engagement less likely and underscores the need for accessible, well organized, and responsive services and it is to this that we now turn.

The treatment programmes

There are two programmes of treatment. The day-hospital programme is outlined in Fig. 5.1. The Intensive Out-patient Programme (IOP) consists of an individual session of 50 min and a group session of one and a half hours per week. A timetable is given to all patients. Individual and small group therapy form the core components of both programmes but expressive therapy,

MONDAY	TUESDAY	WEDNESDAY	THURSDAY	FRIDAY
9.00 AM – O P E N I N G – 9.00 AM				
	9.30–10.30 SMALL GROUPS		9.30–10.30 SMALL GROUPS	9.10–10.00 POLICY MEETING
10.00–11.15 LARGE GROUP	10.45–12.00 CASE CONFERENCE	10.00–11.00 SMALL GROUPS	10.30–11.30 GROUP SUPERVISION	10.00–11.15 LARGE GROUP
11.30–12.30 GROUP SUPERVISION	12.00–1.00 STAFF GROUP		11.30–12.30 POTTERY	11.30–12.45 DEPARTMENTAL BUSINESS MEETING
L U N C H				
1.45–3.15 ART GROUP	1.30–3.00 DRAMA AND GROUP ACTIVITY	1.30–2.45 SELF-HARM GROUP	1.30–3.00 WRITING GROUP	1.30–2.15 Organization of weekend: individual meetings
		3.00 CLOSE		3.30–4.30 SOCIAL
4.30 PM – C L O S E – 4.30 PM				

Fig. 5.1 Halliwick psychotherapy day unit.

accessed according to need and its perceived usefulness as judged by the patient and staff, is part of the day-hospital treatment only. Some patients find art group, writing group, and drama therapy distinctly useful, whilst others experience them as too provocative or without merit. Whilst these reactions are discussed with the patient, attendance at the expressive groups is encouraged rather than required.

In the day-hospital, each small group has 6–8 patients with two therapists but in IOP, although the groups have the same number of patients, there is only one therapist. This has been done for pragmatic reasons related to costs, staff numbers, and patient demand. Using only one therapist allows more patients to be treated and the limiting factor is the availability of individual sessions provided by members of the team. Individual sessions are not provided by therapists from elsewhere, since we believe that it is important for all aspects of treatment to be integrated.

The essential element within the day-hospital programme is the link between all components. The themes within the small groups inform the focus of the large groups and determine the topics used within the expressive therapies. Of course the small groups, of which there are 2 or 3 in the day hospital depending on patient numbers, may be struggling with different issues (although it is surprising how often they overlap) and so the team need to combine them into a single topic that makes sense to both themselves and the patients.

One small group was concerned that the day-hospital was inadequate for their problems, complaining that there was no 24-h emergency contact with the staff. They felt that referral to unknown staff within the general hospital was useless and one patient had read that in another treatment, patients could call their therapists during an emergency. Another small group talked about the intensity of the treatment and feeling overwhelmed by group sessions on three consecutive days. One patient asked if the small groups could be spread out over the week.

In discussing the major themes of dependency and need on the one hand and over-involvement on the other, the staff decided to use a theme of 'too much–too little' for all the expressive groups during that week.

Staff

The selection of staff

Not all staff can work with patients with PD. They need a high degree of personal resilience and qualities that enable them to maintain boundaries whilst offering flexibility, survive hostility without retaliating, and manage internal and external conflict without becoming over-involved. They must be effective 'team players' and comfortable with working in a multi-disciplinary group without insisting on strict, professionally determined, demarcation of tasks. The rigid, narcissistic, self-protective, defensive professional is positively harmful to a team approach. The flexible, reflective, communicative, considerate individual who is clear about personal and interpersonal boundaries and who can tolerate and withstand the emotional impact personality disordered-patients have on himself and a team is a bonus. Characteristics such as these are neither the property of any single professional group nor easily developed solely through training or experience. They relate to an individual's own personal history, security of attachment pattern, and personality, and whilst these characteristics are difficult to assess, they are likely to have an impact on effectiveness of treatment. Improved outcome on thoughts of self-harm and suicide is associated with therapists holding a 'non-pejorative conceptualization' of people meeting the criteria for BPD (Shearin and Linehan 1992) and psychotherapy research suggests that a complementary pattern of interpersonal style is associated with better outcomes (Andrews 1990). Henry *et al.* (1990) found that poor outcome client–therapist dyads were distinguished from good outcome dyads by a pattern of therapist hostility and reciprocal patient self-criticism, possibly because they fail to develop a constructive therapeutic alliance.

It is plausible to suggest that a therapist's previous experience with important others and his ability to form relationships will impact on his capacity to form relationships with borderline patients. Dunkle and Friedlander (1996) demonstrated that therapists who are comfortable with closeness are more likely to experience their alliance with a patient in a positive light but this did not take into account the interaction between patient and therapist styles, which is heavily influenced by transference and countertransference. A further study (Dozier *et al.* 1994) found that case managers with secure attachment styles were able to respond appropriately to patients' underlying needs and to resist patients' pull to behave in a manner that confirmed their preconceived schematic representations of self and others when compared with case managers with pre-occupied or dismissing styles. But the situation is more complex because Tyrrell *et al.* (1999) found that patients work best with professionals who show a different attachment style to their own, suggesting that a complementary but distinct affiliative style may allow a patient to disconfirm rigid working models and develop new ones. The de-synchrony, as long as it is not too disparate, may stimulate greater mentalization on the part of both patient and therapist if the therapist works hard at giving accurate and 'marked' interventions. This is in keeping with Kantrowitz (1995) who found that too much overlap between patient and therapist conflict led to 'blind spots' in therapy, and with Eagle's view (Eagle 1996) that attachment styles are an important variable in therapist ability to understand the mental states of others. Finally, Rubino *et al.*'s (2000) findings that anxious therapists tended to respond less empathically with fearful patients may be of significance in treatment of BPD in relation to drop-out and acting out.

Overall this evidence implies that basic professional training is only one aspect of suitability as a practitioner to treat BPD and the ability to form a therapeutic bond is an essential element if a collaborative relationship is to emerge and the patient is to engage and remain in treatment. It has been suggested that experts in BPD (Kernberg and Linehan) 'meet the patient's emotional intensity or lability head on with a steady emotional intensity of their own. Both therapists give the patient the feeling that they are present, engaged, and indestructible' (Swenson 1989). Stone (1990) suggests that patients with BPD 'have a way of reducing us to our final common, human denominator, such that allegiance to a rigidly-defined therapeutic system becomes difficult to maintain. They force a shift in us, as it were, from the dogmatic to the pragmatic'. At the very least, the mental health professional therefore has to retain the capacity to be steady, skilful, and competent despite provocation, anxiety, and pressure to transgress boundaries.

In conclusion, generic mental health training is a necessary but insufficient preparation for treatment of BPD even if it has focused on psychotherapeutic skills. Practitioners need to show an ability to assess threats of suicide, self-harm, and violence without anxiety, to deal with emotional storms and crises with reflection, to be able to set appropriate boundaries with tolerance, and to have a robust but flexible demeanour. Some of this comes through experience, some by tending to one's own physical, spiritual, and personal well-being, and some through regular supervision, team support, and consultation with others. Once these basic skills and human attributes have been achieved, it is feasible to continue further training in the treatment of PD.

Characteristics of training

Our treatment programme takes a multi-disciplinary team approach and so training needs to be team-focused as well as tailored to the needs of the individual practitioner. Training should be supported by the trainees' organization, be linked to clinical service developments, and be targeted to different levels of expertise. The role of a clinical leader is crucial and particular attention needs to be paid within the organization to his or her level of skill in individual and group therapy, leadership quality, political influence within the services, and ability to motivate and maintain enthusiasm and prevent burn-out. This ensures that a newly-acquired knowledge base has the best chance of being translated into practice.

A framework for the development of basic techniques used in treatment includes an understanding of how to:

- set up and maintain treatment boundaries
- enhance mentalization
- use transference
- bridge the psychological gaps
- retain mental closeness
- work with current mental states
- recognize deficits
- use the real relationship

Sample training materials for these techniques are to be found in Appendix 2.

The team

The first task in developing a treatment programme is to create a therapeutic team. We have already discussed the characteristics of therapists necessary for cohesive team development and for maximizing the likelihood of successful outcome but some specific skills must be held within the team including knowledge of prescribing, ability to manage crises, talent in organization of a multi-component programme, and competence in expressive techniques. It is for these reasons that we use a multi-disciplinary team consisting of nurses, psychiatrists, psychologists, and occupational therapists. Effective teamwork can only take place if the team meet regularly for specific purposes and feel secure to talk openly to each other. Hence within the partial hospital programme, the team meet after every group to discuss the material of the group session and to hear how it may relate to treatment within the individual session. This allows the team to formulate each patient's problems using material from all aspects of the programme. Development of a cohesive team is easier said than done but can be created through staff mentalizing about themselves and each other—practising what they preach! One team rule is that each member has to show within a discussion that they have understood the viewpoint of the others before disagreeing or putting forward their perspective. This peer group meeting is part of a cascade of supervision ranging from informal to the formal which is discussed in the next paragraph.

Within IOP the individual and group therapist meet after each group session so that both are aware of the significant themes of therapy. Their joint understanding of the patient is synthesized into a formulation which informs the next sessions. Again, this forms part of the supervisory process and is discussed in the following paragraph.

The emphasis on discussion and consensus between therapists highlights an important principle of MBT, namely the integration of therapists. This contrasts with integration of therapies in which techniques from different therapies are used in treatment to address diverse problems. We consider the cohesive interaction between therapists to be of singular importance whereas simply combining therapeutic interventions without a coherent strategy shared by all different people involved in a complex treatment leads to puzzlement for the patient and confusion for the staff.

The key worker or primary clinician

Within the day-hospital programme there are five whole-time staff for 25 patients and within IOP, two whole-time staff for 24 patients but all work as a team together to allow cross-cover when necessary. The optimal staff to patient ratio is unknown and needs to take into account patient severity as well as staff experience and training.

The individual therapist is appointed as the patient's key worker whose main task is to oversee the treatment plan and ensure that the patient is kept in mind at all times. Whilst this sounds obvious, it is surprising how often patients can be 'forgotten' for periods of time when staff have heavy workloads. It is our experience that 'forgetting' has significant meaning within the transference relationship and is commonly an indicator of increased risk. Some patients colonize the mind of their key worker to the extent that another patient is pushed out of mind and yet an essential element of our treatment is establishing recognition that 'out of sight is not out of mind'. Consequently the team have a system of going through all patients on a daily basis to clarify where they are and to identify their level of risk (see p. 228).

The additional roles of the key worker are to establish a therapeutic frame, identify social, housing, legal, or other areas of difficulty, to monitor risk, liaise with other agencies, organize the case review, alert the team to developing problems, and to make sure medical notes are kept adequately. The key worker is required to record a weekly-written summary of treatment which must include major themes from group and individual therapy and a statement about risk.

But any important clinical issues and action taken should be recorded on a daily basis. The key worker does not have sole professional responsibility for the patient: this is held by the team and ultimately the Responsible Medical Officer (RMO) who is the senior psychiatrist in the team.

Some argue that the joint role of individual therapist and key worker muddies the therapeutic process and greater purity in treatment would be better. This is an empirical question to which we do not know the answer but it is our practice to appoint someone other than the individual therapist as key worker if a patient has considerable social, medical, or other practical needs.

A patient was referred by his probation officer having been released from prison following a sentence for grievous bodily harm to his former partner with whom he had two children. Liaison with the probation officer was a statutory requirement and the patient was attempting to gain access to his two children, which necessitated regular meetings with legal representatives. It was agreed that the individual therapist should be protected from the practical aspects of these matters so that he could focus on the therapeutic process. This was agreed with the patient and another member of the team acted as key worker.

The responsible medical officer (RMO)

A psychiatrist acts as an RMO for the purposes of the Mental Health Act and it is his duty to consider whether a patient should be detained compulsorily. The Mental Health Act (1983) provides a legal framework for a patient to receive treatment for a mental condition without his consent but confusion remains about the position of PD in relation to this provision and this differs between England and Scotland as well as throughout Europe. The present Mental Health Act in England is often interpreted as excluding those with PD from compulsory detention because of a 'requirement' that the mental disorder be 'treatable' (treatment is likely to alleviate or prevent a deterioration in the patient's condition). Many clinicians have not seen PD as a treatable condition and so patients have been summarily discharged from hospital without follow-up or further support. New legislation is likely to remove this clause, which implies that PD will be brought further within the scope of everyday mental health services.

The problem for specialist treatment services for PD is that someone within the system has to be the nominated RMO. In our treatment programme, this responsibility is not transferred outside the treatment team, even though this clearly brings into the patient–team relationship a dynamic involving power and control which may interfere with the development of a therapeutic alliance and trusting relationship. Some argue that the role should be placed outside the treatment team in a divided-function model (see p. 145) but this presents a problem both for the team and the external psychiatrist who has to take a major decision about a patient's liberty without adequately knowing the patient whilst the group who know the patient well side-step the issue. Of course they may advise the psychiatrist but this is tantamount to detention by proxy and, to some extent, becomes a deception since the psychiatrist is unlikely to go against robust clinical advice from a team who are treating the patient. So, our policy is to have this aspect of the relationship 'on the table' at the beginning of treatment and placed firmly in the context of, first, our major aim to keep patients out of hospital and, second, our requirement that patients retain responsibility for their own lives and their actions and do not transfer it to others. Detention of a patient in hospital is rare and when it occurs it is more likely to be related to a co-morbid problem or an unacceptable increase in risk. Nevertheless, we point out that we have a duty of care to treat patients to the best of our ability and to assess continually the risk they pose to themselves and others which is done with them rather than without them.

A patient was brought to the hospital in the middle of the night by police having been found drunk in the street with a large knife. He was admitted overnight but because he had been detained initially on a 72-hr police section, assessment was required to decide if it should be continued or revoked. At assessment, the psychiatrist in the team noted that this admission followed previous patterns in which the patient had been drinking and then attempted to kill himself. Although exploring how the patient had managed not to harm himself on this occasion, the psychiatrist elicited clear signs that the patient still intended to kill himself. He had planned his suicide, he had written a note, he dismissed his treatment as useless, and he showed some symptoms of depression. The psychiatrist talked to the patient about remaining in hospital until he was able to think more clearly about himself and explained his reasons for continuing the section. At the same time arrangements were made for the patient to continue in the treatment programme, access his therapy sessions, and to see the psychiatrist on a regular basis to address this exercise of institutional power and its meaning in terms of the patient's life and its effect on future treatment.

Some patients attend treatment stating that they have taken an overdose and when advised to attend the emergency department refuse to go. What should the RMO and treatment team do at this point? The legal situation is clear but goes against natural instinct. Under common law a doctor is only allowed to administer treatment when a patient gives consent based on the principle that patients have a right to self-determination and the hardened borderline patient will use our emphasis on self-responsibility to demand his own 'right to die'. A competent adult can reject medical or surgical intervention even if such a decision is life-threatening. In law the patient's wishes must be respected whether his reasons for withholding consent appear irrational, are unknown or even non-existent. But not to insist on treatment and arranging for the patient to go to hospital for emergency treatment seems to contravene the sanctity of life and strike at the very core of treatment. So should the RMO detain the patient? In order to consider this, the RMO must assess the patient's capacity to reach such a decision. A patient can only be considered to lack the relevant mental competence to make treatment decisions if he is incapable of any of the following: 'comprehending and retaining treatment information', 'believing such information', or 'weighing such information in the balance and arriving at a choice'. If a patient is capable of all the three elements, consent or refusal to treatment must be judged as valid and respected and it is of no benefit to detain the patient since the same rules apply. Of course patients with PD virtually always demonstrate competence. Our policy is therefore to continue a dialogue with the patient and to call an ambulance on their behalf and ask them to go to the emergency clinic. The assessment must be done by one of the doctors and another member of the team in order to have third party verification of what has been said to the patient and the existence of competence is recorded carefully in the notes.

The situation in which a patient presents a danger to others is less clear and the ethical and legal issues in England and elsewhere are not clearly established unless the patient shows incapacity. Practitioners interested in treating patients with PD should familiarize themselves with legal cases and official guidance on this matter.

Assessment

All patients are assessed first by a senior member of the team. If this clinical assessment indicates a presumptive diagnosis of PD, a full research interview is arranged and the Structured Clinical Interview for the DSM performed for both Axis 1 and Axis II disorders along with the revised version of the Diagnostic Interview for Borderlines (Zanarini *et al.* 1989). The patient is then seen at least once, more usually 2–3 times, by two members of the clinical team from the day-hospital or the IOP depending on the clinical assessment of severity of the patient's problems. The aim of this series of initial meetings is not solely related to diagnostic assessment but also linked to motivation and engagement of the patient in treatment, clarifying the context of treatment, day-hospital or intensive out-patient, that may be most appropriate, and developing a therapeutic alliance.

Clinical indicators for admission to the day-hospital programme include chaotic lifestyle with unstable housing, serious suicide risk, substance abuse, problems of impulse control which have led to personal danger, frequent brushes with the law, transient difficulties in reality testing, failure to respond to repeated short-term hospitalization and other intervention, and evidence that destructive living and hopelessness has been incorporated into the personality.

One aspect of assessment is to identify those patients who are not suitable for day-hospital or intensive out-patient dynamic treatment. As a rule of thumb, those individuals who show schizoid and schizotypal characteristics can become excessively anxious in an emotionally volatile milieu and treatment becomes traumatic rather than therapeutic. This group of patients is probably best offered less intensive individual therapy. A further group, namely patients with antisocial/dissocial PD can cause considerable problems but many patients are co-morbid for borderline, narcissistic, and antisocial disorders so they are impossible to avoid. In essence, if a patient shows co-morbidity in this way it is important that the team are aware of it and constantly monitor the possibility of the exploitative antisocial patient taking advantage of the more vulnerable borderline patient. The assessment should make explicit the ways in which this may have occurred before in the patient's life.

Finally a brief comment on some of those odd quirks of patients discovered through assessment which seem to have more importance than the textbooks suggest, being common but rarely described. First is the 'mirror sign'. Borderline patients find it inordinately hard to look at themselves in the mirror. We have had patients who had no mirrors at all in their house, patients who have had to shower or bath in the dark to avoid looking at their body, and individuals who could not buy clothes in stores because they had to try them on, be looked at and commented on by the shop assistant, and decide whether the clothes suited them or not. One patient only bought via catalogue and internet shopping. Yet another patient found it difficult to walk through shopping malls because she saw herself reflected in all the shop windows. It seems that borderline patients do not like what they see, are perplexed by their reflection, and that it destabilizes them perhaps because what they see does not map on to their internal image which itself is unstable. Reflection simply destabilizes it more. Second is the 'pink slipper' sign named after the patient who first presented in this way. It is observed when visiting a patient at home or in a hostel for the first assessment. The patient attends the assessment wearing childrens' slippers, for example slippers shaped as animals with large furry ears, zebras with a curly tail, elephants with a trunk, or in the case of the eponymous patient, large pink flamingos. This homely, cosy, diminutive appearance is contrasted with the exposed cuts on the arms demonstrating that self-harm has taken place recently. This juxtaposition probably represents the struggle that so many borderline patients find themselves in as they attempt to maintain their self-structure, wanting to look after themselves and care for themselves but being overwhelmed as they do so. Finally there appear to be two types of patients who self-lacerate and are worthy of distinction during the assessment. The first type is the chaotic cutter who embarks on cutting frenzies all over the arm or leg or other area of the body. This patient's moods are commonly volatile, rapidly fluctuating, and unpredictable. The second is the controlled cutter who makes a single deep cut in a managed and organized way. These patients tend to harm themselves more severely requiring stitches and sometimes muscle repair. Clinically they represent a higher risk group of patients.

Engagement in treatment

It has been shown that drop-out rates of around 40–50% occur in specialist treatment programmes for PD (Gunderson *et al.* 1989) although our drop-out rate is around 25–20% (Bateman and Fonagy 1999). The commonest conscious reasons given by patients for failure to attend are frustration with treatment, lack of social supports, and difficulties attending appointments for logistical reasons. Day-hospital treatment becomes impossible if a patient either lives too far from the hospital or has a difficult journey to get there. In these cases it is probably better to offer intensive out-patient treatment. Patients who find it difficult to sustain everyday social interaction and to meet the demands of daily living cannot travel long distances for treatment. Even if they protest that they can and will do so, it will increase the likelihood of their dropping-out at the point at which their ambivalence or hostility is aroused. Home visits to patients at risk who live far away become increasingly problematic, time-consuming, and impractical.

Few people want psychiatric treatment and most borderline patients have both sought and rejected help over a number of years so their motivation for treatment cannot be taken for granted. To this extent the core of treatment is about engaging the patient in a constructive and progressive dialogue; even when patients seem to be involved with treatment, motivation fluctuates rapidly, sometimes within the course of a day, making it difficult to engage them in a constructive dialogue. At one moment they demand help and yet at another they reject it and this has led clinicians to discharge patients prematurely. It is not appropriate to refuse treatment to a patient simply because they appear to show little wish for change. Ambivalence about change is central to the borderline character structure. The offer of treatment threatens psychological equilibrium and increases anxiety and so is likely to be rejected at some point. The task of engagement is to negotiate constructively any rifts and ruptures in treatment whenever they occur and gradually to establish the therapeutic relationship on a more trusting level.

Non-attendance during treatment not only threatens the viability of the patient's treatment but, if endemic, also can destabilize and fragment the whole programme. Patients organize pre-group meetings or telephone 'conferences' to check who is attending and some patients arrange a boycott of a group. Such destructive activities have to be challenged early and patients asked to talk about their criticisms of treatment in the group or individual session. Non-attending patients are telephoned at home and if this fails to provoke attendance, a letter is sent suggesting the patient attends his next individual session to explore the underlying reasons for his non-attendance. Finally two members of the team visit the patient at home to establish contact and to help the patient return.

The process of preventing drop-out and engaging the patient in treatment starts before the patient enters treatment and continues throughout the programme. The therapist has to be constantly aware that borderline patients may feel compelled to leave at any point and that the impulse to do so may arise suddenly and with little warning and be based on a misunderstanding of something that has been said or alternatively on an inaccurate or accurate recognition of a feeling a team member has about the patient. The development of a relational and working alliance is the most important aspect of the engagement process.

The engagement process involves:

- outlining a pathway of admission to the programme and providing a leaflet about the programme and its 'rules';
- stabilizing social aspects of care, for example housing and benefits;
- ensuring the clinic or hospital at the centre of treatment is easily accessible to the patient and appointments are at agreed times acceptable to both patient and treatment team;
- establishing agreed short-term goals at the outset of treatment;
- defining and agreeing roles of mental health professionals and others, e.g. probation officers, involved in the care of the patient;
- focusing the initial work on a dynamic formulation;
- helping the patient early in treatment to recognize the onset of frustration and to develop ways of reducing it;
- developing a treatment plan during an in-patient admission if the patient is in hospital allowing initial attendance from the in-patient ward.

Pathway to admission

Provision of information

The assessment process is the first point of contact with the patient and consequently is extremely important (see Assessment, p. 156). Prior to admission, two members of staff meet with the patient at least once. More commonly the team meet with the patient on a number of occasions to explore motivation and to provide education about the programme. In addition, exploration of relationships and their transference implications begin at this time but without overt transference interpretation.

This introductory process may take weeks or months in some cases and must include the following:

Clarification of key problems, as identified by the patient

Commonly these include problems with relationships, propensity to suicidal acts and acts of self-harm, difficulties of affect control, distrust of others, drug misuse, and symptomatic distress. They must be clearly identified and agreed with the patient.

Explanation of the underlying treatment approach and its relevance to the problems

In particular it is important to explain to the patient that an attempt is made to recognize how their problems have developed, what current factors are maintaining them, and how this is addressed within both individual and group work. An explanation is given in this context about affect control, effortful control, and mentalization.

Information about individual and group therapy and how it can lead to change

Patients often ask why they have to attend groups but rarely request reasons for individual sessions. Patients worry there will be no time in the group to consider their problems, they will end up looking after everyone else, no one will listen to their difficulties, or that the therapists will be unable to give them enough attention. In contrast the individual session is viewed as a time to focus on oneself, as a place to be looked after and given full attention, and as a refuge from hostility and misunderstanding. Patients need to be disabused of these assumptions and we describe the problems and benefits of both group and individual therapy whilst exploring their anxieties. Our qualitative feedback suggests that group therapy stimulates the greatest anxieties early in treatment but towards the end of the programme, patients believe that their experience in the groups has been rewarding and mutative.

We explain the group as a context in which patients can consider themselves in relation to others in the immediacy of a peer interaction, as a situation in which they can explore their misunderstandings of the motives of others by asking other patients about different perspectives, and as a place in which they can understand how they operate in a group of people to stabilize themselves. It is recommended that patients always solicit others' views of them and be open about their assumptions of others. The individual session is a context in which the patient can form a more intimate relationship to explore more personal themes, their development and their repetition in the present. We discuss transference, its vicissitudes, and its use as a tool to understand underlying anxieties.

The need for regular attendance is discussed. The patient is asked to contact the day-hospital or out-patient team if they are unable to attend on any given day. A copy of the programme is given to the patient. Information on travel expenses, lunch, medical certificates, and the prescription of medication is given (see p. 195).

An outline of confidentiality

The programme operates within a system of team confidentiality. This minimizes splitting, ensures that all staff understand the problems faced by all patients, and enables staff to cover each other effectively during absences, holidays, and other breaks.

The treatment team respects privacy of individual sessions and does not discuss information volunteered in the individual sessions in the groups. However, every aspect of treatment, including the individual session, is discussed within the team. The patient is informed about this team confidentiality and its aim of maximizing safety and the effectiveness of help. Contact with professionals outside the team is agreed with each patient.

All members of the groups are required to keep information on personal issues within the treatment setting.

If a member of the team considers a patient as a threat to himself or the safety of others, he may breach confidentiality and speak to agencies, family, close partners, and others. But whenever possible, the patient's agreement is obtained but if this is impossible the patient is informed of the reasons for the transfer of clinical information to other mental health professionals as soon as possible.

Clarification of some basic rules

Violence

Violence, verbal or physical, to others is not tolerated. In the case of physical violence, the person responsible may be discharged and the police involved. In other cases time-out may be given, the length of which is decided by a minimum of two members of the staff team. However, it is policy that an individual is asked not to return to the unit until he feels safe and in control of his impulses and before he does he should contact the team by phone or letter to state that this is the case. An appointment is then arranged to discuss the situation in more detail.

Damage to the fabric of the treatment setting results in time-out and breakages are charged.

For further discussion of violence see p. 235.

Drugs and alcohol

Patients under the influence of drugs or alcohol are not allowed to remain in a group or individual session. When asked to leave, many patients challenge the therapists and demand that blood or urine samples are taken to prove the veracity of their denial. There is no blood or urine testing. The agreed rule at the beginning of treatment is that if two members of the staff believe that a patient appears to be under the influence of drugs or alcohol, they are empowered to ask him to leave and only to return when his mind is not altered by drugs or alcohol.

Sexual relationships

It is impossible to prevent patients meeting during the evening and weekends and at other times, for example after an out-patient group. Some may meet by chance since they live locally, others feel isolated and lonely and so seek out contact, viewing other members of a group as kindred spirits. The dangers of regular outside contact are discussed during the first few meetings, pointing out that it interferes with the treatment of the individual as well as influencing the whole group. If meetings take place they should be discussed within the group and individual session and not kept secret. Sexual relationships between patients are strongly discouraged.

Stabilizing social aspects of care

There is nothing worse than trying to engage a patient in long-term treatment if social conditions are unstable. If a crisis occurs, the team do not know how to contact or to trace the patient and the patient is unable to think about anything other than how to survive the next night or where he is going to stay. Individuals with severe PD are frequently evicted from housing and rented accommodation and this leads to recommendations for provision of supported accommodation even though such accommodation is often time-limited. Although individuals need to be assessed on a case-by-case basis, the majority of patients find intensively supported accommodation too intrusive and lacking in privacy. The constant personal interactions in group homes lead to anxiety and may induce withdrawal or emotional storms. Withdrawal evokes an opposite reaction from staff who may attempt to coax the patient to interact more; emotional storms undermine constructive relationships and eventually lead to a breakdown of peer and staff support unless handled with patience and sensitivity. Generally it is better if patients are given more responsibility for their everyday living in permanent accommodation. It is therefore necessary to:

- develop close working relationships with housing departments and social services
- ensure information is available about emergency procedures
- invite the housing manager and social worker to case conferences if appropriate and certainly to the admission case conference
- inform social workers of progress of treatment

Assuring the possibility of contact with the patient

Intriguingly, despite the fact that most of our patients are unemployed, the majority have mobile phones. Borderline patients fear isolation and like to maintain contact with friends, support networks, and professional staff and at the same time control the extent of the contact. Mobile phones with their 'number calling' identification facility and their flexibility for 24-hr contact seem to fulfil these requirements. This is a bonus for treatment because it allows the team to contact the patient with relative ease. Even if the patient does not answer the phone, a message enables him to see that attempts at contact have been made indicating that the team are keeping him in mind even in his absence. If a patient is at high risk and fails to answer the phone it may be necessary to call the patient from an unusual number because he may be not be answering phone calls specifically from the hospital number. On many occasions we have found that when we do this the patient rarely refuses to speak although to some extent they have been tricked into answering the phone. This minor deceit is contrary to the general openness and frankness of our treatment approach but it seems a price worth paying if risk is reduced. A further 'trick' is to ring outside normal office times which may reduce risk simply because the patient is astonished but relieved that he is being thought about outside normal times. Being faced with the reality of being kept in mind is startling from a teleological perspective because it means that the team 'care' at a time when the patient believes that nobody is concerned. The action of calling outside normal office times is an acceptable aspect of the 'real relationship' (see p. 216) but should only be done after agreement within the team to ensure that it is an appropriate boundary violation, that its aim is to confront the patient with a positive reality, and that it is likely to reduce risk.

Clear-agreed goals

There is a hierarchy of goals: Initial goals (patient specific); Long-term goals (patient specific); Overall long-term goals (programme specific).

Initial goals are short-term and directed towards

- engagement in therapy
- reduction of self-damaging, threatening, or suicidal behaviour
- appropriate use of emergency services
- stabilizing accommodation
- rationalization of medication
- development of a psychodynamic formulation with the patient

Once a stable platform has been established on which treatment can take place, individual, longer-term goals are negotiated with the patient.

Long-term goals include targets to increase:

- identification of emotions and their appropriate expression with others
- personal integrity
- personal responsibility
- interpersonal function.

Each patient is considered within the framework of the overall long-term goals (see Treatment Aims). A patient-specific formulation is developed, considered in terms of the programme, and discussed with the patient. All long-term aims are developed in a patient-specific or idiographic way and form part of the dynamic formulation agreed with the patient in the early individual sessions. For example, some patients may be better at identifying and controlling emotions than others but find it almost impossible to consider their responsibility in relationships. Others may be overburdened with responsibility, blaming themselves for everything that has gone wrong in their life and yet find it difficult to know how they feel in many circumstances and be prone to violent outbursts.

Defining and agreeing roles of mental health professionals and others involved in the care of the patient

By the time a patient is referred to a specialist treatment service for PD, there are likely to be many mental health professionals involved in their care. Typically these include psychiatrists, community nurses, support workers, social workers, housing officers, probation officers, and others. Often roles are blurred and 'split treatment' has occurred by default with little coherent planning because many of the professionals may have become involved during crises.

At the point of admission to specialist treatment, a case conference is held to which all the professionals currently involved in the patient's care are invited. The patient should also be present at the meeting. The purpose of the discussion is to:

- clarify the role(s) of each professional outside the specialist treatment team;
- determine who is to continue involvement and for what purpose;
- establish who is the named Key Worker;
- formalize emergency procedures;
- agree the level of risk, warning signs, and action to be taken (See sample Crisis Plan, Appendix 3);
- establish who is the Responsible Medical Officer for the purposes of the Mental Health Act and for medical/psychiatric responsibility;
- define the patient's responsibilities.

In particular it is essential that a professional from outside the treatment team who continues contact with the patient is clear about his

- role and responsibility
- level of autonomy about decision making
- interdependence on the specialist treatment team.

A final summary of the meeting is written and sent to all concerned.

History taking

History taking is essential. The task is not to elicit a broad sweep of history but to obtain a comprehensive account of the patient's present and past problems, their development, and their significance in the patient's life in order to inform and guide an overall treatment plan. Relationships with primary attachment figures are explored in detail. Taking a history does not simply involve listing a series of events but requires the placing of important events and relationships into a context of mental experience. The therapist not only wants to know about the patient's affect or behaviour but also about their inner mental experience, their interpersonal context, and the effect on their relationships with primary attachment figures. Without this knowledge, the therapist is handicapped and cannot begin to develop an understanding of the underlying meaning of behaviour and affect. The therapist constantly seeks information that may help formulate the difficulties around the four main target areas, namely affect expression, internal representations, self, and relationships. In order to do this attention needs to be paid to:

- previous emotional storms
- suicide attempts and self-harm
- episodes of violence
- interpersonal behaviour
- intimate relationships
- previous treatments and their outcome.

Interpersonal behaviour and intimate relationships

A pervasive pattern of instability of interpersonal relationships characterized by alternating extremes of idealization and devaluation and frantic efforts to avoid real or imagined abandonment is a defining characteristic of BPD. Early in therapy, it is important to explore the patient's relationships extensively, starting with parental or caregiver relationships. One way to do this adequately is to ask such questions as 'can you give me five adjectives to describe your relationship with your mother/father/partners and then I would like to consider some examples that illustrate each description?' Again it is important here not just to get a behavioural account but to ask actively about the mental experiences the patient believes they had at the time and to foster reconsideration of the experiences from the viewpoint of the present, i.e. 'has your view of the relationship changed over time or is that how you see things now?' In addition, this is the time to start using 'transference tracers' (see p. 208) by asking the patient urbanely if he thinks we all need to be on our guard to prevent similar events happening in the relationship to the treatment programme or to the team, particularly if there appears be a repetitive pattern. It is common to find that relationships with mental health professionals follow the same pattern as personal ones, manifesting idealization and devaluation. This needs to be brought to the attention of the patient and concern expressed about it being repeated in treatment.

Some patients attempt to control their feelings by withdrawal and adapt to their problems by avoiding relationships. This can result in an apparent improvement. Careful history taking will reveal that symptoms arise only when the patient becomes involved in close relationships and recede if withdrawal takes place. For some borderline patients, this retreat is less painful than attempts to develop relationships and there is a progressive withdrawal over time. Inevitably when this has occurred it makes it more difficult for them to join in a programme that actively involves the development of a therapeutic relationship. Recognition of this pattern is necessary to prevent psychological retreat and behavioural withdrawal at those times when emotional turmoil is stimulated by treatment. In addition it is important that the team do not mistake emotional and physical withdrawal and a lessening of symptoms for improvement. Whilst necessary at times as the only way to reduce tension and anxiety, it is defensive and fails to deal with the underlying problems.

Previous treatments and their outcome

Many patients with severe PD have long histories of failed treatments, of which a number will have ended in acrimony, violence, frustration, and sense of abandonment for the patient. As a result, borderline patients distrust or are wary of mental health professionals. This interferes with constructive engagement of the patient in yet another treatment and so understanding of what has happened in earlier treatments is essential if strategies are to be planned appropriately. The therapist should remain neutral about who was responsible for the breakdown of previous treatment even if the patient attempts to recruit him as an ally in criticizing other practitioners or services. What is important is an understanding of the processes that led to the breakdown of treatment and identification of the mental experiences of the patient and his beliefs about the motivations of the professionals involved. Again this should be linked to the possibility that further treatment may have the same end result and a major task of the treatment will be to try to avoid a negative outcome. In order to do so both patient and therapist need to agree likely precursors of a breakdown in treatment and keep them in mind throughout the programme.

Equally important in assessing previous treatments is the identification of interventions that the patient found helpful, the aspects of their problems that improved, and their understanding of how those benefits were brought about. This may help the patient reassess previous treatment and balance its benefits and detriments without deriding and dismissing or idealizing it at all. For the therapist there may be indications of interventions that the patient will find useful.

Formation of relational and working alliance

Patient and therapist form a relational and working alliance with the aim of integrating therapy into a coherent and understandable process. At the beginning of therapy, the therapist needs to help the patient understand the process of therapy and its purpose. Therapy cannot be treated as a black box in which something magical will take place as a result of an active therapist doing something to a passive patient. It is a collaborative process in which the therapist is constantly trying to understand the patient and their mental states and to help them observe themselves. The alliance is often seen as having four components: (a) the ability of the patient to work purposefully in therapy, (b) the capacity of the patient to form a strong affective bond to the therapist, (c) the therapist's skill at providing empathic understanding, and (d) the agreement of patient and therapist on goals and tasks (Gaston 1990). Combining all these elements leads to a relational and working alliance.

The constant finding that outcome of psychotherapy correlates reliably with patient–therapist alliance implies that stronger alliances should be associated with better outcomes. Indeed this seems to be the case (Stiles 1998). There have been a number of studies examining the alliance between borderline patients and their therapists, some of which have noted its fluctuating nature (Horwitz *et al.* 1996). Others have shown a gradual progression of the alliance over time suggesting a correlation with outcome (Gunderson 1997) and the therapy outlined by Stevenson and Meares (1992) in their successful outcome study emphasized the therapeutic alliance. It is within this context that we place a focus on aspects of the alliance early in therapy.

The relational alliance is built up gradually through empathy and validation, reliability, and readiness to listen. Hope in hostility, assurance in affect storms, and the very basic quality of being human are also necessary if a relational alliance is to survive the vicissitudes of treatment. The therapist needs continually to remain calm and to maintain hope especially when being relentlessly criticized or denigrated by the patient. Affect storms can rapidly undermine a working alliance and leave a therapist feeling unappreciated, misunderstood, and hurt.

Empathy and validation

Empathy is a demonstration of the therapist's attunement to his patient and, although often wordless, may take the form of statements such as 'you seem to feel really hurt when talking about how you were treated in that way'. In empathy, the initial emotional resonance in the therapist is followed by an empathic abstraction using conscious knowledge based on earlier understanding of the patient and personal experience. This is used to create a transient role identification with the patient in order to understand his reality. The representation of reality in borderline patients is restricted and remarks made to the patient must take this into account.

A patient was complaining about a friend who failed to turn up to a meeting. Listening to the tone of the complaint the therapist said 'you sound as if you feel he didn't want to see you'. The patient answered by saying 'if he had wanted to see me he would have been there. He just wanted to hurt me by saying he would be there and then not turning up'.

In this example the patient is unable to think of alternative explanations for his friend's absence and his mind can only work according to the visible outcome, which was his friend's failure to turn up, rather than on an understanding of his motivations, which may have been to make the meeting.

Whilst the therapist may have to work on this empathic understanding early in therapy, the aim is not just to make empathic remarks but to develop affective attunement which, in contrast to empathy involving cognitive processes, takes place outside consciousness. Affective attunement is unconscious emotional resonance (Hoffman 1978), illustrated by situations such as one person shouting 'aaaagh' and sucking their finger when someone else hits theirs with a hammer. However, developing affective attunement does not constitute a treatment in itself. Understanding how their finger came to be hit and how to avoid it in future are equally important processes although this will take place later in therapy. It is only in early sessions that the development of affective attunement is more important to ensure formation of a constructive relational alliance.

In the example above, the therapist does not challenge the explanation given by the patient about his friend's failure to arrive. His empathic remark validates the patient's experience, which is accepted at face value. It is important not to invalidate the patient's experience, which is usually understandable from their teleological point of view (see p. 61). Later in therapy, the therapist may help the patient identify the feelings and the accompanying mental experience and relate it to therapy itself in an attempt to move the patient from a teleological stance to an intentional mode.

Towards the end of the treatment, the therapist arrived late for the individual session. When he arrived he apologized to the patient and, knowing the patient quite well, said 'I guess you may have thought that I didn't want to see you today'. The patient confirmed this feeling and an exploration of the feelings and mental experience began. In fact the patient had become increasingly angry and hurt thinking that the therapist not only did not want to see him but also his preference was to be at home with his family. This had led the patient to think about leaving the building himself and 'scoring' some illicit drugs. The therapist said 'I can understand how you would think I would prefer to be at home with family and how that could lead to you feeling angry and hurt (empathic validation) but the problem is that it leads you to feel that you have to do something harmful to yourself. Because of everything that has happened to you, you see me as malicious in the same way as your father and find it difficult to think of me as a different person. You want to harm yourself when you are thinking about harming him' (transference interpretation).

In this example the therapist tries to expand the patient's view of reality through transference interpretation. This can only be done when the relational alliance is secure.

Reliability and readiness to listen

The whole programme should be organized so that sessions are dependable and the patient can trust that they will take place at the allotted times. We have already emphasized the borderline patient's tendency to judge motivation on outcomes so it is imperative that if a group, additional session, or review is planned and a time agreed with the patient that it takes place; if it does not the patient will presuppose the staff did not want to see him, embryonic trust will be eroded, and the therapeutic alliance ruptured. The regularity of the individual session is part of the overall reliability of the programme and must be organized so that the patient understands its purpose and can rely on its structure. The therapist should not underestimate the importance of the individual session to the patient even though he may deride it at times. Chaotic use of the sessions by a patient should not be mirrored by disorderly organization. This will serve only to increase the patient's anxiety, especially if it is part of an unresolved countertransference response in the therapist. In all our qualitative feedback, patients emphasize the value of the individual session as a place in which they feel they can talk more freely and consider their relationships with others, particularly in the groups, and with friends outside. The reliability of the therapist makes them feel that the session is theirs.

Readiness to listen is more than sitting silently. It is a state of mind in the therapist which is represented to the patient and links with the mentalizing stance discussed on p. 203. The therapist is ready to listen from the patient's perspective and he refrains from promoting his own view. Only when a patient feels sure that a therapist can listen from his point of view is it possible for the patient to be 'ready to listen' to the therapist's standpoint. To this extent transference interpretation is done carefully and sensitively early in treatment and it is only later in treatment that transference perspectives become fully meaningful to the patient.

Dynamic formulation

The dynamic formulation is developed in the individual sessions, may take a variable length of time, and should only be attempted once all the information described earlier has been explored. The purpose of developing a dynamic understanding of the patient's problems is to place feelings and behaviour within an individual context and to commence the development of a coherent interpersonal and developmental narrative. Frequently, borderline patients have an incoherent narrative that makes little sense to them, leaving them unable to explain their personality development with any lucidity. They become schematic and categorical, linking specific events with explicit problems.

The development of the formulation is the beginning of helping the patient to understand himself by exploring his personal story. Each identified theme should be linked to the programme to demonstrate how treatment can address the problem, thereby increasing the patient's understanding of the rationale behind the programme. It cannot be assumed that patients will comprehend the reasons for different aspects of the programme or that they will entrust themselves to the process of therapy unquestioningly in the belief that it will help them. Too often there have been previous failures of treatment. Similarly it cannot be supposed that patients will understand a formulation written in technical language. It is more likely to alienate them and to make them feel suspicious or misunderstood. Any formulation must be jointly developed and be understandable to patient, therapist, and team. It is written down as a working hypothesis rather than a veridical truth established by a therapist and is reviewed throughout the treatment programme.

Example of formulation

Jo Bloggs is a 22-year-old man who presents in a confident and articulate manner but who feels that his problems have never been taken seriously. He said that he has known there is something seriously wrong with him for some years now, but that his parents refused to recognize it when he was younger. He was contemptuous of his previous psychiatrists, saying that it would have helped if most of them could have spoken English, although he felt that one psychiatrist had been good at establishing his diagnosis. In this respect, Jo had visited various Internet websites on BPD, the criteria for which he felt described well his sense of himself, except for impulses towards self-harm and suicide. He could not understand what motivates others to do this 'because it hurts'. However, he described problems with relationships in which initial desire and passion soon turns to devaluation and a feeling that people are not good enough for him, an intensity of emotions that fluctuate rapidly and sometimes uncontrollably, frequent outbursts of temper, and some paranoid feelings.

Jo was the youngest of two children. His parents were divorced, separating when he was 12. His older brother, now 24, did well academically, having gone to University. Jo spoke largely contemptuously of both his parents, who he felt covered up that there was something seriously wrong with him. He seemed to be slightly more forgiving of his mother. The one consistently positive figure in his life he says is his brother, although he acknowledged feeling envious of his brother's comparative success with women, but he dismissed his brother's long-standing girlfriend as stupid, which seemed to be motivated by feelings of competitiveness for his brother's attention.

When asked in more detail about the very difficulties he feels have been dismissed by others, Jo elaborated on his deep sense of mistrust of others, which he described as paranoia, feeling that everyone is first and foremost self-serving. He also spoke of his lack of confidence, although he openly described how he can swing between feeling unconfident and vastly superior to everyone else, adding that most people experience him as arrogant. He described how he struggles in social situations, often finding it difficult to connect with groups of people, or know how he should be in this circumstance. In these situations, he has been prone to 'black-outs' when he suddenly feels absent, as though everything is going on as if he was not there. He was clear that this happens when he feels he is not getting enough attention. Furthermore, Jo spoke of the intense fits of rage he is prone to experiencing when he wants to smash something over the head of the nearest person. He was initially unforthcoming about describing what happens to him in these moments, giving me anonymous examples, such as when someone accidentally bumps into him in the street.

However, in our second meeting he disclosed more freely about more personal circumstances. In particular, Jo spoke of a rival male at work who he felt was very similar to him in that he was terribly arrogant as a way of dealing with deeper insecurities. This rival belonged to the Rugby Club that Jo joined in his first year in order to boost his self-confidence. He would apparently make teasing comments and put-downs about Jo which would leave him feeling consumed with rage. Jo described on one occasion how he had picked this rival man up by the scruff of his collar and slammed his head against the wall. He alluded to other occasions when his rage had led to him hitting friends, although it seems he has never got into trouble with the law for his violence.

Jo gave numerous examples of situations in which he has felt let down, dismissed, or not given enough attention or credence by others. This has often occurred in the context of seeking the favour of women over and above that of male acquaintances. In these situations, Jo has shown a ruthlessness and cruel vengefulness. He described one situation as a teenager whereby he had socially crippled a boy who he had considered to be his best friend, by telling everyone this boy's embarrassing secrets. This was a response to this boy having won the favour of a girl that Jo had liked. Moreover, he had been somewhat surprised that this friend should feel very annoyed with him, passing it off as something his friend should have just got over. In the other examples that he gave, it seemed that he had no qualms about discarding anybody whom he felt wronged by.

In this respect, I was concerned by the apparent lack of inner conflict Jo experienced regarding his behaviour, and wondered how much he felt his problems would improve if people simply treated him better. Thus, the point of most concern for him seems to be the point at which he experiences any injury to his self-image, and that in these moments there seems to be nothing more important than re-establishing this image, regardless of the consequences for others. This fragility of his sense of self is consistent with borderline and narcissistic personality difficulties, whereby any such damage to his self-image evokes unbearable feelings of shame and humiliation, which he feels compelled to discharge. However, his need to put those feelings back into the other, and his cruel use of others in order to shore up his self-image suggest, as I have stated, antisocial traits.

On the positive side, Jo does seem to have maintained a constructive relationship with his brother, and his ownership of the deep insecurities that underlie his difficulties, as well as his recognition of how isolated he has become, may enable him to reflect on the agency he might have in his difficulties.

Based on this outline and our initial individual sessions we have agreed on the following questions and areas of importance and identified where they can be addressed:

1. his short-lived relationships may be repeated in therapy with passion and enthusiasm for therapy transforming into dismissal, disappointment, and hurt. This may lead to drop-out—individual and group therapy;
2. concern that people do not take him seriously—all staff to be aware and Jo to let us know if he feels something is not being taken seriously;
3. beware of envy of peer group (like brother, friend's girl-friend) and defensive responses such as denying the importance of their success, its meaning to them, or devaluating them—group therapy;
4. emotional withdrawal when not getting enough attention—group;
5. reversal of roles may occur with him being angry and dismissive when fearful that others are likely to do the same to him. Linked to parental relationship—individual session;
6. provocation of rage when others put him down. Beware of violence and need to 'walk away' until able to address what happens—group;
7. understanding the mental collapse and instability that occurs when people tease him which leads to violence. Did you feel that this man failed to consider you and your feelings, i.e. mentalize about you?—individual;
8. is a core problem his need to protect his self-image—people have to see him as he wants them to see him.

These areas of importance will be re-evaluated in three months in the case conference with the patient and the team.

Expressive therapies

The aim of expressive therapies in the day-hospital programme is to offer an alternative way of promoting mentalization. The use of art, writing, or other expressive therapies allows the internal to be expressed externally so that it can be verbalized at a distance through an alternative medium and from a different perspective. Experience and feeling is placed outside of the mind and into the world to facilitate explicit mentalizing. Under these circumstances mentalizing becomes conscious, verbal, deliberate, and reflective. In effect, patients generate something of themselves outside which is part of them but separate and so at one moment represents an aspect of themselves and yet at another is simply a drawing or essay. To this extent the therapy creates transitional objects and the therapists have to work at developing a transitional space within the group in which the created objects can be used to facilitate expression whilst maintaining stability of the self.

Patients find expressive therapies produce less anxiety, particularly early in treatment, than reflecting internally on themselves in relation to others. In expressive therapy, an aspect of the self is outside and so less dangerous, controlling, and overwhelming. Feelings become manageable and the understanding of oneself and others is more tolerable.

We do not purport to be experts in the delivery of art therapy and other expressive therapies requiring formal training and so we outline here specific aspects of our approach in relation to mentalization. The techniques can be applied within the frame of most types of expressive therapy.

General strategic recommendations

The general approach to patients in expressive therapy is no different from other aspects of the programme. In the expressive therapy the therapist needs to:

- ensure that the focus of the expressive therapy is related to the themes of the group therapy;
- allow patients to contribute to the development of the topic to be used in the expressive therapy, e.g. theme to be painted, feeling to be written about;
- focus on the expression of affects, their identification, and their personal and interpersonal context;
- ensure patients consider the meaning of the expressive efforts of others;
- help patients recognize that others may see their work in a different way to how they see them.

Organization

Expressive therapies are organized in small groups of 6–8 patients who gather for 15 min with the therapists to discuss the theme of the therapy. After the topic is decided and agreed, the patient group disperse to work alone on the task for half an hour and the group then reconvenes for an hour to discuss each patient's work.

Specific recommendations

The therapists need to ensure that they give equal attention to each patient's contribution. Our general pattern is first to ask one patient to describe what he feels another patient is expressing in relation to the agreed topic and to relate this to his knowledge and experience of the patient. An attempt is made to include all patients within this process of discussing the meaning of others' work before asking each patient to outline their own ideas about their own work and to consider whether other patients' understanding enriches or detracts from what they have done. It is important that therapists continually bring back the discussion to the theme under examination rather than follow other avenues of exploration. It is our intention to increase the patient and therapist's ability to attend to a task without being diverted by other themes in an attempt to increase effortful control (see p. 86). Often patients will be distracted by emotional reactions and will fail to attend to the dominant theme and find themselves pre-occupied with sub-dominant themes.

Common problems

Drop-outs

Not all patients engage in treatment or find the programme beneficial and, as a result, either drop out of therapy or ask to be referred elsewhere. Under both these circumstances, the team are trained to explore the underlying reasons for dissatisfaction, to refrain from attempts to persuade the patient to stay, and to encourage the patient to talk about his wish to leave in group and individual therapy before a final decision is taken. The patient needs to understand that his decision is not irrevocable and the key worker makes sure that leaving the programme is negotiated with compassion in the hope that a patient can ask to return without feeling ashamed and humiliated—the door should always be left open. Patients are allowed to re-refer themselves rather than accessing treatment through another agency and every patient who drops out or leaves early is offered a follow-up appointment after 1–2 months to re-evaluate their decision. The purpose of this meeting is to promote mentalization by considering the decision to leave from a distance. The mental and interpersonal context at the time of leaving is explored, its consequences defined, contingency plans made for crises, and a further appointment given if appropriate.

Staff are asked to monitor countertransference responsiveness with additional care when a patient might drop out because patients place therapists in specific roles in order to justify their decisions. Countertransference reactions commonly include relief that the patient is leaving, desperation to keep the patient, personal humiliation and anxiety about therapeutic ability, and beliefs that leaving is a suicidal equivalent and the patient will be unable to manage without the therapist. All these reactions need understanding in terms of the patient's personal history, current mental state, and his transference relationship with the team and therapist.

In-patient care

In-patient care in the management of crises should be patient-determined. But for patient-determined admission to be effective, a trusting relationship has to be developed between the treatment team and the in-patient staff. Failure of either group to understand the approach of the other leads to misunderstanding, splitting, undermining of treatment aims, and likely deterioration in the patient. The key worker should liaise carefully with in-patient staff and be able to explain the exact reasons for admission, agree contingency plans for untoward events such as self-harm, and whenever possible set up an admission meeting between members of the teams and the patient to minimize misunderstandings.

A patient requested admission for herself because she knew that her suicidal impulses were becoming dangerously compulsive and so the intensive out-patient team helped her contact the in-patient unit to request admission. Admission was arranged the same afternoon and because the ward was geographically close, the therapist accompanied the patient. At the meeting with the admitting nurse, the patient said that she wanted to go out that evening to a pre-arranged meeting with her friend. This conflicted with the in-patient protocol of not allowing suicidal patients off the ward for 24-h to allow the staff to make their own assessment. The therapist thought that it was safe for the patient to go out as long as she knew that she could return to the ward. Eventually it was arranged that the patient would contact her friend who would come to the hospital and accompany the patient outside and return with her to the ward at the end of the evening. This enabled the in-patient staff to feel 'safe' and the patient to retain responsibility for herself to some degree which was important for her work with the psychotherapist.

The team need to train in-patient staff not to attempt to 'treat' the patient. Treatment is best done within the specialist programme and the purpose of in-patient admission is not to address underlying problems but to give respite. This can be difficult for in-patient staff who may feel devalued and used and yet their role in managing a patient in a safe and minimally restrictive environment, preventing regression, and encouraging responsibility cannot be overestimated. The attitude of the in-patient staff needs to be one of fairness and neutrality towards the patient whilst promoting a brief admission without being rejected. Decisions about discharge should be passed back to the patient and treatment team or agreed within a meeting of all staff involved with the patient. Sudden discharge by staff or immediate self-discharge by the patient is to be avoided.

Supporting the team

Team morale

Patients with PD can sap team morale for a number of reasons.

First, borderline patients are emotionally challenging, at times picking on staff members, finding their weak spots, threatening them, undermining their therapeutic zeal, evoking negative countertransference and other feelings, inducing frustration, and becoming dismissive of their work. Second, change in PD is slow and, at times, staff and patients have to recognize that considerable work is repeated without obvious benefit; working through the same problem within different contexts is common place and necessary. Whilst repetition might seem disheartening at first, and it is not uncommon to hear statements from staff such as 'we've been here before', 'this is the same old pattern', it is also a chance to re-visit the problem when it is 'hot', allowing another opportunity of change and development. Third, splits within the team, whether arising from problems within the patient or in the team itself, commonly manifest themselves as disagreements which may become polarized making it hard for individuals not to blame each other for management or treatment difficulties. Fourth, the fluctuating nature of the problems of the borderline patient and the intermittent crises can lead to an onerous workload and constant anxiety about risk. Finally a suicide of a patient not only has a profound effect on the individual caring for the patient but also on the whole team who blame themselves, feel that they will be blamed by others, and have to face a psychological autopsy in which all aspects of the treatment of the patient is reviewed. The effect that all these factors have on the individual and team is determined in part by the function of the team itself. A team working cohesively looks after its members, protects them, helps them understand what is happening or has happened, gives a member a rest when necessary, allows time for further training, and ensures that any one individual is not overburdened with high-risk patients.

A team needs constant attention to maintain smooth functioning and consideration should be given to how it is structured. Leadership is needed at different levels. Within the team it should come from the most experienced and senior professional whose task is to preserve the structure of the treatment programme, support staff, supervise on an everyday basis, and treat the more problematic patients. Leadership of the service rests in the person who is best placed to offer expert supervision, who can negotiate within the system, and who has the respect of all staff. Leadership is given rather than taken or assumed because of professional identity. The qualities of a good leader are not specific to any one professional group and are related more to some of the personal qualities identified earlier that are important in treatment of PD.

Sustaining team enthusiasm and morale is primarily through an admixture of serious work with supervision, provision of time for private learning, and the development of a space to laugh and cry together. The latter is rarely discussed openly but there is no doubt that a team that can laugh together and be sad with each other about their professional trials and tribulations as well as some of their personal concerns when appropriate will function supportively and effectively. The humanity of a team will create a secure atmosphere within the treatment milieu allowing disagreement between therapists to take place in safety, for example during a group, and the facilitation of a questioning culture.

In group therapy, one of the therapists made an interpretation in the group that was followed by silence. The other therapist sensed that the patients had not understood the interpretation at all and in fact he had not done so himself. He said to the therapist 'I didn't understand a word of that, do you think you could try again to explain what you were trying to say'. The therapist laughed and said 'I wasn't sure that I understood it either as I was talking and so maybe it is a good idea to start again'. This allowed the group to confirm their belief that sometimes staff did not know what they were talking about but also demonstrated that it was possible to question things constructively and to stimulate further thought rather than to dismiss or ignore what is said.

Supervision

It is impossible to maintain team morale and to deliver effective treatment without supervision. It is all-too-easy for treatment to become chaotic, for staff to develop extreme or idiosyncratic views, individual members to feel victimized, patients to turn into scapegoats, and mistakes to be made involving boundary transgressions. Supervision reduces the likelihood of these events and is organized on a group and individual basis as an intrinsic part of the programme.

Supervision needs to be considered in terms of the team itself. We consider the team meetings which occur after each group to be supervision by and for the peer group. The participating therapists report on the form and content of their recent group and discuss it with the team. This ensures that all members are updated on each patient and his activities within the group as well as allowing discussion of therapist interventions and other aspects of treatment. Formal supervision to the team about the groups occurs twice a week and is provided by the leader of the service which brings with it the danger of a closed system outside the scrutiny of others. To prevent the development of self-serving attitudes, the insidious formation of unquestioned beliefs, and the creation of a 'corporate delusion', each team member has individual supervision outside the treatment programme with a senior member of the wider psychological therapies service even if that supervisor is not trained within our particular techniques. It is important that each therapist feels secure to discuss his own views, the problems he is having with a patient and the difficulties he may be having with his own feelings about the patient or with implementing therapy. It also gives a chance to explain what he does, why he does it, and what happens in sessions, and for his therapy to be questioned by an expert therapist using an alternative perspective. Findings from the individual supervisions are brought together and considered within the framework of our treatment in a further team supervision run by the service lead.

Supervision has a number of overlapping aims. First, it is a method to ensure that therapists keep to the model of therapy and apply it appropriately and with fidelity and we have a therapist adherence scale (see p. 315) to monitor this aspect of treatment. But it is important that therapists do not feel over-scrutinized and criticized when they deviate from the model. Divergence is inevitable because it is easy for a therapist to become drawn in to non-therapeutic interventions, for example sharing aspects of his own life with the patient, or viewing the patient as a friend. Second, it is a place where the therapist should feel free to discuss the major evolving transference themes along with his countertransference responses to the patient. Third, supervision needs to support and to challenge. Simply giving encouragement does not increase skill and may even perpetuate bad habits; so a secure atmosphere in which both the supervisor and supervisee can confront and question each other is necessary. Fourth, the supervision can be used to understand the patient–therapist relationship although supervision itself is not therapy for the therapist. The relationship that the therapist makes in supervision may, in part, reflect the underlying problem in treatment itself.

One supervisee became very challenging in supervision expressing concern that nothing that the supervisor said seemed to help him orientate his mind to tackle the next session. At first, the supervisor tried to make more and more suggestions until he realized that this may be exactly what was happening in therapy—the therapist was giving more and more support to the patient but felt that it was increasingly ineffective. This was discussed in supervision and understood in terms of the patient's envy of the therapist who was of similar age and successful in contrast to the patient who felt unsuccessful with none of her talents realized. The patient was endeavouring to undermine the therapist in the same way that she herself had been by her family. The envy towards the supervisor by the therapist was also a problem that had to be discussed in supervision but this was done later when the therapist felt more confident with the patient.

Finally, supervision is part of in-service training and the validation of a therapist's skills. How often supervision occurs will be dependent on level of training and experience but all therapists, even the most experienced and best trained, should have individual supervision at least once a week and participate in group peer–peer supervision. New staff will need more support and guidance after completion of a training programme.

It will be apparent from this discussion that being a supervisor has its own set of skills and not all experienced clinicians are good supervisors. From our perspective, the supervisor has to be able to demonstrate a capacity to mentalize if he is to provide an anchor for the therapist. Mentalizing is a core method of re-establishing self-stability in borderline patients and is equally a key aspect of restoring stability in a therapist who may have crumbled under attack or become depressed and hopeless after being undermined by a dismissive patient. If the therapist feels hopeless, it is the task of the supervisor to identify the reasons for this state and he does this by considering the patient–therapist relationship and the therapist–supervisor interaction by asking himself mentalizing questions—why is the therapist telling me this now? Why is he expressing it in this way? Does this have something to do with the patient's problem and if so, what? Eventually it is important to formulate the problem in a way that is understandable to the therapist and to discuss techniques that may be useful in moving therapy along. After supervision, the therapist should leave knowing how to address the challenge presented by the patient and feeling re-invigorated to face the next challenges.

Care programme approach

The Care Programme Approach (CPA) is the foundation stone of current policy for mental health services in England and Wales and so this section may have a particularly parochial feel about it. However, one aspect that forms a cornerstone in our programme is 'user' involvement in the CPA to ensure that it is not something that is done 'on' or 'to' a patient but done 'with' the patient. The CPA arose out of concern about the inadequate follow-up care for people leaving psychiatric hospitals. It emphasizes various elements of good practice including: the assessment of the user's health and social care needs by a multidisciplinary team; an agreed plan of care and treatment; the allocation of a 'key worker' with responsibility for maintaining contact and monitoring the implementation of the plan; and regular reviews. All these aspects are part of the framework within which our treatment is given. It has previously been mentioned that we make careful assessments, develop a formulation that is shared with the patient and modified according to further discussion with the patient, the individual therapist acts as the nominated key worker, and that there are regular reviews with the patient and whole team. However, in our modifications, the patient also has responsibilities for the effective implementation of the treatment plan and this is in accord with guidance about involving users and carers which has been stressed in successive government documents on the implementation of the CPA. Users should be involved in discussions about their proposed care programmes so that they can consider different treatment possibilities and agree the programme. Carers often know a great deal about the user's life, interests, and abilities as well as having personal experience of the user's mental health problems and should be involved in the CPA. The guidance we use for our three-monthly reviews (see p. 164) is as follows:

The key worker should consider:

- involving users, carers (family, friends, or care staff from residential homes), an independent advocate (if requested), mental health professionals and others, e.g. police;
- recording users' and carers' views on their involvement with the treatment programme, other mental health services, housing and social care, and admission to hospital if occurred;
- identifying and recording separately the users', carers' and professionals' views on problems and needs and aims, and noting disagreements;
- formulating action plans designed to meet problems and agreeing timing of subsequent review arrangements;
- providing specific information about treatment and its rationale;
- ensuring the patient has full information about any medication;
- obtaining explicit agreement (by signature) of all parties to the treatment plan.

These recommendations should be used flexibly and creatively.

One patient treated in IOP was the lead singer in a pop group and the other members of the band acted as her primary carers—she called them her 'family'. After discussion with the patient, they were invited to the initial case conference and involved in development of a treatment plan which had to take into account logistic problems when the band were on tour. Arrangements were made for the patient to return each week for her group and individual session and where possible 'gigs' were not arranged the night before those sessions.

Adherence

The whole point of a treatment manual is to guide a therapist in procedures, techniques, attitudes, therapeutic manoeuvres, and actions which are specific to the therapy in the hope that this will limit the variability in treatment delivery, allow replication of research findings, and help bridge the gap between research and clinical practice. Yet if this is to be the case, an essential requirement for all clinicians is to ensure that the treatment itself is applied with integrity, that is that the procedures are carried out as intended. There are a number of interrelated concepts within the frame of treatment integrity including differentiation from other treatments and therapy competence, that is its application with a particular level of skill. But it is treatment adherence that is the most central. We have therefore developed an adherence scale (see Appendix 4) to measure whether MBT is being given as suggested. In general this scale measures only gross aspects of treatment but we have tried to include more detailed aspects of treatment because it is the more subtle departures from delivering treatment as intended that are more problematic. They can be difficult to detect and yet undermine treatment altogether even when the overall frame seems robust. The adherence scale is for use in rating video or audio tape but can also be used in verbatim reporting of sessions during supervision.

We are indebted to John Clarkin for his suggestion that practitioners can be validated as competent by asking them to watch video tapes of sessions by other specialists, which have already been rated for adherence level by senior practitioners, and to rate them for adherence. Their reliability can be used as a measure of their understanding of the treatment itself and may represent their ability to implement this in clinical practice. Rating is not an all-or-none phenomenon and practitioners should be within an acceptable range on most measures but assessors of adherence must be more subtle than simply counting the interventions or monitoring the framework. Adherence to treatment is influenced by transference and countertransference and what may be more important is not whether a practitioner is 'off-model' at a specific point but whether he can return to the model within a reasonable time within the session. If a practitioner is continually pushed off-model within a session and yet returns to 'base' quickly, he is likely to be adhering to treatment and applying it with considerable skill. This should be taken into account. Competence of practitioners is not simply a matter of adherence. All interventions can be given with commensurate skill or appalling clumsiness especially in terms of their timing, subtlety, emotional quality, and sensitivity. This is difficult to measure but one way that can be considered is to use information from patients who are asked to report on the therapist's behaviour after, say, an individual session.

Conclusions

This detailed description of our treatment organization is best considered as a series of clinical recommendations rather than as prescriptive advice and should not be implemented without question or modification when developing services. The manner in which we engage the patient, stabilize social aspects of care, maintain basic rules etc. may be done in other ways depending on resources and context. But there are some characteristics of treatment that we consider as essential features of mentalization-based treatment and which should not be varied. They are necessarily, although easily, transferred to different contexts and settings. Without them, treatment of borderline personality will be compromised and so we devote the next chapter solely to a discussion of these critical organizational aspects of MBT.

6 Transferable features of the MBT model

In our review of the literature (Bateman and Fonagy 2000) we concluded that treatments shown to be effective with borderline personality disorder (BPD) had certain common organizational features:

- high level of structure;
- consistent and reliable implementation;
- theoretical coherence;
- taking into account the problem of constructive relationships including the formation of a positive engagement with the therapist and the team;
- flexibility;
- intensity according to need;
- an individualized approach to care;
- good integration with other services available to the patient.

Our approach adheres firmly to these general features of treatment and, in our view, any treatment method for BPD needs to ensure that these requirements are met. We are not alone in this belief. The Practice Guideline for the Treatment of Patients with BPD issued by the American Psychiatric Association supports our view (American *et al.* 2001). The way in which we maintain and adhere to this set of principles in MBT is the subject of this chapter. Each characteristic is discussed in turn according to its underlying principle, the rationale behind it, and how it is implemented.

Structure

Principle

Structure is needed to form a framework around therapy that is neither intrusive nor inattentive and which, much like a benevolent uncle, can remain in the background but be around to catch things when they get out of control.

Structure describes the way in which a programme is put together, how it is implemented on a daily basis, how it is organized over the longer term, how predictable it is, and how clear its boundaries are in terms of roles and responsibilities. Inconsistency, lack of co-ordination, incoherence of response, unreliability, and arbitrariness are all antithetical to structure. But structure is not simply a 'how' phenomenon but also a state of mind in which both patients and therapists are able to think about aspects of treatment from a shared base. To this end, patients and therapists need to understand therapy, its purpose, and the reason for each of its components. This enables therapists to respond to common clinical problems consistently and fairly.

Rationale

It is generally accepted that borderline patients receive fragmented, inconsistent, unreliable, and reactive rather than proactive treatment within most psychiatric services. This is a result both of inadequacies in the services themselves and of the way that borderline patients interact with those services. For example patients commonly demand immediate help when distressed. This is rarely forthcoming and so their behaviour escalates with threats of suicide, self-harm, or violence. Initially these may be resisted by mental health professionals but gradually, almost imperceptibly, staff reactions become inconsistent and driven by panic with some offering intervention such as hospital admission whilst others refuse to consider it. In effect, services become unpredictable to the patient, mirroring the unstable self with which the patient is struggling and reinforcing unconstructive ways of managing crises. Just as the patient feels in danger of fragmenting, so the service splinters into uncoordinated bits of care with no stable core. Instead of presenting a view of the internal world of the patient which is stable and coherent—a major aim of our treatment so that it may be adopted as the reflective part of the patient's self—a chaotic and inconsistent view is offered which leads to confusion and further panic in the patient. A common response to this is to make a contract with the patient but this is rarely effective in maintaining structure of treatment (see p. 125) and simply acts as another hurdle through which the patient has to jump to obtain treatment.

Boundary violations

The gravest danger of failure to sustain treatment structure is of boundary violations. Establishing structure militates against regression and it is regression, along with unprocessed countertransference responses, which can stimulate transgression of patient/therapist boundaries. Regression in BPD remains a topic of debate and some practitioners suggest that the capacity for borderline patients to regress can be therapeutic. This belief has its origins in the work of

Balint (1968) Winnicott, and others, whose response to regression in patients was to provide a 'corrective experience'. In the analysis of Margaret Little, Winnicott is said to have extended sessions, held her hand, visited her daily at home during prolonged times of regression, and cradled her head to help her relive her birth. In our view there is no place for such actions in the treatment of borderline patients and maintenance of structure is as important for therapists as it is for patients, although if applied too rigorously it can become antitherapeutic. A balance needs to be struck which allows some regressive process but not enough to encourage acting-out and destabilization which in turn can lead to boundary violations.

A trainee psychiatrist became concerned about his relationship with a patient and so asked for supervision. He had offered to see a borderline patient once weekly for a maximum of 6 weeks following her discharge from hospital. The purpose of the meetings was to help her cope with the move from a long in-patient admission on an acute psychiatric ward to independent living. During session 4, the patient requested an extension to her sessions and he agreed to 2 additional meetings. At session 6 she reported suicidal feelings and stated that she felt the psychiatrist was the only person who was keeping her alive and without the sessions she would kill herself. His response was to suggest that the sessions could continue for as long as they were needed. Gradually the psychiatrist found himself offering the patient longer sessions since it was felt that more time was needed to help her understand what had happened to her prior to her admission to hospital. In order to accommodate the longer appointments, he gave her a regular time at the end of the clinic. Shortly afterwards, she refused to leave the clinic and lay on the floor crying, requiring him to spend a further hour talking to her to persuade her to leave. Eventually she agreed to leave if he picked her up and soothed her by holding her hand as she walked out of the building. Reluctantly he did this since it was late and there were no other staff in the clinic to help. He became more concerned when the patient stated that she realized that he loved her and stood outside his home. At this point he came for supervision.

This vignette demonstrates how the initial aim of sessions can be subverted and how inexperienced practitioners may fail to recognize this. The boundary of the original agreement had been crossed without patient or therapist understanding the potential consequences. The distinction between the tasks of the therapist and demands of the patient were further eroded as later and longer sessions were offered. This was the slippery slope that can lead towards a catastrophic boundary violation of a sexual relationship between patient and therapist. The initial agreement of 6 sessions should have been adhered to. If further help was necessary, for example because of suicidal feelings, this should have been discussed separately and appropriate treatment offered. Further, the trainee was working alone and without support and his offer of sessions should have been in a context of a carefully-considered treatment plan. With the more complex borderline patient it is important that practitioners do not work alone.

Gabbard (2003) describes a miscarriage of psychoanalytic treatment in which a suicidal borderline patient induces a belief in the analyst that only he can save her and as he becomes more frantic about her suicide risk and decides not to admit her to hospital, he agrees to allow her to spend a night at his house. Inevitably this leads to a sexual encounter and yet even though wracked with guilt the analyst continues to believe that 'at least I saved her from suicide'. Gabbard suggests that boundary transgressions such as these are directly related to the mismanagement of aggression and hatred. The analyst is determined to demonstrate that he is completely unlike abusive parents and that he can compensate the patient for her tragic past. In order to do so his analytic posture disavows any connection to an internalized representation of a bad object that torments the aggressor. He has named this 'disidentification with the aggressor' (Gabbard 1997). From our perspective it is an aspect of the patient's alien self which is lodged in the analyst but goes unrecognized and takes up occupation like an abscess that has to be drained. As the analyst becomes the alien self, there is a collapse in mentalization. The capacity for secondary representation and the 'as if' analytic process is lost; frequently enactment becomes inevitable, as a result of an omnipotent belief that the analyst can save the patient. Team approaches to severely suicidal borderline patients reduce the likelihood of boundary violations resulting from unrecognized countertransference responses and a collapse of mentalization.

Implementation

Structure is inherent in our treatment within its organization, its daily implementation, and over its longitudinal trajectory. On a daily basis, group and other therapeutic sessions start on time, therapist holidays and study time are arranged in advance, phone calls to patients are returned within the agreed time and so on. Use of a team approach protects against boundary violations and minimizes chances of therapist excess.

Structure starts with information. Each patient should be given written information about their treatment, their responsibilities, and therapist and team commitments (see Appendix 5). This is helped by patients themselves contributing to an introductory leaflet, perhaps by giving a personalized account of what treatment is like. Rules and regulations should be clear. It should not be a surprise to a patient that they are asked to leave treatment if they overtly threaten or act violently towards another person in the unit. Threats to people outside are a different matter and may become a focus of therapy rather than being a reason for discharge.

Treatment is structured around three phases: engagement in treatment, psychological work within a therapeutic relationship, and leaving treatment. Each phase requires a different approach from the therapist and the team. At the beginning of therapy the team is active, continually attempting to clarify problems, and engaging the patient. Individual sessions are structured with a primary aim of developing a formulation of the problems although a balance is maintained in sessions between therapist activity and patient freedom to explore.

Transference tracers (see p. 208) are used as a method to stimulate awareness in the patient of the patient–therapist relationship as a conduit for understanding wider problems. During the period of psychological work, the middle phase, the team allow more exploration using transference and countertransference, confront acting out, and challenge misunderstandings. At termination of treatment the anger, sense of abandonment, disappointment, and anxiety about finishing need to be sensitively explored and given meaning in terms of the patient's current and past life.

Consistency, constancy, and coherence

Principle

It is crucial to maintain consistency, constancy, and coherence of treatment because individuals with PDs detect and exploit inconsistency. Occasionally, this may be conscious and part of an attempt to fulfil personal desire.

A voluntary patient who was on an acute psychiatric ward following concerns about suicidal impulses met with her therapist saying that she was no longer suicidal but had no wish to return to her hostel accommodation because she did not like the other residents. She also admitted that she had continued to suggest to the nurses that she remained a suicide risk. After discussion about the underlying causes of her dislike of the others and her deception of the nurses, and exploration of how she might tackle the problems, it was agreed that she would leave hospital that day and make the appropriate arrangements with the nurses. However on return to the ward she told the nurses that it had been agreed that she was to remain for a further 3 days. This deception only came to light when the therapist contacted the ward later to arrange a time with the nurses to review the patient's progress and management on the ward.

Rationale

Although in the instance above there was no dispute between the therapist and the other mental health professionals, it transpired that two of the in-patient nurses had disagreed about the patient remaining in hospital. When disagreements occur more time can be spent on calming inter and intraprofessional disputes than on treating the patients themselves. From a psychodynamic perspective, inconsistency arises when 'splitting' occurs within teams. Splitting is regarded as arising for a number of reasons and, whenever it occurs, the most important point is to try to establish its meaning. Sometimes, externally-manifested splitting may simply be a result of poor team communication whilst at other times it may be a representation of the internal processes of the patient. Yet at other times splitting within therapists or teams can result from their own unresolved transferences and have little to do with the patient. An understanding of these processes will enable the team to offer consistency and will allow each member to be constant in their approach, since as long as the underlying reasons are understood, a mismatch between cause and intervention will be avoided. Different causes of splitting need different interventions. Splitting arising in the context of unresolved transferences needs teamwork rather than patientwork but splitting emanating from projections of the patient may need clinical discussion within the team followed by dialogue with the patient.

Inconsistency of therapists, for example in reactions to crises, management of acting out, and response to patient demand, is fuelled by incoherent and incomprehensible theory. A therapist who does not have a good grasp of the underlying theoretical basis of interventions is not able to think quickly and effectively during treatment and tailor interventions, within a coherent framework, to the uniqueness of each and every clinical situation. It is imperative that therapists work together to ensure that they all understand the process of treatment, the reasons for interventions, and how to implement them. Confusion within therapists will engender panic in the patient which in turn will lead to instability in their representational system. This is not to suggest that therapists should simply become rigid and firm whenever problems arise but that they need to maintain a stance of mentalization and consider the problem from that standpoint.

Implementation

Restricting the number of people involved in a patient's care to those whose roles and tasks are carefully defined reduces the chances of creating inconsistency. This needs to be done at the beginning of treatment via the professionals' meeting (see p. 164). Minimizing the number of individuals involved in the care of the patient may be difficult if treatment for the PD is separated from the psychiatric care although a 'divided functions' (see p. 145) approach with good collaboration in the context of a carefully-crafted treatment plan between therapists and psychiatrists is possible. Nevertheless consistency is likely to be improved by a specialist team approach.

As well as restricting the numbers of therapists, it is helpful to avoid changes wherever possible. This is of particular relevance in the treatment of BPD in which change in therapist is experienced as a re-enactment of earlier loss and abandonment and can lead to despair and subsequent drop-out. Senior, experienced figures who show few changes over time are clearly preferable and are likely to be able to work more effectively with problematic presentations of patients with PD than trainees who move posts at regular intervals.

As soon as any other professional becomes involved in the care of a patient, the new role and how the individual links with the core treatment team need to be discussed. This applies, for example, when the patient is admitted to medical or psychiatric hospital, the criminal justice system is involved, or housing support is necessary.

A patient in treatment was arrested for credit card theft and subsequent fraud. Reports were requested, the resulting sentence suspended and the individual placed on probation. The probation officer was invited to the next full review of the patient and his role discussed. It was agreed that the probation officer would fulfil his obligation to the patient and the courts by seeing the patient every two weeks to ensure that he understood the likely consequences of further criminal acts. For our part it was agreed that we would focus therapy on the underlying processes that had contributed to his criminal behaviour and address his difficulty of understanding the effects of his actions on others. Clear channels of communication were agreed between the probation service and the treatment team and it was agreed with the patient that the probation officer was to be included within the 'team confidentiality'.

Relationship focus

Principle

Because PD is characterized by problems in forming and maintaining constructive relationships, a primary focus of treatment has to be on an understanding of relationships.

Patients' difficulties in forming and maintaining constructive relationships are re-enacted in treatment between patient and therapist, between patient and team, between patient and patient, between team members, and between the team and the system within which they work. Even behaviour that interferes with continuation of therapy must be placed within a relationship context. It is inadequate to focus merely on the behaviour itself. In order to focus on the relationships within the treatment, setting a detailed understanding of the quality of other relationships made by the patient is necessary, including not only those with intimate partners but also those with housing and support workers. It is these relationships that often betray the patterns of interaction that create difficulties for the patient and others.

Rationale

Difficulty with forming stable relationships arises from problems in mentalization and reflective function. Impairment in these areas can be rectified through a focus on the relationship between patient and therapist. The juxtaposition of need for support and understanding from others with fear of intimacy and distrust of their motives leaves the borderline patient beleaguered and insecure. Relationships become unstable and rapidly changeable and a supportive friend can suddenly be experienced as malevolent and dangerous. Therapy must therefore attempt to embody a secure base and not to repeat this pattern of interpersonal interaction.

We have already discussed the tendency of borderline personality-disordered individuals to become non-reflective and impulsively reactive in emotionally-charged intimate relationships. Consequently, the therapist has to make considerable effort to monitor the level of reflectivity within the therapy relationship, especially when it becomes emotionally charged. Without a focus on the relationship, the essence of the patient's problems will be missed along with the chance of the patient making longer-term changes. For example a patient who acts violently may do so because they are unable to monitor their own internal state and are unable to take the perspective of the other who is considered hostile until proven otherwise. If there is only a focus on the violent act itself, the underlying mental processes that led to the outburst will remain unchecked and unaltered, ready to fuel the next action.

Implementation

The therapist maintains the focus on the therapeutic relationship by adopting a mentalizing stance (see p. 203) and carefully considering the transference and countertransference processes that become apparent within the treatment. These include not only the transferences manifested in the relationship with the individual therapist, but also those aroused within the groups and towards the service as a whole. The team seek to understand the atmosphere created by some patients, the feelings engendered in others, their own reactions to the patient, and to use this understanding to address the myriad relationships the patient has with others within the system of treatment. For example the relationship of the patient to the administrative staff may be as informative for treatment as that to the therapist.

A volatile patient was persistently hostile to his therapist, insulting her about her abilities and frequently commenting adversely on her appearance. This was in contrast to his contact with the reception and administrative staff to whom he was polite and friendly. In fact they only became aware of the difficulty of his hostility and threatening behaviour when typing a letter about his clinical treatment. They reported how pleasant he was to them and this led to a more detailed discussion in the clinical team about the patient's need to use hostility defensively in more intimate relationships. His relationship to the reception staff was civil because of its sociability in contrast to that to the therapist which was based on a closer attachment. This understanding was discussed with the patient and led to recognition on the part of the patient about his problems of experiencing warmth towards others.

Flexibility

Principle

The typically unstable lifestyle of patients with BPD indicates the need for flexibility in treatment.

Instability in lifestyle evinced by patients with BPD is inevitably manifested in relation to psychiatric services. Appointments are missed, treatment advice is disregarded, motivation to get help fluctuates rapidly, and professionals are regarded as wonderful at one moment and useless and ineffective at another. Such attitudes and actions should not be interpreted as indicating that the person does not want help, nor taken as an opportunity to discharge the patient, nor be seen as evidence that the treatment is working, nor used to fuel the narcissism of the therapist. What they do indicate is the need to be flexible. Initial attempts to engage a patient in treatment must be flexible, and once treatment itself has commenced, the team need to show willingness to compromise over the detail of treatment for a short time.

Rationale

Without flexibility, the borderline patient cannot be engaged in treatment. Their tenuous grasp of personal identity is weakened by any interpersonal encounter. This includes discussing their problems in detail with mental health professionals. Once their representation of themselves in relation to another becomes confused, their response can only be either to leave the apparently threatening situation or to resort to rigid representations of themselves in relation to the other. Both solutions stabilize their sense of self but at the same time undermine motivation for treatment. Treatment becomes dangerous and something to be avoided whilst at the same time being the very thing that they wish for. It is necessary for the therapists to ensure that the patient's sense of self remains stable during the early stages of treatment. Only later is the therapeutic relationship likely to withstand the panic associated with destabilization.

Implementation

In order to sustain a posture of flexibility the therapist needs to be aware of what not to do as much as what he should do. The borderline patient's tendency to default to rigid role assignment when representations are destabilized can easily be reciprocated by the therapist. The more the patient challenges the therapist, perhaps accusingly, or insists that the therapist has a particular state of mind, the greater the chance that the therapist will take an opposing view or will even take on the very state of mind of which they are accused, and thus become equally entrenched within a rigid system. This will lead to a battle that only the patient can experience as being won, even though it is a Pyrrhic victory since it usually heralds a breakdown in the relationship. Flexibility is maintained through the mentalizing stance of the therapist in which the task is an attempt to understand the state of mind of the patient at any given moment and to represent that understanding to the patient whilst at the same time ensuring countertransference responses are considered.

Flexibility needs to be built in to treatment delivery. A patient may be excessively anxious about group sessions and fail to attend on a regular basis but come to all his individual sessions. In this situation the flexible therapist focuses on the underlying anxieties leading to non-attendance at the groups. The inflexible therapist issues ultimatums about discharge from the programme for non-attendance at part of the programme. Permissiveness in this respect is a virtue as long as the aims of the sessions are clarified with the patient. In this example the anxieties of group interaction would become the focus of the individual sessions. If there was no return to the group within an agreed timescale, a review of treatment would become necessary since the individual therapy would be deemed ineffective in its purpose of helping the patient return to the group.

Intensity

Principle

In general, borderline patients require a level of care of sufficient intensity to stabilize social chaos and reduce dangerous and impulsive behaviour. The principle to follow is that patients should be given enough time to consider their problems and their treatment on their own but not too much to induce panic about what happened in the sessions or to leave them feeling abandoned during crises.

Intensity refers to the concentration of treatment in terms of frequency of sessions, depth of psychotherapeutic work, and the need for a comprehensive package of care. It needs to be balanced with length of treatment. Some patients may need high intensity for short periods and others low intensity for a longer time. The partial hospital programme and out-patient treatment are for 18 months but are of different intensities with the partial hospital (PH) treatment being organized on a daily basis over a week and the intensive out-patient (IOP) care being offered on a two-session-a-week basis.

It is almost impossible to gauge whether a borderline patient needs a high (in-patient), moderate (out-patient), or low (out-patient) level of concentration of care. Some patients need in-patient treatment, the most intensive level of care, during which individuals devote their whole time to treatment, often leaving their families and social supports. However, we do not yet know which patients benefit from which level of care (Chiesa *et al.* 2002*a*). Paradoxically, it may be individuals with less serious problems that benefit from such a high intensity of care whilst those that have the greatest need benefit from a lesser level of intensity of care. Borderline patients feel trapped in situations that require high levels of interpersonal interaction. Specialist in-patient units can be so frightening that a patient whose defences are brittle and whose sense of self is unstable may have to leave precipitously in an attempt to restabilize. In contrast those patients with greater stability can adapt to the situation and use the milieu to their advantage.

Rationale

Partial hospital and intensive out-patient care can probably provide an appropriate balance between need, safety, and dependency on the one hand and autonomy, risk, and self-reliance on the other. It is neither too much nor too little. Titration of intensity of interaction is problematic for borderline patients who have a tendency to become over-involved and so drive off the very person they want to be with.

A 28-year-old female patient started a relationship with a man who shared similar interests with her. She was aware of her tendency to demand too much and tried to control her urges to contact him excessively. However, on one occasion that she rang up he was not at home when she expected him to be so she started to 'text message' him every few minutes. Getting no response she sat outside his house all evening and when he returned home she demanded to know his movements, who he had been with, and what he had been doing. She became so insistent and threatening that eventually he called the police to have her removed.

As a result of the moderate intensity of treatment in partial hospital treatment, patients can test their assumptions and understanding about a situation very quickly as they attempt to reduce the volatility of their emotions. Difficulties can be reconsidered the following day within the PH programme or within a few days in the out-patient treatment. In addition, problems encountered within one setting can be discussed within another enabling the patient to link different aspects of treatment and to recognize that problems encountered in one setting can be reduced by working on the problem elsewhere. Often borderline patients believe that they have to tackle a problem head-on when in fact reflection elsewhere on the problem may produce the solution and reduce emotional volatility. Patients learn this quickly and commonly discuss problems encountered within group therapy during an individual session. This can easily be generalized. In the example above, it may have been better for the patient to discuss the situation with a friend before she acted on her intense feelings. Later during treatment this patient, who was then in another relationship, was able to manage her feelings and to discuss them within group therapy before she acted on them.

Implementation

Level of intensity is intrinsic to the programmes. Nevertheless, it is important to ensure that patients have adequate time between sessions to reflect, to rest, or to distract themselves. In the PH programme, some patients find that the time in between groups, say between a morning and an afternoon group, allows them to have a psychological rest whilst others feel it is wasted time and would rather have more to do, demanding a greater intensity of treatment. Overall demand for greater intensity is as likely to be defensive as it is a wish to change.

Individual approach to care

Principle

Each patient must be considered as an individual with his or her own problems and not seen as someone who has to fit in to a fixed treatment programme.

At the beginning of treatment, therapists have to use the programme flexibly, be flexible themselves, and not attempt to insist that the patient fits into all aspects of treatment immediately. Early in treatment, patients may find that attendance at groups provokes anxiety and, as already mentioned, we take a permissive stance to this problem as long as the anxiety is being addressed in the individual session. In addition, the group therapist may see the patient outside the group to discuss the patient's predicament.

The mentalizing stance taken by a therapist is intrinsically one in which all patients are considered as unique with their own history, their own development, and their own compromises. Within this stance the therapist has to ask how will this patient join in with this aspect of the programme, what may prevent him doing so, how can he be helped to participate given his individual circumstances and how can this be reconciled with the programme itself? On the other hand, it is important to ensure that individual care does not lead to excessive self-aggrandizement, special rules, or interference with the overall process of treatment, and all aspects of the programme should be given equal importance.

Rationale

Borderline patients do not like being considered as simply another one of many, any more than other patients, and indeed in many ways they have been subjected to more neglect and abuse than others so it is not surprising that they demand individual care. What they seek is attention and responsiveness from a person who is not pre-occupied with their own problems or whose 'mind is elsewhere'. Borderline patients rapidly recognize a therapist who is more involved with their own problems than with attempting to understand theirs and some will mercilessly attack such a therapist for repeating with them the very situation that they feel has led to their neglect—a carer who failed to have them in mind. Engendering an experience in a patient that their problems are the focus of an interview or discussion creates a situation in which the patient can realize that their mind and its processes are important and not secondary to the mind of others. Their minds have been ignored or become an extension of another mind so often that they have no sense of themselves. Individual attention can ameliorate this and be part of the process of change.

Implementation

Attentiveness, listening, challenge, and responsiveness need to be ever present in the interactions between staff and patient. Individual therapy enables a degree of personal attention to be provided, allows time to focus on specific problems of the person, and is a place for detailed exploration of more intimate aspects of difficulties. In qualitative feedback, patients, almost universally, report that the individual sessions are the most prized part of the programme during the early stages of treatment but are equally clear that the group sessions become more important during the later stages of treatment. A balance needs to be maintained throughout treatment with the individual care being offset by the group therapy. Borderline patients not only have to focus on their own mind but on that of others. It is the latter with which they may have more difficulty. Individual therapy on its own can become an enclave within which they take refuge, ruminating on themselves in order to protect themselves from the minds of others. Stability and progress is more apparent than real and it is all too easy to engage with patients in pretend mode (see p. 218). This ever present danger of the 'enclave' in individual therapy is tempered by the addition of group therapy and is part of our rationale for a combination of joint individual and group therapy rather than either alone.

Use of medication

Principle

Medication is an adjunct to psychotherapy. It enhances the effectiveness of psychotherapy, improves symptoms, stabilizes mood, and may help patients attend sessions. Prescription needs to take into account transference and countertransference phenomena and therefore needs to be integrated into the programme itself.

Rationale

Borderline patients experience volatility of emotion. Symptoms of anxiety and depression can be replaced rapidly by anger and elation; clarity of mind can be substituted by bewilderment and fragile grip on reality. This roller-coaster ride of rapid mood change and sudden perplexity which is particularly evident at the beginning of treatment may respond to medication. Symptom control by appropriate prescription in the context of the relationship with the treatment team may be instrumental in engaging a patient in treatment. The use of medication in BPD is well-reviewed by Soloff (1998) and summarized in the APA Guidelines (2001). Our prescribing practice follows those recommendations. Overall, the clinician needs to determine whether the primary symptoms are related to problems of affect control (lability of mood, rejection sensitivity, 'mood crashes' e.g. inappropriate, intense anger, temper outbursts; chronic 'emptiness', dysphoria, loneliness, anhedonia; and social anxiety and avoidance), impulsivity and sensation-seeking (risky, reckless behaviour; cognitive impulsivity—no reflective delay, low frustration tolerance; impulsive-aggression: recurrent assaultiveness, threats, property destruction; impulsive binges: drugs, alcohol, food, sex, spending; recurrent suicidal threats, behaviour, some self-mutilations), or cognitive perceptual disturbance (suspiciousness; paranoid ideation; ideas of reference; odd communication: vague, 'muddled' thinking, magical thinking; episodic distortions of reality: 'micro-psychotic' episodes, derealization, depersonalization, illusions, stress-induced hallucinations) and prescribe accordingly.

Whilst the evidence base (reviewed in Chapter 2 p. 50) suggests that medication may control the different groups of psychiatric symptoms of BPD, prescribing in practice is more complex.

Implementation

Medication is prescribed by the psychiatrists within the team but is discussed by the whole team. If the psychiatrist is the patient's therapist, medication is considered by the other psychiatrist.

In nearly all trials of medication in BPD drop-out rates are high and non-compliance with dosage and frequency is common. These findings concur with clinical experience. Borderline patients take medication intermittently, fail to follow prescribing guidance, and may use prescribed medication in overdose when in crisis. These facts alone suggest that prescribing needs to be done carefully and only within the context of a trusting therapeutic relationship. The use and effects of medication need to be discussed with patients prior to prescribing, the target symptoms clearly identified, an agreement made about how long the drug is to be used, and a method to monitor its effect on symptoms established. Most important is the patient's agreement to take medication in the first place and the role of the doctor is initially to provide information and to remain neutral about whether the patient takes medication or not. This is not the same as declining to give a recommendation of a specific drug for an explicit reason. After information has been given to the patient, the prescriber may make a recommendation but should not become overly engaged in persuading the patient to follow advice. The more a prescriber attempts to convince a patient to take a drug the greater the patient's resistance may be, feeling that their moods and behaviour have become intolerable to the treatment team. Often it is helpful to explain to a patient that medication may help him use therapy more effectively, that it is an adjunct to therapy and not a replacement, and that if it does not help over an agreed period it can be reduced and stopped.

Borderline patients seek quick results, yet effects of medication may take some time to become apparent, so it is necessary to maintain their co-operation even if they experience little initial benefit. The best way to do this is to take an interest in how the patient responds to the tablets and to arrange regular meetings to discuss symptom change, side-effects, and changes in dose. In general we expect patients to take medication for a minimum of 2–4 weeks unless there are intolerable side-effects and this 'rule' is agreed when medication is started. Only then will we consider the use of another drug assuming the patient has taken the original drug according to prescription. If the patient stops the drug before the agreed time no other drug is prescribed until the 2–4-week-period is completed. This reduces the demand for drug after drug when no effect occurs within a few days and prevents 'creeping' polypharmacy. Soloff (Soloff *et al.* 1993) has suggested that the exception to these kinds of rules is antipsychotic medication such as haloperidol and that the benefits may occur rapidly but wane within a few weeks. Discontinuation may therefore be appropriate after a few weeks although there remains little information on the use of newer antipsychotics. Discontinuation of medication needs to be done carefully and many clinicians believe that borderline patients are more sensitive to side-effects and withdrawal effects of medication than other patients although there is no evidence that this is the case; nevertheless reducing medication slowly whilst implementing another is probably the best course.

Maintaining sensible rules is harder than it sounds because patient demand and clinician judgement are influenced by transference and countertransference phenomena. For this reason, we integrate prescribing into the treatment programme and ensure that other channels of obtaining psychotropic medication are blocked, for example from the general practitioner. If patients obtain medication elsewhere it becomes a split off part of treatment, which the patient can idealize when therapy is difficult and use to dismiss therapy as useless.

Equally, the reverse may occur and medication may be denigrated at times of positive transference. Both medication and psychotherapy are important for effective treatment of BPD.

If transference and countertransference are not taken into account, the psychiatrist will prescribe when it would be better to help the patient manage his own symptoms or not prescribe when it would be of benefit to the patient. On the one hand, borderline patients may demand medication in the context of an attack on the therapist using it as a way of expressing dissatisfaction with therapy and yet on the other, they may use it as a transitional object representing a continuing relationship with the treatment team or doctor which helps retain stability during breaks. When it is recommended, they may refuse to consider it even when furnished with all the information, feeling that it is to be used to control their mind; they may use it defensively to sedate themselves so that they 'can't think and feel'; or rely on it excessively believing that they have not developed the capacity to control or reduce their own symptoms. In all cases it is important to understand the meaning within the context of the transference and countertransference relationship because all these reactions are determined by the state of the patient–therapist relationship. If the patient idealizes the psychiatrist, medication is more likely to have a beneficial effect than if he is denigrated but transferences of the borderline patient are rarely so straightforward and an idealization of one team member may be accompanied by dismissal of another which complicates prescribing further.

The psychiatrist is not immune from countertransference responses even if his task is solely to look after medication. He may himself find it difficult to process his feelings and prescribe in a desire to 'rescue' the patient or in a vain attempt to 'do something'. These reactions may account for the high number of medications borderline patients take over time even though polypharmacy is rarely recommended. Zanarini (personal communication) found that at 2, 4, and 6 years after an index hospitalization 90% of her borderline sample were taking at least 3 medications at each time point. A patient who is anxious or suicidal may become demanding and make the psychiatrist anxious which in turn makes him prescribe—his capacity to mentalize is eroded. Conversely the patient who wishes to stop medication may be persuaded to continue it because of the psychiatrists' fear of relapse. Often it is patients who ask to reduce the number of medications that they are taking and many patients begin taking tablets on an intermittent basis without telling their psychiatrist for fear of causing disappointment.

In order to reduce the ill-effects of transference and countertransference and to increase their positive effects on decisions about the use of medication, any initiation of medication should be discussed within the team, the reasons for its use defined, and a plan of implementation developed. The psychiatrist should not act unilaterally. Rarely is medication best prescribed in an emergency. At those times it is best to work with the patient's current mental state and to understand it in terms of recent interpersonal events, the individual therapy, and the group work.

Following a group, a patient demanded to see the team psychiatrist to discuss her medication. She had been referred to the unit recently and, in common with usual practice, her medication had not been changed or discussed in detail until both she and the team felt that they 'knew' each other better. She was taking an SSRI, an antipsychotic, a mood stabilizer, and night sedation. In the discussion she asked for something else because she felt that the medication was not working. She 'felt awful, depressed, and anxious' and the psychiatrist found her to be oversensitive with some paranoid symptoms. The history of medication use was confused and the patient was unclear about when she had started different drugs and which was helpful. It was apparent that she had been on many different medications over the years, most of which she dismissed as useless. As the doctor discussed each drug she said that she did not want to stop it and it became evident that she wanted to remain on her present medication but have something in addition. Feeling annoyed and frustrated and wanting to end the interview, the doctor began considering changing the antidepressant but realized that this was more out of annoyance with the patient's attitude and his impotence to suggest anything helpful. In keeping with our treatment and considering his countertransference the doctor asked her if she had suggested changing her medication because she, herself, had felt upset in the group and did not know what to do about it (the patient's frustration and annoyance). The patient did talk about her distress in the group and her own feelings of not knowing how to cope with them but still wanted some medication. The doctor agreed that this would be discussed by the whole team and that he would see her again the following day.

Some clinicians attribute deceit, cunning, and dishonesty to borderline patients. If this is their prevailing attitude they should not treat them. More complicated is a situation when the treating therapist or psychiatrist feels that a patient is being deceitful and may, for example, appear compliant but is actually hoarding medication whilst developing a suicide plan. Initially this should be discussed in the sessions and be reported to the psychiatrist who may feel that the evidence of stockpiling is adequate to stop prescribing altogether. Even more problematic are cases where the patient continues to deny the concern of the team, maintains a questionable innocence, and takes the medication at a lower-than-prescribed dose so that some can be accumulated for a later overdose. This must become a focal aspect of therapy sessions, particularly in terms of deceit, secrecy, and suicide planning.

Summary of guidelines for psychopharmacological treatment

- consider the primary symptom complex e.g. affect dysregulation, impulsivity, cognitive-perceptual disturbance; and current transference and countertransference themes;

- discuss implementation of medication within the treatment team;
- educate the patient about reasons for medication, possible side-effects, expected positive effects;
- make a clear recommendation but allow the patient to take the decision and do not try to persuade the patient to take the medication;
- agree a length of time for trial of medication (unless intolerable side-effects) and do not prescribe another drug during this time even if the patient stops the drug;
- prescribe within safety limits, for example giving prescriptions weekly;
- see the patient at agreed intervals to discuss medication and its effects. Initially this may be every few days to encourage compliance, to monitor effects, and to titrate the dose;
- do not be afraid to suggest stopping a drug if no benefit is observed and the patient experiences no improvement.

Integration of modalities of therapy

In Chapter 3 we discussed the importance of the attachment relationship in the formation of an unstable self-structure and the development of BPD. Disruption of early affectional bonds sets up maladaptive attachment patterns and undermines a range of capabilities vital to normal social development, of which affect regulation and mentalization are of overriding importance. Activation of the attachment system in therapy results in dramatic, unpredictable shifts in the patient's emotional state and construction of himself and others. The borderline patient wants a relationship for both comfort and safety from emotional pain but also fears it, viewing it as malevolent and dangerous. This dynamic nature is particularly acute within psychoanalytically-orientated therapy in which the intimacy of the process can rapidly activate desires and anxieties. The intensity and disorganization of the interaction compromises mentalization, emotion becomes uncontrolled, and the patient either closes down his mind or leaves therapy. The strength of this reaction may explain the high drop-out rate in many programmes. Provision of individual and group therapy allows splitting of transference, softens the emotional intensity, and protects the patient from the consequences of too powerful an activation of their attachment process. The patient can take refuge within individual therapy when group therapy becomes frightening or seek sanctuary in the group when individual therapy becomes too difficult.

The simultaneous provision of group and individual therapy is an ideal arrangement within which to encourage mentalization. A patient who is excessively anxious and aroused in group therapy will be unable to explore his problems within that context and so the individual therapy session becomes the place of safety where he can reflect critically and thoughtfully about himself in the group. At these times, the individual therapist ensures that the patient concentrates on his problems within the group, the interpersonal context in the group that may be driving the anxiety, and how his fears relate to current and past aspects of his life. This requires careful co-ordination between the individual and group therapists to minimize adverse consequences of splitting of the transference and to make certain the patient moves towards mental balance rather than continuing to manage anxiety through splitting, idealization, denigration, and withdrawal.

The danger of patient and therapist unwittingly slipping into pretend mode is discussed in Chapter 7 (see p. 218). The combination of group therapy and individual therapy protects against this development because patients who try to take refuge within individual therapy continue to be challenged within the group by other patients who rapidly detect pretence and confront anyone who hides behind intellectual defences and false understanding.

Conclusions

The essential organizational features outlined here are not definitive features of MBT but characteristics of a well-organized and thoughtful programme of treatment. They are easily transferred to different settings to provide a framework for the application of more specific treatment intervention and there is little dispute about their importance as an essential aspect for effective intervention. But it is equally probable that they are insufficient for good outcome. In the next chapter we will consider more specific interventions used in MBT.

7 Strategies of treatment

The overall aim of our treatment is to help the patient to establish a more robust sense of self so that he can develop more secure relationships. For this to happen, group and individual therapy need to be co-ordinated, interventions require focus, emotional expression must be brought within a normal range, and coherence created within a patient's personal narrative. But most of all, as we have continually emphasized, patients have to develop a capacity to mentalize if there is to be a buffer between feeling and action, impulses are to be caught before they become overwhelming, and motivations of self and other can be monitored and understood. In order to achieve these aims, four core strategies are recommended—(1) enhancing mentalization, (2) bridging the gap between affects and their representation, (3) working mostly with current mental states, and (4) keeping in mind the patient's deficits. Many therapists recommend the use of the 'real relationship' in addition to the therapeutic relationship in the treatment of borderline personality disorder (BPD), despite its dangers, and so this topic, including working with recovered memories, is discussed at the end of the chapter.

Enhancing mentalization

The mentalizing stance is an ability on the therapist's part to question continually what internal mental states both within his patient and within himself can explain what is happening now.

A therapist needs to maintain a mentalizing stance in order to help a patient develop a capacity to mentalize. Why is the patient saying this now? Why is the patient behaving like this? Why am I feeling as I do now? What has happened recently in the therapy or in our relationship that may justify the current state? These are typical questions that the therapist will be asking himself within the mentalizing therapeutic stance. Understanding aspects of these questions will allow the therapist to link external events, however small, to powerful internal states which are otherwise experienced by the patient as inexplicable, uncontrollable, and meaningless. The therapist needs always to try to understand what is confusing to the patient, how to make some sense of it, and how to clarify it. In effect the mentalizing stance enables the patient and therapist to develop a language that adequately frames and expresses the complexity of relationships, motivation, and internal states.

The challenge for the therapist is to maintain a mentalizing therapeutic stance in the context of countertransference responses that may provoke the therapist to react rather than to think. In fact countertransference enactments are inevitable and it is necessary to be permissive (non-self-persecutory) about them whilst trying to guard against them. The therapist has to accept that in order to stay in mental proximity with a patient he must occasionally find himself acting with the patient in a manner that would normally be uncharacteristic of him (e.g. be critical of the patient, lose his or her temper, become excessively familiar etc.). He enacts, becomes the vehicle for, an 'alien' part which is located within the self of the patient (see p. 89). If the therapist is to be any use to the patient, he has to become what the patient needs him to be. Yet it is clear that if he becomes that person, he can be of no help to the patient. The therapist's aim should be the achievement of a state of equipoise between the two—allowing himself to do as required yet trying to retain in his mind a clear and coherent image of the state of the mind of the patient i.e. maintaining a mentalizing stance, and remaining able to communicate that state of mind to the patient in an understandable way without forcibly pushing parts of the alien self back to the patient too quickly.

A focus on psychological process and the 'here and now' rather than on mental content in the present and past is implicit in this approach. An important indicator of underlying process and the 'here-and now' is the manifest affect. Therapists need to develop an awareness of prevailing affect if they are to be able to grasp the internal struggle of the patient. Identifying affect is an initial step and is best done through exploration of current emotions. There is no place for a therapist telling the patient how he feels even if the therapist believes that he knows how his patient feels. Telling a patient how they feel will confuse the patient who will become uncertain about whose feeling it is that is being described. Is it theirs, the therapist's, or someone else's? This type of interaction will lead to instability of the patient's self-structure, resulting in panic, the use of projective mechanisms, denial, or even withdrawal from the session. Patients have to become aware of their own feelings and accompanying representations, describe them bit by bit, and build a context in which they can make sense of them, if they are to feel that they are theirs. The therapist must avoid becoming an iatrogenic agent who creates affects in the patient and then explores them in terms of the patient. Only after an affect has been identified accurately by the patient within the therapeutic relationship can exploration begin of the psychological processes being mobilized to manage its mental and physical effect.

Bridging the gaps

There is a gap between the primary affective experience of the borderline patient and its symbolic representation. This gap has to be bridged in therapy if the reflective process is to develop with a view to strengthening the secondary representational system.

The core of psychological therapy with individuals with severe personality disorder (PD) is the enhancement of reflective processes. The therapist must not only help the patient understand and label emotional states but also enable him to place them within a present context with a linking narrative to the recent and remote past. The gap between inner experience and its representation engenders impulsivity. The therapist needs to create a therapeutic milieu in which the experiences of the patient can be transformed from confusion to meaning, especially in terms of interpersonal understanding. This is achieved not only by interpretations of moment-to-moment changes in the patient's emotional stance but also by focusing the patient's attention on the therapist's experience. This enables an exploration of a mind by a mind within an interpersonal context.

The patient comes in looking somewhat agitated and frightened, sits down and remains silent.
Therapist: 'You appear to see me as frightening today'.
Patient (challengingly): 'What makes you say that'?
Therapist: 'You had your head down and avoided looking at me'.
Patient: 'Well, I thought that you were cross with me'.
Therapist: I am not aware of being cross with you so it may help if we think about why you were concerned that I was.

Here the therapist has rightly focused on a simple interchange that shows how he believes the patient is experiencing him, and has avoided describing a complex mental state to the patient in one large interpretation. Interpreting a more complex psychological process, however accurate or inaccurate it may be, is likely to destabilize the patient who will become more and more uncertain and confused about himself as the contradictions and uncertainties are pointed out. The result will be an attempt by the patient to adhere to a rigid, schematic representation of the relationship between patient and therapist, which in this situation is likely to have a paranoid flavour. It is equally important not to focus on a patient's conflicts and ambivalence (conscious or unconscious). Change is generated in borderline patients by brief, specific interpretation and clear answers to questions. In this example the therapist identifies simply and straightforwardly why he had suggested that he thought the patient was frightened of him. The next move in the session is to consider why the patient has become concerned that the therapist is angry with him but only after it has been made clear by the therapist that he is not.

To explore aspects of the patient's experience without this being apparent is experienced as persecuting and cruel, especially at the beginning of treatment, and exploration can only be done in this way when a transitional area has been established in therapy.

The ever present danger in trying to 'bridge the gap' is that when the therapeutic relationship intensifies through confrontation and complex interpretation, this highlights a patient's difficulties in creating a distance between internal and external reality. So, the therapist's task is in some way analogous to that of the parents who first make the situation secure and then create a frame for creative play—except in this case it is thoughts and feelings that need to become accessible through the creation of such a transitional area. In the move towards mentalization, the therapist must get used to working with its precursors, namely mind states in which internal is identical with external, ideas form no bridge between inner and outer reality, and feelings have no context. The task is the elaboration of teleological models into intentional ones, psychic equivalence into symbolic representation, and linking affects to representation. Integrating the dissociated modes of the patient's functioning where sometimes nothing feels real (certainly not words or ideas) and at other moments words and ideas carry unbelievable potency and destructiveness can seem an awesome task. Yet progress is only conceivable if the therapist is able to become part of the patient's pretended world, trying to make it real, while at the same time avoiding entanglement with the equation of thoughts and reality.

Entanglement leads to the activation of the inevitable destructiveness often found in borderline patients in relation to the therapeutic enterprise. It is rarely adequately dealt with by confrontation or interpretation of aggressive intent. Rather, comments are more helpfully aimed at the emotional antecedents of enactments—the emotions that cause confusion and disorganization. The therapist has to remain calm under fire, whilst at the same time being able to demonstrate that words, thoughts, and discussion are eminently more expressive than behaviour. In order to do this, the therapist may have to show something of himself at certain moments, for example through humour or irreverence.

In this way the patient will experience the relationship as a place in which ideas can be played with. In the transitional area thus created, thoughts, feelings, and ideas neither belong internally nor externally and so their power to overwhelm is lost—they are no longer either the therapist's or the patient's, but shared.

Failure in the transitional area in borderline patients receives some support from attachment theory which has stressed the common characteristic, shared by the ambivalently attached/pre-occupied and borderline groups, 'to check for proximity, signalling to establish contact by pleading or other calls for attention or help, and clinging behaviours' (Gunderson 1996). All these phenomena imply a difficulty in maintaining a stable representation of the other and the need to use the therapist as a transitional object, an extension of the patient who lacks separate identity and feelings (Modell 1963). The importance of transitional relatedness in these patients is also demonstrated by striking histories of using transitional objects (Morris *et al.* 1986) as well as bringing such objects to hospital more frequently than patients with other psychiatric disorders (Cardasis *et al.* 1997).

Transference

With borderline patients, transference is not used in the clinical situation as a simple repetition of the past or as a displacement and should not be interpreted in this way. Transference is experienced as real, accurate, and current by the borderline patient and needs to be accepted by the treatment team in that way.

In order to clarify our use of transference we shall use a somewhat artificial contrast between 'classical', and 'modern' (or 'contemporary') practice and thought. The most straightforward 'classical' definition of the dynamic aspect of transference may be summarized as a process by which the patient transfers onto his therapist those past experiences and strong feelings—dependency, love, sexual attraction, jealousy, frustration, hatred—which he used to experience in relation to significant persons such as his mother, father, or siblings earlier in life. The patient is unaware of this false connection and experiences the feelings not as if they are from the past but as directly relevant to the present. This viewpoint suggests that interpretation of the transference uncovers and allows the re-experiencing or reconstruction of the past in the present and, once insight into it has been achieved, helps to overcome past trauma; it emphasizes reconstruction of the past. It is important to understand that we do not use transference with borderline patients in this way.

In contrast the 'modern' view sees transference not so much as the inexorable manifestation of unconscious mental forces, but rather as the emergence of latent meanings and beliefs, organized around and evoked by the intensity of the therapeutic relationship. In clinical application there is a de-emphasis on reconstruction. Present-day wishes, character formations, and personal expectations are seen as being influenced by the past but not simply representing it in a straightforward way. Transference has thus become a much wider concept involving the interplay between the patient and therapist, representing the conflicts of the mind and reflecting the interactions of the internal object representations; it is a medium through which the individual's internal drama is 'played out' in treatment; a new experience influenced by the past, rather than a repetition of an earlier one.

In this modern view, the dynamic is in the present, often only remotely influenced by an infantile constellation from the past. Further, transference is seen as a positive therapeutic force, not simply as a representation of the past that if interpreted can lead to insight, but as a probe used by the individual to elicit or provoke responses from the therapist or others that are essential for a stable representation of the self. Transference is an interactive process by which the patient responds to selected aspects of the treatment situation, sensitized by past experience.

In summary, in borderline patients it is important to understand that:

- transference is not used in the clinical situation as a simple repetition of the past or as a displacement;
- interpretation of transference as a repetition or as a displacement should not occur;
- transference is experienced as real, accurate, and current by the patient and needs to be accepted by the treatment team in that way;
- transference is used as a demonstration of alternative perspectives—a contrast between the patient's perception of the therapist or of others in the group and that of others.

Interpretation in a direct manner simply makes the borderline patient feel that whatever is happening in therapy is unreal. This leads to a dissociative experience and a sense that their own experience is invalid. If such transference interpretations are made, the patient is immediately thrown into a pretend mode and gradually patient and therapist may elaborate a world, which however detailed and complex, has little experiential contact with reality. Alternatively, the patient either angrily and contemptuously drops out of therapy feeling that their problems have not been understood, or mentally withdraws from treatment, or establishes a false treatment which looks like therapy but is in fact two individuals talking to themselves.

It is important that exploration within the transference is built up over time. At first, reference to different perspectives and internal influences that may be driving them should be simple and to the point. There is no place for complex statements implying a veridical truth as seen by the therapist. Both patient and therapist have to start from a position of 'not knowing' but trying to understand. In order to build up this exploratory aspect to the therapy, we use transference tracers.

Transference tracers:

- are interventions used early in therapy that highlight problematic areas, especially about different perspectives;
- gradually focus on the relationship between patient and therapist to highlight patterns of behaviour and ways of relating to others;
- do not attempt to define and explore in detail alternative perspectives;
- are not used as a confrontation.

Their purpose is to light the night sky, point the way, give a subtle hint of alternative perspectives, and not to confront or to challenge.

In an initial assessment, a patient told the therapist about a number of incidents in which he felt that people failed to understand him. He detailed numerous encounters with mental health professionals in which he had dismissed their attempts to help him as futile and pathetic, often walking out of meetings. The assessor asked about other relationships where he might have behaved in a similar manner and it turned out that his relationships commonly ended with dismissal of others and this had included his mother whom he described as 'unbelievably stupid'. The assessor pointed out that in treatment, his feeling that someone in the team was stupid would be important to watch out for since it might herald a breakdown in the therapeutic relationship.

This statement by the assessor is a transference tracer linking previous experience to future action. The therapist does not invoke links to the historical past, for example by including the mother.

After 3 months the patient persistently told his therapist that he was stupid and eventually walked out of the session. The therapist followed the patient out of the room and suggested 'you seem to think that I am stupid whenever you feel let down; maybe that is your way of dealing with feeling so disappointed in me'.
Patient: 'Too bloody right I am disappointed in you.'
Therapist: 'Then tell me what it is that is so disappointing'.
Patient: 'Why should I? You should know but you are too stupid to realize'.
Therapist: 'That is why I am asking you to tell me. You may remember that when we first met that we realized that at some point you would feel I was stupid and that we would have to understand how accurate that was if we were not to repeat the pattern of your previous treatments'.

The therapist has not focused on the destructive component in relation to the therapeutic enterprise by confrontation or interpretation of aggressive intent. The patient's actions and dismissal are best understood as self-protective and interpretation is aimed at the emotional antecedents of the enactment and the emotions that cause confusion and disorganization. If the initial suggestion that the patient's dismissive attitude is related to feeling let down is rejected, the therapist should accept the dismissal and not challenge it further, although he may suggest to the patient that this remains an important area to explore by saying—'you know, that feeling you have that I am stupid seems to apply to others as well and it may be important that we think further about it at some point'. The therapist should not push the theme early in therapy; rather, the task in initial sessions is to identify dominant relationship themes and tentatively link them to therapy and the treatment process. Initially, relationship themes may be best defined by exploring the patient's relationships outside the treatment setting or towards the hospital itself or perhaps the treatment team rather than directly exploring the relationship between patient and therapist. Direct statements about the relationship between the patient and therapist may stimulate anxiety and be experienced as abusive. Only towards the middle or end of therapy when stable internal representations have been established is it likely to be safe to use the 'heat' of the relationship between patient and therapist in a more direct way to explore different perspectives. Even then it needs to be remembered that change is generated in borderline patients by brief, specific interpretation.

We are not suggesting therapists avoid transference, which is essential for effective treatment, but that their use of it is incremental and moves from distance to near depending on the patient's level of anxiety. Most patients with severe BPD rapidly become anxious in intimate situations and too great a focus on the patient–therapist relationship leads to panic which is manifested as powerful and, sometimes uncontrollable, expressions of feeling.

Retaining mental closeness

Retaining mental closeness is akin to the process by which the caregiver's empathic response provides the infant with feedback on his or her emotional state to enable developmental progress. The task of the therapist is to represent accurately the feeling state of the patient and its accompanying internal representations.

We have already discussed the concept of 'mirroring' (see p. 64) as being a crucial interpersonal interchange within an attachment context. It is through this process that the child acquires a sensitivity to self-states and eventually the states of others. This sensitivity is an essential element in the development of the representational system and is dependent on the internalization of the caregiver's mirroring response to the infant's distress—the caregiver's empathic response provides the infant with feedback on his or her emotional state and, as long as it is marked as representing the child's mental state and is reasonably accurate, it leads to developmental progress. Retaining mental closeness is akin to this process and the task of the therapist is to represent accurately the feeling state of the patient and its accompanying internal representations. In addition, the therapist must be able to distinguish between his own experiences and those of the patient and be able to demonstrate this distinction to the patient—marking (see p. 66). Fortunately for the therapist, the accuracy of the identification of the patient's feeling state need only be 'good enough'. A slight mismatch or discrepancy between the representation of the patient's state by the therapist and the actual state of the patient may be a main driver of psychological development. A mismatch compels patients and therapists to examine their own internal states further and to find different ways of expressing them if communication is to continue. In addition, the therapist has to be able to examine his own internal states and be able to show that they can change according to further understanding of the patient's state. In this respect countertransference is crucial.

Countertransference

There are different types of countertransference that need consideration in the treatment of borderline patients. Countertransferences are generally considered as emotions that arise within the therapist as a result of the patient's treatment of him as an object of one of the patient's earlier relationships. However, other countertransferences are different and akin to empathic responses, based on the analyst's resonances with his patient rather than resulting from an evocation of earlier object relationships. These 'concordant' countertransferences (Racker 1968) are extremely common in treatment of patients with PD and link with affective attunement (Stern 1985), empathy, mirroring, and a perspective that aspects of all relationships are based on emotional identifications between individuals. The therapist 'reads' the patient's behaviour and responds in a complementary manner, which is in turn 'read' by the patient. One feeling state has been knowable to another and both sense that the transaction has taken place without the use of language. In our terms this is 'implicit' mentalization with clear marking of the experience by the therapist, which will be met by an equally 'implicit' response on the part of the patient.

In order to retain a mental closeness, the therapist has to maintain a benign split within himself to allow a constant interplay between thinking and feeling, between himself and the patient, between his experience and the events the patient is talking about. Sandler (1993) uses the term 'primary identification' for an equivalent process and regards it as similar to automatic mirroring. Thus, if the therapist has a direct emotional reaction to a patient's actions or behaviour, and this reaction is not one that he is being unconsciously pushed into, then this should be seen as primary identification. If such identifications stimulate unresolved unconscious wishes within the therapist, conflict arises, which results in the mobilization of defences, the formation of blind-spots within therapy, and a distancing of the therapeutic relationship. For example feelings of inadequacy or importance engendered in the therapist by the patient may lead to annoyance or overzealous attempts to help the patient.

A therapist reported that he had recommended to a patient that she should not attend group therapy whilst he was away since he believed that she was terrified that another patient would threaten her and he would not be there to support her. In supervision it became clear that he had begun to believe that his skills were necessary to protect the patient when, in fact, the group therapist was perfectly capable of ensuring that the patient's anxieties within the group were managed appropriately. Following discussion and exploration of the therapist's wish to protect the patient it seemed that the patient's apparent vulnerability had evoked a feeling in the therapist that was related to his own need to protect vulnerable young females.

This example illustrates how retaining mental closeness has its dangers and yet is necessary if therapy is to be effective. It also underscores the need for supervision to ensure that therapists remain 'on task' and do not become 'entangled'. Every therapist is prone to failures of mentalization, countertransference enactments, and formation of blind spots and there is no doubt that borderline patients may suddenly evoke strong feelings which, if unprocessed, can lead to a mental collapse in the therapist.

Working with current mental states

There can be little therapeutic gain from continually focusing in the past. The focus needs to be on the present state and how it remains influenced by events of the past rather than on the past itself. If the patient persistently returns to the past, the therapist needs to link back to the present, move the therapy into the 'here and now', and consider the present experience.

This is often easier said than done. Many patients are, themselves, lost in past traumas, ruminating about abuse, fantasizing about revenge, and demanding retribution. Particularly during states of intense emotion, the patient may be unable either to hear the therapist's comments or recognize their attempts to address the situation.

A patient began screaming at the therapist, declaring that no one understood how the abuse by her father when she was 8 years old had ruined everything. She stated that there was nothing that anyone could do since her body had been interfered with and he had 'got away with it' since no one had believed her. Her father was a well-respected member of the local community and so when she had told her teachers her claims were dismissed. Whilst saying all this, the patient began walking around the room and hitting her chest saying 'see, see, see, there is no body left'. The therapist suggested that he was trying to listen to how she felt the abuse had ruined her life so that they could work on how to stop the trauma being so powerful in her life now. The patient just screamed at him and continued hitting herself so he continued to talk about ensuring that there was some session left otherwise her feeling that no one understood the effect of the abuse would remain.

In such an emotionally-charged situation, the therapist needs to continue to talk to the patient as calmly as possible whilst keeping to the task of the session, which is to help the patient to control emotion so that the exploration can carry on. Gradually this may increase the patient's capacity to reflect on herself in the present, even when experiencing powerful feelings either from or about the past. The therapist's brief statement about wanting to have some session left is not translated into an extensive interpretation, for example taking the abuse that the patient is inflicting on him as representing the abuse that she suffered from her father. Borderline patients find such a mental leap extremely difficult and will become confused, wondering what the therapist is talking about. It is much better to focus on the current problem, which in this example is the effect on the session of the patient's overwhelming emotion.

Simple statements such as the one given here, even though verging on use of metaphor (see below) by linking the body with the session, are more effective than extensive interpretation.

Anger and other strong emotions about the past have to be re-orientated towards the present. Most people bring anger and other feelings about earlier situations into their present life and in therapy it is necessary to look for the target of the feeling in the present rather than leave it hanging in the past. The target is often the therapist, once a therapeutic alliance has been forged, but it is not necessarily so and the therapist must also consider others in the patient's current life before linking the feelings solely to some aspect of the therapeutic relationship.

In order to work closely with the current mental state it is always necessary to consider which elements of the patient are projected, which are not, and whether, at any particular time, the therapist is maintaining a mentalizing stance and able to consider their own mental state as well as that of the patients.

A patient said that he was not going to say anything to anyone because he could not be bothered. The therapist responded by saying that he himself could be bothered to talk and it struck him that the patient often responded by withdrawing when he felt that people did not like him. The therapist gave an example of how the patient had believed only a day earlier that other patients in his group did not like him (illustrating the transfer between therapists of information from one aspect of treatment into another) and yet he had denied having such feelings. The patient said 'so what'? The therapist answered that the 'so what' was that it could be easier for the patient to insist that others did not like him than it was to accept that he did not like others. In effect he could remain stable and unconcerned if it was nothing to do with him but it left him feeling empty—'there was nothing to say'. This statement led the patient to think a bit more about who he did not like and why and whether this was linked to his feeling of emptiness. Nevertheless the session ended with the patient continuing to feel that nobody liked him but this is to be expected since the exploration of the patient's perspective and its discrepancy with that of others needs to be repeatedly reconsidered within many other current contexts before both patient and therapist can be confident about whose feeling is whose. Only when this aspect is clear can the therapist begin to address the dispositional aspects of the psychological process.

- Use of metaphor, conflict, and interpretation of unconscious phantasy

In working with current mental states it is essential to avoid using metaphor as the primary discourse with a patient. Borderline patients have a poorly-developed ability to use secondary representation and limited symbolic binding of internally-experienced affects so the use of metaphor is relatively meaningless to the patient. Rather than heightening the underlying meaning of the discourse, use of metaphor is more likely to induce bewilderment and incomprehension.

A patient talked in a group about how the roof of her house was leaking and there was a slow drip of water causing her carpets to get wet and become saturated. She was angry about it and did not know what to do and asked the group for help. Another patient asked if she had demanded that the Housing Association came and fixed it but she said that they did nothing and that each time she had asked them to fix a problem they had never taken it seriously or done anything. When she had told them about the leak, the Housing Worker had said that he would come round but he had not which she assumed meant that he did not like her. The group continued to discuss possible avenues of redress until the therapist asked another patient why he thought that the patient herself believed that non-attendance meant that the Housing Worker did not 'like her'.

The therapist could have taken the material immediately as a metaphor for the patient's 'leaking' psychological state, her vulnerable sense of self, her saturated feelings, and her experience that the team are failing to fix her problems but in the first instance it is safest to take the material at face validity and ask other patients about the problem. From a teleological point of view the patient herself can only feel that something has been done in the group if she is left with clear ideas about potential solutions. Unless this occurs to some extent, the patient will believe the group dislike her in the same way that the Housing Worker does since they too have not taken her seriously which is something that can only be judged from the physical outcome—in the case of the Housing Worker this is of course mending her roof and stopping the leak but in the case of the group it is actually giving her practical solutions or even someone, perhaps the therapist, offering to mend the roof himself. Only after possible solutions are established, is it sensible to consider the material in relation to the group itself, for example by considering saturation of feelings in the group, lack of protection, and a therapist who is experienced as failing to fix psychological problems.

Conflict interpretation also detracts from a focus on current mental states. Borderline patients cannot easily hold more than one idea, desire, or wish in mind at a time and have little access to alternative states. So, conflict interpretation is likely to be meaningless and confusing. Some practitioners interpret unconscious phantasy and conflict directly to borderline patients using part–object body language. The lack of secondary representation in the mind of the borderline patient, however, leads patients to react to terms such as breast and penis not as metaphors but as the objects themselves. One patient became terrified in a group when another patient stated that she had had chicken breasts for supper the previous evening. The patient left the group rapidly saying that no one should eat breasts.

Bearing in mind the deficits

Borderline patients may appear to be capable, thoughtful, sophisticated, and accomplished and yet it is well-known that their unemployment rate is similar to that seen in schizophrenia (Gunderson *et al.* 1975). Whilst it is important to recognize the strengths of all patients, it is equally vital to understand their deficits, otherwise therapists develop unrealistic expectations, anticipate rapid improvement, and set inappropriate goals.

Deficit in the capacity for mentalization can be masked by an apparent intellectual ability that lures therapists into believing that borderline patients understand the complexity of alternative perspectives, accept uncertainty, and can consider difference. In fact at one moment a borderline patient may hold a particular view and yet at another time maintain the opposite is true, in one therapy session a patient may describe a feeling that holds special significance but which is later denied as being relevant, and continuity of feeling, belief, wish, and desire may be lost between therapeutic sessions. Constancy of belief and consistent experience of others elude the borderline patient, resulting in idealization at one moment and denigration the next. The task of the therapist is to establish continuity between sessions, to link different aspects of a multi-component therapy, to help the patient recognize the discontinuity, and to scaffold the sessions without holding the patient to account for sudden switches in belief, feeling, and desire. The borderline patient does not lie but is unable to hold in mind different representations and their accompanying affects at any one time. All are equally true, and the therapist must accept the balance between opposing perspectives and work with both even though they appear contradictory.

The teleological function of borderline patients requires therapists to ensure that they do what they say they will do. Motivation of others is judged by outcome. A letter to an employer, support for a College application, completion of income support forms must all be done within the agreed time; offers of additional sessions should be honoured and the team must show consistency and equity in dealing with all patients. Whilst a neurotic patient may accept that a therapist has forgotten something and accept an apology or the offer of an alternative explanation, the borderline patient believes he has forgotten because he does not like him or wants to punish him.

A patient phoned to ask for an emergency appointment. It had been agreed within her care plan that she would be seen within 24 hr by someone if both patient and team member felt that the underlying reason was urgent and no alternative way of dealing with the crisis was agreed on the telephone. When asked the reason for the urgency, the patient became abusive saying 'if you have to ask then you don't want to see me; I'll have to manage on my own' and put the phone down.

A partial hospital patient spent her spare time between groups doing complicated jigsaws that took a number of months to complete. When one of the jigsaws was near completion, another patient knocked the table resulting in some of the jigsaw falling on the floor. Although he apologized saying it was an accident, the patient attacked him and a serious fight ensued. The staff were unable to determine whether knocking the table was deliberate or accidental and so each patient was seen alone and both were sent home and asked not to return until they felt safe to talk to each other.

In both these examples, the motivation of the other is judged and responded to according to the outcomes. The fact that the therapist asked the patient about her underlying reason for an emergency appointment meant that the desired outcome of a rapid appointment was being rejected when in fact the question was the first stage in a process to decide on the best course of action. In the second example, the fact that the jigsaw ended up on the floor meant that the 'table-knocker' patient had wanted to destroy the jigsaw and by extension part of the patient's self-structure. Whilst this understanding of the patient's motivation may have been correct, the violent response suggests that no alternative understanding was available to the 'jigsaw' patient and she was profoundly destabilized by the event.

A primary aim of therapy is to help the patient move from a teleological understanding of motivations. If this is to be successful, therapists must ensure that they themselves do not become caught within the teleological system by proposing simple explanations for complex processes. For example it is common to hear non-attendance of patients explained on the basis that it means the patient does not want to come. It is more likely that the patient does want to attend sessions but is too anxious and struggling with a persecuting representation of the therapist. Further complications arise if the therapist begins to believe that actions are curative and many borderline patients convince therapists to do things on the basis that actions have real meaning—'I would really believe that you cared about me if you cuddled me'. Yet this is the area of boundary violations (see p. 184) and a belief in the 'real relationship' in which the therapist accepts that their actions are the only thing that will result in improvement or, worse still, that they can 'save' the patient by offering love and affection.

Real relationships

Borderline patients crave therapeutic relationships that are emotionally charged, supportive, compassionate, accepting, special, and personal. There is a danger that the therapist may respond to these demands either by withdrawing from the patient or by allowing the difference between the relationship of therapy and intimate relationships outside to disappear.

The therapist may counteract the borderline patient's demands for intimacy for fear of transgressing professional boundaries by becoming distant, uncaring, cold, unresponsive, and indifferent which simply fuels patient demand for contact and responsiveness. A destructive interaction develops which, if left unchecked eventually leads to a breakdown in treatment. In contrast some therapists unwittingly and almost imperceptibly attempt to make the therapeutic relationship 'real' which for many patients means narrowing the difference between the relationship of therapy and intimate relationships outside. Patients begin to ask personal questions, attempt to find out about the therapist's private life, even become involved in activities linked to the therapist, and disclosure of information by the therapist increases. Justification for exchange of information is often based on the collaborative nature of therapy and a belief that the patient needs a 'healthy', normal relationship if the abusive, destructive relationships of the past are to be remedied.

There is no place in treatment for either reaction and when they occur, supervision is necessary to understand the reasons driving the development and to restore the therapeutic relationship. It has already been mentioned that such developments are common in treatment of borderline patients because of the teleological stance and countertransference responsiveness (see above) but some aspects of the 'real' relationship are more complex than simply being considered as a boundary violation. Patients need their therapists to 'do' something at particular times and the therapist must differentiate between a push from the patient to cross a boundary and their need to have believable evidence for their own internal state.

A patient in the intensive out-patient programme was distressed that her therapist was going on a training course for 10 days. Shortly before the therapist's study leave it became clear that she thought her therapist was really going away because he 'couldn't bear her anymore' and that he 'wouldn't give her a second thought although she would be thinking of him all the time'. The day before his leave the patient wrote a brief note to the therapist saying that she had decided to leave therapy. After discussion the team agreed that the therapist should send the patient a postcard and on it mention the date and time of the next session.

This unusual action was agreed because of our view that the patient's sudden termination of therapy, turning passive into active, was linked to her terror that the therapist would lose her from his mind which would lead to instability of her self-structure. The physical reality of the postcard would validate an alternative belief that the therapist continued to have her in mind even though he was absent. Of course at another level of significance the postcard provided gratification, but this could be explored further in treatment if necessary.

Working with memories

In Chapter 3 we presented some of the evidence about retrieval of memory and cautioned against assuming its accuracy. So what should the therapist do when confronted by clients' requests for validation of their memories of maltreatment? Some advise absolute acceptance, maintaining that one should always believe the client's version (e.g. Williams 1987); others offer direct assistance in the process of reconstruction of the past (Schuker 1979; Bernstein 1990); yet others express the general presumption that the patient's fledgling memory is likely to be veridical (Dewald 1989). Davies and Frawley (1991) go so far as to suggest that the therapist should enter rather than interpret the dissociative experience, as a doubting stance would be a 'secondary betrayal' of the patient whose original experience was ignored. All these strategies manipulate the patient's material to some degree. The error lies in the therapist allowing his or her preconceived ideas to shape the evolution of the patient's free associations.

While the interpersonal situation created by those patients who desperately need external validation is certainly difficult, even for experienced therapists, it must be wrong to collude with the patient's attempt to use the therapist to reduce the unknowable to a fact. From our point of view the task of the therapist is to contain the patient and to show both genuine understanding of his state of uncertainty and the resulting hopes and conflicts. It is far more difficult to empathize with the patient's not knowing than to reduce uncertainty by pretending to know. Ultimately, confirming a reality basis for the patient's vague sense that something inappropriate might have happened is the same sort of technical error as direct reassurance.

Through giving reassurance, the analyst not only colludes with one side of a patient's ongoing conflict, but also communicates an inability to withstand the patient's demands for false certainty. In this way, his own incapacity to tolerate uncertainty is communicated. The patient is then obliged not only to live what may be a false reality, but, perhaps even more damaging, to support what he unconsciously perceives as the therapist's psychic fragility. Paradoxically, many therapists intend such interventions to show the patient something quite different—that is, an inner strength in facing up to unbearable images and to think the unthinkable.

Hyperactive mentalization and pretend mode

Borderline patients have knowledge but not belief. Their beliefs are changeable, fragile, fleeting, and contradictory and this is countered by seeking out others who appear to have beliefs and understanding. In doing so they take on others' beliefs as their own, becoming excited by them, adept at developing them and applying them to themselves. This is especially true of psychological understanding of the human condition which offers the hope of bringing explanation and understanding to the inexplicable and mysterious. Patients become only too ready to engage in discourse about themselves in relation to others, their past history, and their motivations, thoughts and feelings. Inevitably this is characteristic of the more high functioning borderline patients who can fool even experienced therapists into thinking that they are psychologically minded and have high level of understanding of themselves in relation to the world. But this is pretend mode in which ideas appear to have meaning but in fact have no links to other ideas, no depth, and no personal value.

There are a number of clues that make it clear that this evident high degree of mentalization is more apparent than real. First, it has an obsessive character. Patients begin to spend most of their waking life thinking about themselves, give over all other activities to therapy, talk incessantly to friends about their problems and the underlying causes, and even consider training as therapists or counsellors themselves. Second, it becomes apparent over time that there can be dramatically different mental models of things which are readily exchangeable. Thoughts and feelings show no stability and each time the same personal theme is elaborated a mental image and understanding is presented which is very different from previous images. The patient appears unaware of this contradiction and expresses surprise if challenged by the therapist. In general it is best not to confront the patient with inconsistency, at least initially, since, in pretend mode, they have no access to their previous understanding of others. Third, their elaboration is overly rich and frequently assumes complex and improbable unrealistic aspects. Talking to them about their own thoughts and feelings leads to rapid agreement without obvious scrutiny and when reflectiveness occurs it doesnot seem to have any ramifications. Finally, there is no felt feeling. The patient talks about affect but it is not felt at the same time. The sessions become empty.

The involvement of the therapist in this process stabilizes the patient who then becomes 'addicted' to therapy and can never leave because his identity is part of a complex 'psychoanalytic identity' which is two-dimensional rather than developmental. Experience of mental states has no implications so there can be a hyperactive feeding on itself, a generation of ideas, a complex interweaving of scenarios, a stage play that at the end seems to have gone nowhere. Not surprisingly these patients find separations from treatment problematic and they break down rapidly at the end of treatment.

For an individual therapist whose aim is to increase mentalization, challenging pretend mode in which mentalization seems well-developed raises the possibility of embarking on a strategy which invalidates the aim of therapy itself. First the therapist has to avoid encouraging hyperactive or pseudomentalization. To do so some techniques should be avoided. The therapist should never talk about complex mental states but keep his interventions brief and to the point. Sessions should be focused rather than discursive and patients not encouraged to elaborate too much and the therapist has to keep in mind the apparent mentalization as a deficit rather than a strength. In our programmes the juxtaposition of group and individual therapy may protect against excessive meaningless mentalization. Patients do not have the brief of enhancing other patients' mentalization and so are free to challenge.

A patient talked a great deal about herself and her understanding of what had happened to her. She monopolized groups and found it difficult to listen to others. Often other patients would give up trying to interrupt and simply sit back and go to sleep. Eventually one patient interrupted her and said 'you have gone a long way on all this bullshit but I sure as hell hope that you are nearly running on empty'. At this point a number of the other patients awoke and began a concerted attack. The group therapist intervened and suggested that whilst it was clear that 'more gravel was needed to deal with the possible bullshit that it needn't be thrown around'.

Conclusions

The strategies described here and the use of transference form the core of MBT. Together they establish a mentalistic, elaborative stance on the part of the therapist which ultimately enables the patient to find himself as he really is, first in the therapist's mind and later in his own as he integrates this image as part of his sense of himself. For the patient, enhancing mentalization, encouraging affect representation and preventing escape into pretend mode gradually transforms a non-reflective mode of experiencing the internal world, which forces the equation of the internal and external, to one where the internal world is treated with more circumspection and respect, separate and qualitatively different from physical reality. The therapist's respect for minds generates the patient's respect for self, respect for other and ultimately respect for human narrative. But these overall strategies have to be reinforced with the use of specific techniques and these are the subject of the next chapter.

8 Techniques of treatment

In the previous chapter we stated that the general aim of mentalization-based treatment (MBT) is to help the patient to establish a more robust sense of self so that he can develop more secure relationships and we elaborated the underpinning strategies of treatment, emphasizing the mental attitude to be taken by the therapist in all clinical situations. We now turn to more specific technical recommendations for achieving this overall psychological aim. For clarity, these are organized around four major psychoanalytic treatment goals which form a hierarchy of overall treatment aims. These are:

- identification and appropriate expression of affect;
- development of stable internal representations;
- formation of a coherent sense of self;
- capacity to form secure relationships.

The initial task is to stabilize emotional expression because without improved control of affect there can be no serious consideration of internal representations. Even though the converse is true to the extent that without stable internal representations there can be no robust control of affects, identification and expression of affect is targeted first simply because it represents an immediate threat to continuity of therapy as well as potentially to the patient's life. Uncontrolled affect leads to impulsivity and only once this is under control is it possible to focus on internal representations and to strengthen the patient's sense of self.

The four overall treatment goals overlap and may be sub-divided into a number of smaller objectives that are targeted throughout the treatment programme within group and individual sessions. In this chapter, we discuss how to translate them into clinical interventions within each of the principal therapeutic contexts of the programme, namely group and individual therapy.

Identification and appropriate expression of affect

General principles

Rationale

Borderline patients become overwhelmed by feeling and are unable to differentiate between affective states at times of high general arousal. Their capacity to regulate their manifest emotional states appears impaired. This has been generally recognized as a core symptom of the disorder. Within the current programme we conceive of the failure of emotion regulation as a consequence of a general difficulty with understanding the emotions that arise, their conscious and non-conscious determinants, and labelling affect states in appropriate ways. Our intervention therefore focuses on helping patients understand their intense emotional reactions in the context of the treatment setting. Intervention is primarily necessary at times when failure of affect regulation leads to irrational behaviour and inappropriate responses to others. Commonly this can result in impulsive actions including acts of self-harm, suicide attempts, and altercations with others. With appropriate intervention, the risk of such enactments can be substantially reduced.

General strategic recommendations for identification of affects

Throughout the treatment programme it is necessary to:

- continually clarify and name feelings;
- understand the immediate precipitant of emotional states within present circumstances;
- understand feelings in the context of previous and present relationships;
- express feelings appropriately, adequately, and constructively within the context of a relationship to the day-hospital team, the individual session, and group therapy;
- understand the likely response of the team member involved in an interaction.

Individual session

The individual sessions provide the primary context within which key features of the collaborative understanding of the model can be developed. The process of enhancing the patient's capacities of understanding their affect states starts in this part of the program and is subsequently continually reinforced in other contexts. During every individual session it is necessary for the therapist to:

- ensure that key affects are identified;
- explore the antecedents to the feeling;

- review the consequences both for the patient and for others;
- challenge dissociative states.

Often the therapist needs to examine events that may have occurred in other components of the programme during an individual session. For example difficult interactions with other patients or with the therapists in group therapy may need examination. But simply looking at a feeling and its antecedents and consequences is not enough.

The patient must

- consider who engendered the feeling and how?
- ask 'what feeling may I have engendered in someone else even if I am not conscious of it that may have made him do that to me'?
- explore whether the feelings have occurred or are connected to events either in the immediate or longer-term past;
- assess the appropriateness of the feeling to any given situation in terms of others' understanding of them;
- establish the appropriate locus of these feelings within current relationships either past or present in terms of mechanisms of defence (particularly projection and displacement).

The therapist needs to:

- identify whether the feelings are relevant to the transference relationship;
- link the past with the present and to the here and now or vice versa;
- help the patient consider alternative explanations of events whilst maintaining neutrality about which explanation is right and which is wrong;
- consistently understand and explore paranoid or other massive distortions that may be leading to rage or uncontrolled aggression.

Group psychotherapy

Once the focus on affects has been established within the individual session, the three-times-a-week group sessions can be used firstly to reinforce the focus on exploring the interpersonal context within which strong feelings tend to arise and, secondly, to evolve a routine pattern for confronting and dealing with these. Affects experienced by individuals in the group and by the group itself are identified during the course of group therapy. It is necessary for therapists to recognize personal feelings of patients and to differentiate them from the feeling within the whole group. For example, whilst the feeling of a particular individual may be depressed, the overall affect within the group may be angry. This helps sensitize the patient to the feelings of others and to differentiate them from their own. Patients have a tendency to overgeneralize their own subjective state to others around them (externalization).

The therapist must therefore ensure that group affects are:

- identified and agreed by the group;
- explored and understood by the group;
- where appropriate related to group transference to the therapists;
- recognized as being the responsibility of the group.

This allows each individual to develop a sense that the affect within a group of people is more than the feelings that they themselves are aware of. In order to ensure this understanding, the therapist must pay attention to the conscious and unconscious emotional reaction of individuals to the group. The patient can also profit from the help which other individuals receive from having their feelings identified and how these impact on the group, and how they, as members of the group, respond unconsciously to the intense feelings of another member before these are made explicit by the therapist.

The therapist must therefore ensure that individual affects are:

- identified within the group and by the group;
- verbalized and explored in relation to others within the group;
- recognized as having influenced others in the group;
- recognized as having been induced in oneself by beliefs about others' reactions and motivations;
- that, as far as possible, feelings, however intense, do not spill over from the group to other settings in the hospital.

Impulse control

General principles

Rationale

Impulsive acts commonly take place in the context of high emotional arousal. We view them, in part, as the result of failed attempts to control emotional states or come to terms with interpersonal interactions. Many authors have identified this as a secondary effect of inadequate emotional regulation. Others consider the acts to have meaning, with which we agree. But we take a view that first it is important to help the patient to understand the precursors that led to their impulsive action. It is considered inevitable that these episodes will occur, regardless of attempts to minimize the risks, because self-harm is consequent on dysregulated arousal from social challenges within the normal range. It is therefore important that staff should be free of a sense of personal responsibility for another person's life. Guilt and anxiety about impulsive acts can powerfully interfere with other aspects of the therapeutic strategy. While there is little value in attempting to impart meaning to an act at a time of high emotional arousal, it is absolutely essential to make use of episodes to help patients achieve a better understanding of the way in which their inability to understand their own internal states or those of others can provoke them to desperate actions and to use these experiences to deepen their understanding of their states of mind.

In order to tackle impulsivity effectively the therapist has to move through a series of steps with the patient, each of which has to be consolidated. First he must ensure that the patient becomes aware of a distressed state as a problem which he can do something about. Second the patient needs help to identify the feeling state and place it in an interpersonal context if he is to establish freedom of movement to the extent that he can think about himself and others without recourse to action. This may be facilitated by getting the distress out of the head and into the world through drawing, writing, and art which helps the patient move from enfeebled, implicit mentalization to explicit mentalization.

General strategic recommendations for dealing with problems of impulse control

- staff need to be constantly alerted to the possibility of serious and potentially fatal impulsive acts;
- they need to prepare for this possibility by being familiar with individual patterns of self-harming behaviour;
- when confronted with the possibility of impulsive acts, the essential requirement is to engage the patients in discussing their action, to establish communication about it, and to attempt to maintain this communication for as long as possible. Additional time may be given outside the programme;
- in the course of this conversation a systematic attempt is made to place some of the responsibility for the patient's actions back with the patient with an aim of re-establishing self-control. It needs to be made clear that the staff are able and willing to respond to the emergency;
- when possible and appropriate staff may attempt to identify and elaborate with the patient the immediate interpersonal and affective antecendents to their impulse;
- no attempt is made initially to interpret the patient's actions in terms of their personal history and the putative unconscious motivations or their current possible manipulative intent;
- following the impulsive act the experience must be thoroughly reviewed in a number of contexts including individual and group therapy.

Suicide attempts and self-harm

A picture must be developed of episodes of attempted suicide and self-harm not only by itemizing the antecedents and outcome of the episodes but also by identifying the concurrent mental experience at the time and the exact context. At least three episodes of suicide and self-harm are detailed in this manner along with a further three episodes in which no self-harm or suicide attempt took place even though the context and mental experience were similar and the impulse was present. The therapist may ask the patient 'Are there other times like these when you have felt like harming yourself but have not done so?' The purpose here is to understand small but important differences in mental state that enable the patient not to self-harm or to attempt suicide, since this may give clues to the level of risk a patient represents as well as providing hints about how to help a patient decrease the likelihood of suicide attempts and self-harm.

A patient reported that she ritualistically organized her suicide attempts by laying out a small table with tablets and razor blades. The compulsion to do this commonly started hours before. One evening she had completed her preparatory ritual and was just about to take an overdose of paracetamol, cut her wrists, and lay in a warm bath when the telephone rang. She had asked a friend to phone at exactly 8.00 pm which was the same time that she had planned to kill herself. The phone call interrupted her suicidal pathway and she packed away the tablets and razor blades. This allowed the therapist to become aware that there was a time delay between thinking of suicide and attempting suicide, the pathway could be interrupted even at the last minute, and the patient herself unconsciously wished to survive.

A common theme linked to suicide attempts and self-harm is fears of abandonment and the therapist should ask specifically about episodes in which the patient has either feared or experienced abandonment, starting as early in life as the patient can remember. Borderline patients' self-coherence is realized through relationships and dependent on them. Aspects of themselves, specifically the alien self (see p. 89), are externalized and lodged in the other in order to form a bearable, but fragile, self-representation, which is experienced as life-saving by the patient. Potential abandonment by the other threatens this tenuous stability and suicide and self-harm are seen either as a way out of unbearable collapse of the self-representation or as a last-ditch attempt to re-establish the relationship which supports the alien self. An additional element relates to the child's experience that only something extreme would bring about changes in the adult's behaviour, and that their caregivers used similarly coercive measures to influence their own behaviour. This coercive interaction must be avoided in the therapist–patient relationship.

A significant complication of self-harm and suicide attempts is the countertransference and emotional responses of staff. Suicide attempts and self-harm are often experienced by staff as an attack representing an aggressive communication. Indeed patients often insist that the self-harm is visible to the therapist by wearing a short-sleeved T-shirt or that the suicide attempt involves others.

During the first few weeks of treatment a patient took two overdoses, one during the evening and the other at the weekend. On each occasion, before doing so she phoned the day-hospital leaving a message on the answer machine about her actions. She began the message by saying 'by the time you listen to this I will be dead' and went on to thank the staff for trying to help her. She then started taking tablets ensuring that the act was audible on the tape. A later phone message revealed her to be drowsy and she accused the staff of not being available when she needed them.

Whilst these actions cause anxiety in staff and may be experienced as a direct attack on treatment and the staff themselves, they are in fact an attack on the alien self and an attempt to stabilize the self-representation at a time when the patient experiences a sense of abandonment, in this example evoked when the day-hospital was closed for the evening or for the weekend. Rarely are they directed specifically at a therapist. From a teleological perspective absence of the therapist, closure of the day-hospital, breakdown in a significant relationship, means abandonment and failure to care which threatens the return of the alien self. Once a patient experiences its return, the alien self has to be projected into someone or something if stability is to be re-established. Many borderline patients use their body as a receptacle for unwanted aspects of themselves and self-harm is an attack on the alien self. If the therapist takes it as a personal attack, he will be unable to mentalize about the act, fail to retain mental closeness, and inappropriately focus on the action as an attack rather than as an attempt to maintain stability.

A further common emotional response to suicide attempts is of escalating anxiety on the part of the therapist which may have countertransference aspects but is more often an evocation of the therapist's own professional concerns. Self-destructive acts may evoke considerable panic in others leading to a destructive cycle in which a patient's actions are responded to with panic. The therapist feels he has to 'do something'. The arousal in the patient and therapist overwhelms their mentalizing capacities with the result that actions are taken more to reduce the concern of the therapist than to help the patient. It is at these times that a failure in 'marking' (see p. 66) of emotions may occur and the therapist attributes his own anxiety to the patient which only serves to leave the patient feeling misunderstood. To protect against inappropriate actions during crises on the part of staff and failures in marking of emotions, any structural decisions, for example compulsory admission of the patient to hospital, must be agreed by two or more members of the team.

It is important to distinguish between suicidal acts and those of self-harm. Often they are seen as lying along a continuum but in fact they are behaviours that probably represent different psychological states albeit with some aspects in common, have distinct meanings, and require different interventions. As a general rule we consider any life-threatening event as a suicide attempt irrespective of conscious motivation until proven otherwise. Equally a non-life threatening event is seen as self-harm even if the patient states that their conscious intent was to die. These cannot be hard-and-fast rules because clarifying motivation, conscious and unconscious, can only take place in group and individual therapy over time and some apparent acts of self-harm are in fact suicide attempts even when the patient denies the intent and the converse may also be true.

Suicide

We take an individual approach to suicide risk and each patient is assessed in relation to acute and chronic risk factors. Overall we operate a high-risk approach and only take over responsibility for a patient if his life is acutely and severely endangered.

Chronic risk is defined in terms of the way in which a patient relates to his interpersonal world over a period of 2 years or more and is divided into high, medium, or low. Patients classified as high-risk show a persistent pattern of suicide attempts whenever they experience a set-back, rejection, or obstacle to their wishes and desires. Those at medium risk show some capacity to accept frustrations and may damage property but do not immediately resort to suicidal acts whilst those at low risk rarely make attempts on their life and have found other ways to deal with problems which must include using social support at times of crisis if they are to be classified here. The long term or chronic risk of a patient is categorized at the beginning of treatment using evidence from assessment interviews and the initial individual and group sessions. Information gathered from these sources is pieced together with other clinical details in the admission case conference (see p. 164) and the long-term risk defined as low, moderate, or severe through clinical consensus. Both team and patient have to accept chronic risk as a baseline of treatment and anticipate that, regardless of classified level of chronic risk, acute risks will develop. In fact those at a low level of chronic risk may present a sudden, unpredictable, high risk after all their strategies to manage a crisis have been exhausted. Chronic risk is managed through the treatment programme itself and does not require specific intervention. It is part of the reason that the patient is in treatment. Responsibility remains with the patient and this should be made clear at the outset of treatment. Challenges within psychotherapy may make a chronic risk worse for a short time and even precipitate an acute crisis but this should not be a reason to avoid confrontation.

Unless a distinction is made between chronic and acute risk, therapy may become iatrogenic because strategies targeting acute risk, such as hospital admission, are inappropriately implemented for chronic risk. Hospital admission does not reduce chronic risk. Anxiety in staff about a patient's continuing suicidal thoughts may lead to defensive, self-protective medicine in which 'special' nursing on a one-to-one basis, over-use of medication, and prolonged hospital stays are used, all of which increase rather than decrease the chronic risk of a borderline patient. In-patient admission should be reserved for acute suicide risk not contained by other measures, homicide risk, treatment of co-morbid disorder, respite for the patient struggling with impulsivity, and uncontained anxiety within the team. It should be brief—only 2–3 nights if possible—have clearly defined goals, be low key, voluntary, patient determined, have defined boundaries and be with a planned discharge irrespective of deterioration on the basis that if a patient gets worse it is likely to be the damaging effect of the hospital on the patient.

A chronically suicidal patient may need a crisis protocol (what to do when a member of the team is not available, who can be reached, what arrangements need to be made) which outlines clearly the role of the patient and the therapist when suicide threats and suicide attempts occur. No 'suicide' contract is made (see p. 125). Responsibility is left with the patient and not transferred to the therapist whose task is to maintain a reflective stance, to provide appropriate support for the patient to access in-patient services if necessary, and to ensure that responsiveness does not feed into a cycle in which the therapists' actions provide gratification to the patient thereby escalating the problem. Over time some patients become aware that suicide threats open a pathway to rapid care although this is rarely the underlying motivation for the threat since the care evoked is inadequate, ineffective, and often found to be unsatisfactory. Escalating threats eventually lead to staff taking increasing levels of responsibility for the patient, even though clinical consensus about suicide risk in BPD suggest the greater the degree of staff responsibility for the patient the worse their clinical state becomes. Determining the level of responsibility to be taken by staff for a patient's life requires confidence, skill, clinical knowledge, and support of the treatment team and the wider structure within which treatment is taking place.

If a patient reports suicidal impulses or is believed to be acutely suicidal, an assessment of risk is made in a 'crisis' meeting with the patient as soon as possible. A member of the team other than the individual therapist participates in this meeting. Response to risk is via the team rather than the individual therapist to minimize the gratification a patient experiences from the extra attention, staff concern, and additional contact. Suicide threats are not allowed to become the currency which buys care and concern, additional individual sessions, extra resources, and further psychiatric intervention. If this occurs it is important for the team neither to respond rapidly to threats nor to arrange a crisis meeting but to encourage the patient to attend the normal programme to discuss their suicidal impulses. Under these circumstances no additional sessions are offered and the responsibility is placed firmly back with the patient.

In the crisis meeting an assessment of risk is made and a plan developed to reduce the suicidal level. Previous episodes, their circumstances, and outcome are taken into account along with the present situation, the degree of patient attachment to the team, and the explicability of the threat. Differentiating life threatening and non-life-threatening statements of suicide is problematic but is improved by team discussion, clinical experience, knowledge of the individual patient, and awareness about the general literature on precursors of suicide. If indicators suggest that a suicide attempt is likely, the assessor explores the patient's desire to die in the context of recent events in the patient's life, including events in the day-hospital or out-patient programme. An affect analysis is performed asking when the patient first became aware of feeling increasingly suicidal, under what circumstances, who was present, what was their reaction, what was the underlying feeling and how has it changed over time? This is interpreted in relation to the group and individual therapy when possible and suggestions made about how to address the experience within those contexts.

A patient telephoned feeling desperate and suicidal having failed to attend a group session the day after he had spoken a lot about himself. He was asked to come in to discuss it. When asked about the onset of the desperate feeling he reported that he had started to feel hopeless and suicidal after talking to his mother two days before who, during his childhood, had been emotionally neglectful. She had been enthusiastic about his successful application for a College evening course but paradoxically this had made him feel uncomfortable, a feeling that later became desperation. He had then talked to the group about her interest in his achievement but this had served to increase rather than decrease his discomfort apparently because the group had also expressed pleasure in his accomplishment of obtaining a College place. The therapist questioned his reaction to his mother and the group, recognizing that the patient's equilibrium had been disturbed because of his need to see others as neglectful and disinterested in him. This had been challenged by the reaction of both his mother and the group and threatened the return of a neglectful, cruel, alien self which was experienced as being within his mother and the group rather than himself. The team member interpreted this and asked the patient to consider whether being seen so quickly to discuss his suicidal feelings might even contribute further to his problems and actually increase his suicide risk because it, too, challenged the perception of others as neglectful. The patient began to understand that his perception of others needed questioning and he agreed to return to the group to discuss the problem. The team member agreed that he would discuss it with the group therapist to ensure that support was forthcoming in the group the following day.

Self-harm

'There is a link between hurting yourself and getting support and treatment. It is hard to resist self-harming behaviour when you know if you do it, you will get treatment' (DoH 2003).

'I bang my head over and over again and don't care about the blood. The more blood the better because it shows that there is something really wrong. People can see the blood but they don't see the pain when it is inside your head.'

'Nobody wants me. Nobody cares about you when you have a personality disorder and they don't recognize the pain. When it gets too bad I start using my Stanley knife to make some marks and sometimes I write words on my arm like hate and slut. Then if that doesn't work I cut deeper and deeper until I get some relief.'

Self-harm is associated with dissociative experiences and patients report the onset of a bewildering feeling which rapidly escalates out of control, becomes unbearable, and is relieved only when cutting takes place. Relaxation and distraction techniques are of moderate benefit because they reduce anxiety but it is necessary to explore the underlying meaning to a patient if the compulsion to self-harm is to lessen. Episodes must be placed in an interpersonal context within treatment, treated within the usual frame of group and individual therapy, and not given undue importance and significance. The patient is encouraged to think about the episode and to talk about it in the next available group or individual session. Feelings stimulated by the group and individual session which may have precipitated the self-harm must be explored.

A patient who cut his abdomen at times of distress talked to the group about his father and the difficulties that he was having in continuing to live with him in the same house. The group discussed his inability to live alone and identified that he felt trapped, not being able to leave and yet wanting to get out. The patient seemed to listen to this and said that he would ask some friends if he could stay with them. After the group the patient left the day-hospital and began drinking and the same evening cut his abdomen so severely that it needed five stitches.

The following day the other patients were outraged that he had cut himself and felt attacked by him after all the work they had done in the previous group. The therapists had to work actively to get the group to think about other perspectives to the self-harm including discussing the instability that had been induced in the patient by talking about leaving his father whose presence was necessary as a repository for the patient's alien self. Thinking about leaving his father had become tantamount to actual leaving and this destabilized the patient.

The team must neither take over the responsibility of trying to stop the self-harm nor react by giving increasing amounts of attention to the patient. Some individuals become addicted to self-harm, integrate it into their lifestyle, and gain pleasure in a secret ritual in which they use razor blades to cut their arm, thighs, or other areas of the body, often carrying razor blades or special knives to provide reassurance wherever they go. We understand this as arising from their recognition of the fragility of their representations which cannot be 'called forth' at times of anxiety. Cutting provides proof of existence and makes their unbearable feeling bearable. The addictive quality of some self-harm may be related to the release of endogenous opiates which has led some practitioners to use naltrexone, an opiate receptor antagonist, to break the addictive cycle (Roth *et al.* 1996). It has met with limited success probably because of the powerful psychological factors dominating self-harm.

In view of the importance of attempted suicide and acts of self-harm in the treatment of borderline personality disorder they form an important focus of both individual and group sessions.

Individual therapy

While individual therapy may not be the context within which an episode of self-harm occurs, where possible the therapist should play a role in establishing contact with the patient at a time when they are threatening self-harm.

This may not always be possible and at other times may not be desirable, for example if a patient utilizes the threat to punish the therapist. The therapist making additional effort at that time may be seen as collusive. However, in terms of reviewing the patient's experience, the individual therapy plays a major role. There may be a tendency to collude with the patient to overlook the episode in all contexts of the programme. This should be resisted. The individual session is the best place for the patient to review their actions and to begin to accept responsibility for the sequence of internal events that led them to do it. It is also the key area in which the pattern of self-harm is established. For example it is necessary to distinguish those individuals whose self-harm cannot be anticipated from those in which it gradually develops over time and follows a predictable sequence of events and feelings.

Therefore the individual therapist should:

- take a detailed history of suicidal acts and acts of self-harm to establish a pattern of these actions for the individual patient during the first few sessions;
- obtain a history which enables the therapist to provide a detailed description of affect states and situations related to suicidal acts and self-harm;
- work out a formulation about suicide attempts and self-harm which is understandable to the staff team and to the patient;
- work with the patient collaboratively on strategies that may be of assistance to the therapist and the staff team to engage the patient at times of emotional arousal when potential episodes of self-harm are more likely;
- place previous acts within a context, commonly a context of problematic emotional relationships;
- link recent acts within the relationship of the patient to the day-hospital or to the therapist within transference;
- show the patient that his actions are understandable given his feelings immediately prior to the act of self-harm, his current inability to deal with these feelings, and his past experiences;
- help the patient to modify his response to his multiply-determined feelings
- explore the affective changes since the previous individual session linking them with events within treatment.

Group therapy

It is important that all threats and actual acts of self-harm or attempted suicide are discussed in the group. Firstly, this allows the individual patient to identify how their actions and impulses are perceived by others and in appreciating others' perceptions they are forced to come to a more complex and realistic understanding of their own actions, their effect on others, the precipitants and their role in coping with their current problems. Secondly, the understanding that other patients bring to bear on impulsive acts in others is likely to be of benefit to themselves by enhancing their own generic capacity to think about their own impulses. This may take a long time in some patients who are able to see things in others but have extreme difficulty in seeing things in themselves. As soon as a therapist is aware of or the patient makes the group aware of intent to self-harm, the action is fully explored in terms of the details of the plan or act, its immediate precursors, the act itself and its likely impact on the patient and others involved, and on the group itself. The aim is to use this information to elaborate the action in terms of the functions it serves for the individual at that specific time either as a way of avoiding thinking or feeling about particular issues or as a way of inducing specific thoughts and feelings in others.

Thus the group therapist both with regard to plans and completed actions has to:

- establish them as topics for discussion within the group;
- ensure the whole group define them as problems (patients find self-harm comforting and need first to define it as a problem);
- explore their obvious precipitants and help the group identify common themes if these exist;
- help the group in identifying the thoughts and feelings that provoked the act or the plan;
- assist the group in exploring the effect of acts on others both within and without the group;
- encourage expression of feelings about the acts within the group including resentment of the patients actions;
- help the group to explore the effect of acts or planned acts on the group process;
- relate any suicidal acts to processes within the group that may have stimulated the thoughts of self-harm. This may, of course, be because the group failed to recognize some aspect of an individual's distress.

Other challenging affect states

General principles

Rationale

In addition to the general points about affect regulation there are specific affects that need to be addressed in both group and individual therapy. Certain affects are found to be particularly challenging both for patients and therapists for different reasons. These include paranoid and passive aggression, envy, idealization, hate and contempt, sexual attraction, love and attachment. It is the interpersonal aspects of these affects that make them particularly challenging. Situations that arouse them are the most common triggers for the disturbing symptoms of BPD such as suicidality and self-harm. Coming to understand the nature and function of these emotions and the reasons for them is therapeutic for these patients.

General strategic recommendations

Throughout the programme the staff:

- give priority to discussing challenging affect states and on these occasions help the patient label and attribute the affect to a specific interpersonal situation;
- identify specific challenging affect states and identify their interpersonal context and reach agreement with other staff concerning their centrality to the patient's problems;
- ensure that the challenging affects do not disrupt interaction at the individual level or within the group;
- show the patient how the affect is interfering with their personal and interpersonal functioning;
- explore how the affect relates to other conscious and non-conscious thoughts and feelings;
- explore with the patient the reasons that they find certain affects difficult to admit to, or to identify, or consciously experience;
- monitor their own role in inducing specific affect states in patients.

Aggression related to paranoid anxiety

A number of patients are aggressive, particularly at the start of the programme, and consciously very angry, often feeling victimized, rejected, and distrustful. The aggression is easy to arouse and may be stimulated simply by talking to the patient or asking a question. The aggression may be verbal or behavioural. The staff need to understand that the aggression is aroused defensively to deal with a perceived threat to the stability of the self, commonly a threatened or actual humiliation, and this occurs because the intention of the other is poorly understood or the person feels threatened by their own state of mind. For instance, a patient may feel intensely and constantly self-critical and be unable to ward off such self-criticism. The result is intense anxiety, which results in projection of the criticism onto the other who is then attacked, leading to the overt aggression.

A patient who was estranged from his partner and 3-year-old son had his visiting rights removed following a row about access. In a group session he described his upset and anger about the level of inappropriate control his former girlfriend had over his role as a father and about her lack of understanding of his function. A female patient said that she would like to have a child but she wanted to become pregnant via artificial insemination so that she could do without the problems of fathers. She then laughed and stated that men were no longer necessary in the world and the sooner they realized that the better. This led the patient to become angry and to become strident about the importance of fathers in the up-bringing of children. The female patient dismissed his reasoning and so he stood up in the group, threatened her, and smashed the glass in the door as he left the room.

In this example the violence arises from the patient's experience of being dismissed and humiliated by both his former partner and now the patient in the group. His fragile sense of fatherhood and manhood becomes unstable as his self-regard is undermined, his own fears of being unimportant are verbalized by another patient, and the return of an alien self becomes a possibility. In this case the alien self is an impotent irrelevant self that he does not recognize as part of him because he experiences it as inaccurate and not his own. He himself was constantly humiliated by his own father who used to taunt him about the size of his penis and he needs to retain a self-representation of himself as a father and man to remain stable. When it is threatened his reaction is viciously to dismiss the group member and the group itself to restabilize himself.

Many borderline patients at the severe end of the spectrum show co-morbidity with narcissistic and antisocial personality disorder (ASPD). Antisocial features increase the patient's tendency to control and manipulate the other with scant regard for their rights and independence of mind. The moment the other person shows some independence of mind, radical action has to be taken and violence becomes possible. Independence of mind not only may be represented by a partner 'doing his own thing' but also by a partner wanting a more intimate and closer relationship. For the borderline patient with antisocial features, both represent danger. This has consequences for therapy since it is inevitable that the therapist will show independent mental existence by attempting to explore more emotional aspects of problems and pointing out different perspectives, all of which may endanger him physically if the patient has developed some dependence on the relationship. Initially the patient may terrorize the therapist to see the fear within him since this will reassure the patient that the externalized alien self remains firmly embedded in the relationship. At this point the therapy may need to become organized around the patient's dangerousness and indeed it is important that therapy both in the individual session and in the groups is done with safety in mind. Part of the function of a detailed history is to predict the possibility of violence and to address it practically and psychologically right at the outset of treatment and before it is too late. The patient may believe that discharge is inevitable because of his threats and, if so, he will try to control his aggression. Yet this prevents exploration of the forces determining the potential violence so a number of steps need to be taken. First it can be pointed out that discharge does not occur because of threats and it is only actual violence that leads to discharge.

Second the therapist has to ensure that he maintains a mentalizing stance and shows that to the patient. An increase in risk arises if the patient experiences his alien self being forcibly returned to him. This destabilizes his self-state and violence becomes a last desperate bid to destroy it and prevent its return. So, finally, the therapist should retain the 'alien self' and not try to return it through forceful interpretation. Understanding of the violent impulse takes place gradually when a crisis is over and risk reduced. Patient and therapist need to think about what happened once some distance has been placed between the threatened confrontation and its apparent resolution.

In the assessment and initial sessions of therapy, a detailed history of violence or threatened violence is obtained. All episodes should be explored in detail. Again what is important here is not just the cataloguing of acts of violence but the causal chain of events linking mental experience and violence. Without this, it is impossible to assess accurately the ever-changing level of risk during treatment. In particular, episodes in which the patient may have misread others' intentions or been oversensitive to criticism or reacted violently to actual criticism should be identified. These can inform the therapist and members of the team of the interpersonal interactions that may inflame a situation, allowing them to de-escalate tension, in a group for example, as quickly as possible. Crucial to interpersonal dynamics in narcissistic and ASPD is anticipated or actual humiliation, which is the most potent threat to the self. In the absence of full mentalization, the shaming experience is felt as actually potentially annihilating (see Gilligan 1997 for a comprehensive psychological model of violence) not an 'as if' experience but one where the psychological experience of mortification comes to be equated with the physical experience of destruction, or 'ego-destructive shame' (Fonagy and Target 2000).

Individual session

Aggression is most commonly aroused in relation to the individual therapist. The patient might verbally or occasionally physically attack the therapist. In the latter case a serious boundary violation has occurred and, after ensuring therapist safety, the session should be ended immediately and the situation discussed with the whole team. In order to understand the former situation the therapist must monitor his most immediate previous communication with the patient. Often the patient will not have understood what was being said or asked and misinterpreted the motivation of the therapist. The therapist should rapidly reflect on this and rephrase the communication whilst reducing the tension within the interaction. The aggression is not tackled directly but noted within the next communication from the therapist, which should clarify the comment that has led to the aggression. As soon as the patient has calmed down, the patient and therapist may explore what was behind the aggression. Once the relationship between the individual and his therapist is on a more secure setting, the therapist is able to bring to bear past experiences of aggression to inform the understanding of present aggression.

Thus in the individual session the therapist should:

- be alert to aggression as an indicator of anxiety and threatened instability of the self;
- not react to personal aggression, for example by being aggressive in response;
- ensure that communication is not disrupted, and keep the dialogue open;
- identify the source of the anxiety in the preceding communications;
- continually self-monitor to identify what he may have said or is saying that might arouse anxiety and consequent aggression;
- educate the patient about the process leading to anxiety and subsequent aggression which must include the therapist's own role in this process;
- early in treatment the therapist should help the patient understand that the final outcome of aggression on his part was stimulated by the therapist.

As the sessions progress, the therapist:

- highlights the relationship between anxiety and aggression and focuses on anxiety as the central problem rather than the aggression;
- uses past instances of aggression to clarify further the present anxieties;
- helps the patient reflect on the situation and helps them to achieve a realistic appraisal of events;
- interprets the underlying dynamic of feared humiliation and its developmental antecedents.

Group therapy

The therapists must be aware of those patients for whom aggression is a central area of their difficulties. Aggression may emerge towards the group therapists or towards the other members of the group. The therapist needs to marshal the whole group to deal with the problem whilst ensuring that the group do not counter-react with uncontrolled aggression themselves. An important part of this is that the group needs to explore its role in provoking the situation and identify the anxieties that may have been aroused in the patient leading to the aggression. Highlighting states of mind that lead to anxiety and aggression is an opportunity to recognize similarities in the ways that patients respond to anxiety.

When the whole group reacts towards the therapists with paranoid anxiety the therapists' responses are similar to those given to an individual patient. In these instances collaboration between the co-therapists may be critical and helps to identify provocative behaviour on the part of one of the therapists.

The therapists need to:

- monitor continually the overt and covert expressions of aggression within the group;
- challenge and draw attention to aggression when it occurs if the group do not question it;
- ask the group and patient to reflect on what has happened that might have made the patient/group anxious and subsequently aggressive;
- highlight the recurrent features within the group that lead to aggression in each individual;
- recognize with the group the precursors which have in the past led to aggression from one of the members of the group or from the group as a whole;
- challenge the group if the aggression gets out of control;
- monitor each other and occasionally challenge each other for reacting aggressively to provocation.

Passive aggression

As well as being overtly aggressive, patients may also manifest destructive, disabling aggression in apparently passive ways. Prototypically, passive aggression is expressed in an overt refusal to cooperate with the treatment team by for example persistently failing to engage in an interpersonal interaction.

A patient spoke a little about herself but when asked to elaborate on her beliefs and events in her life she persistently said there was little to say. The more the therapist asked questions the more the patient said 'I don't know. There is nothing to say really. I don't think that my life has been very interesting'. In fact the patient had led and continued to live an eventful life having travelled extensively, been in prison in the Far East for drug offences, and was currently making suicide attempts. Inevitably the therapist became frustrated about continually asking questions and receiving monosyllabic answers. Using this experience the therapist was able to identify the patient's own frustration about no one listening to her worries or responding to her demands. As a child she had found that stubbornness and quiet refusal to answer had resulted in people reacting to her even if it was often a violent response.

Sometimes the refusal to cooperate is somewhat more subtle. A patient may show compliance and participation but careful observation reveals that he actively undermines a treatment process by for example continually dismissing helpful suggestions, or superficially agreeing with formulations but identifying himself as an exception. Aggression becomes manifest not in the patient but in the frustration and despair of the staff.

Individual session

Unlike aggression related to paranoid anxiety, passive aggression is not immediately noticeable but will become evident to the therapist over a number of weeks.

The therapist might first of all notice that interventions, however straightforward, do not lead to further dialogue or that they are quickly met by reasons why they are inapplicable. Gradually the therapist becomes concerned that any intervention seems futile and he may become demoralized and concerned about his abilities as a therapist. In discussion with the team the therapist often feels bereft of therapeutic skill and powerless to help the patient. Eventually overt feelings of anger about the patient's attitudes may be expressed to the team. The staff need to recognize that the continual undermining of interventions is defensive and aimed at distancing the therapist. It arises from the patient's belief that they will not be helped and they need to pre-empt feelings of disappointment by taking active control. It protects them from a profound sense of loss of self. To accept help and risk disappointment destroys a fragile but life-saving sense of identity.

In the individual session, the therapist should:

- be alert to repeated negative responses;
- initially monitor their frequency and note them;
- ensure that countertransference feelings are constantly clarified by self-monitoring and by discussion with the team;
- identify specific instances when interventions have obviously been undermined, rebutted, and relate them to a range of previous examples;
- help the patient recognize that continual undermining of the therapeutic process or distancing the therapist is a way of controlling anxiety;
- attempt to explore what feelings the patient experiences as being uncontrollable which make him need to control the therapist;
- identify that ultimately the patient needs to believe that any treatment will fail in order to protect their sense of self.

Group therapy

Passive aggression rapidly distorts or destroys the group process and may dominate the atmosphere to the extent that all the group members may begin to feel that there is little point in the group itself. Communication from both patients and therapists is actively undermined. For example the group members and the therapists may work hard on trying to engage a patient in a dialogue but the patient persistently fails to respond or answers only monosyllabically. In contrast to the individual session, the group therapists have to act quickly to counteract the destructive potential of this process. They cannot wait since the pernicious nature of the attack can lead to a fragmentation of the group which interferes with the treatment of all patients in the group. Some patients who themselves are actively aggressive may join the attack on the group but more often they attack the passive–aggressive patient. It is important that the therapists do not facilitate or allow such an attack by one patient on another.

The group therapists should:

- explicitly state that one member of the group appears to find the group unhelpful;
- identify specific ways in which the group member expresses their dissatisfaction;
- identify the destructive way in which the member tackles the problem and encourage the group to consider the detail of the interactions that lead to personal dissatisfaction;
- enlist the help of other group members in recognizing these instances whenever they arise;
- help the group assess the veracity of the complaints and consider how they are to be addressed constructively;
- rapidly intervene if group members attack the patient;
- continually monitor the effect of the passive–aggressive attack on the group.

Envy

Envy is a paradoxical emotional reaction which entails an attack on something which is felt by the patient to be helpful or useful. It is perplexing to an observer because the attack seems to make little intuitive sense. It seems to be against their own as well as everyone else's interest. A patient may ask for additional time from staff, be offered some time, and then not attend; a member of staff who is particularly appreciated by a patient becomes the target of unwarranted complaints. The target of envious attacks may be the clinical team and there is a danger that a patient becomes victimized by the team. This can be guarded against by careful team discussion when attacks occur.

Individual session

Envy may be manifest in the patient's description of their life. Constructive relationships seem to breakdown rapidly or to be undermined. Anything good, such as expression of care and concern, seems to be spoiled. The patient experiences obtaining good or pleasurable things as having been forcibly extracted and only as being offered reluctantly. Good things are seen as being in the other person's control; they cannot have them just because they wish for them, so it is better not to have them or to want them at all. It is better for them to be destroyed and therefore not available. Helpful sessions may be followed by missed sessions or sessions in which the patient is particularly critical of the therapist. These reactions are not the same as aggressive attacks related to paranoid anxieties but they are more a result of the inability of the patient to maintain envious feelings, as with all other feelings, within reasonable bounds. Sometimes the therapist will have recently reported that the patient appears to be making progress only to find that at the next session the patient seems to have returned to their former state.

In the individual session the therapist should:

- ensure that the detailed history of the patient's life identifies the exact circumstances of the break-up of personal and professional relationships;
- not be disheartened by apparent relapse and re-emergence of earlier ways of relating;
- identify that the patient feels that what they had experienced as good in fact feels as though it was bad in an inexplicable way;
- recognize that when something is felt to be partly bad it can become completely and irretrievably bad. It is therefore worthless and meaningless and need not be mourned or missed for its good aspects;
- identify the spoiling effect this has on progress and how it prevents the patient experiencing any benefit from treatment;
- help the patient understand this process without inducing excessive self-criticism or guilt.

Group therapy

Envious attacks occur in groups but in this situation the therapist needs to distinguish them carefully from jealousy or other types of triangular relationships. Jealousy is a more sophisticated emotion than envy and requires a capacity to recognize complex interpersonal processes. It is therefore more likely to arise at the end of treatment, when patients can express feelings concerning the level of attention paid towards certain patients and the perceived unfairness of this favouritism.

Expressions of envy occur throughout group treatment and the commonest manifestation is an attack on another patient who is perceived as having gained benefit or made some progress. The whole group can at times enviously turn upon the therapists shortly after they have made an intervention which was helpful for the whole group. More unusually, following the suicide of a member of the group, patients can express envy of the dead member in a manner which is of course profoundly destructive in character and creates the illusion that death is good and to be embraced as a desired solution.

The therapist should:

- recognize the envious attack and immediately help the 'attacker' identify what it is that they assume that the other person possessed that they could not have. This could be an achievement, a possession, a benefit. But in all these cases it is likely to be rooted in an assumed subjective state which the attacker imputes (often erroneously) to the victim;
- identify the attack as an attempt to destroy the subjective state in the victim rather than an attempt to take possession of the envied object;

- understand that it is for this reason that the continued existence of the envied object is of no relevance;
- enlist the group to help the patient see the objectively meaningless nature of their destructiveness;
- establish the effect of the attack on the victim to ensure that the group understand that envy can have a profound effect on the subjective state of the other;
- consider with the group the possibility that if someone is seen as having received something, perhaps from a therapist, it may be possible for others to have it too without it having to be destroyed.

Idealization

Idealization results in a patient experiencing the treatment programme, the team, or a particular member of staff as having unrealistic powers and abilities. They are imbued with greater goodness than is appropriate and the patient considers the programme or a member of the team to have the answer to all their problems. No areas of weakness are considered. Idealization enables the patient to take a passive and helpless role and feel looked after by the idealized object, sometimes believing that the therapist is going to provide the secure parenting that they missed during their earlier development. This state of mind arises from a need for the patient to split off any consideration of failure of therapy, of poor responsiveness of therapists, or of inadequacy of the treatment. To do so threatens the stability of their sense of self. The patient solicits contact with the therapist and team and requests answers to difficulties but when these are not adequately forthcoming they escalate the demand. This may lead to a sudden reversal of the patient's state of mind and devaluation and denigration may occur, particularly when a therapist has not responded as expected. The team or therapist can do nothing right and treatment can be in danger of breaking down. At these times the patient is unaware of their previous state of idealization. The fluctuation between states of idealization and denigration may be rapid and frequent. The apparently contradictory nature of their state of mind, over a single group or individual session, passes unrecognized by the patient.

Individual session

Idealization of the individual therapist within sessions is obvious. The patient takes everything the therapist says as being helpful, providing new insight into problems, and as having a quality which is neither found in other treatment settings such as the group sessions nor in previous treatments. The therapist may be trusted with private information, evidently not given to others, and may be asked to keep it secret. The therapist may be tempted to do so but it is important to remind both patient and therapist that information given in the individual session is shared with all members of the team (see p. 161). The therapist may begin to feel that they have a special relationship with the patient and become overprotective and believe that they have the answers and understand the patient better than anyone else. This needs to be challenged within team discussions and the therapist should be helped to challenge the patient's idealization gently. Idealization should not be interpreted directly too early but continually alluded to and its dangers, such as the loss by the patient of the chance to develop their own solutions to problems, pointed out.

In the individual session the therapist should:

- clarify that the patient appears to think the therapist has all the answers or that the treatment programme is the solution to all his problems;
- explore previous relationships in which the patient believed someone had all the answers. This should include detailed discussion of the state of mind of the patient when embarking on previous treatment;
- recognize with the patient that giving others special abilities commonly leads to a breakdown in the relationship;
- relate the understanding of the need to idealize in different situations to the present therapeutic relationship;
- consider with the patient some of the advantages of the idealization for treatment. For example it may be the only way a patient can attend regularly without excessive anxiety;
- recognize the defensive aspects of idealization which may serve to cover hostility or other feelings that destabilize the individual's sense of self.

Group therapy

Patients may idealize the group itself but more often idealize one of the group therapists. Commonly this is at the expense of the other group therapist who is either ignored or actively devalued. For example when the idealized group therapist is away the patient does not attend the group. Sometimes the idealization of the individual therapist is expressed in the group rather than in the individual session itself and the group devalued. On yet other occasions one patient may idealize another patient within the group, although this is rare. Some level of idealization in a patient may be appropriate, particularly early in treatment, and may balance hostility from other patients.

The group therapists should:

- recognize when one of them is being idealized and be able to discuss this with each other, initially outside the group, but later within the group itself to ensure that the therapist 'couple' is not split;
- draw the patient's attention to their tendency to listen attentively and respond to one therapist's interventions whilst seemingly not recognizing the usefulness of the help offered by other members of the group or by the other therapist;

- explore within the whole group the consequences of attributing prestige and the answer to all problems to one other person or to the group or treatment programme;
- on occasions challenge the idealization by identifying clearly some therapeutic errors or inadequacies of treatment;
- interpret how members of the group may be encouraging a patient to continue idealizing a therapist in order to protect him so that their own attack is experienced as less dangerous.

Sexual attraction

Patients commonly experience sexual feelings for their therapists or psychiatrists; less often reported but probably equally common are sexual feelings in therapists for their patients. These feelings are part of the underlying basic humanity of patient–therapist interaction which is essential for borderline patients who are acutely sensitive to rejection and feelings of abandonment. But in clinical practice it is important to distinguish between erotic feelings and a non-erotic desire to be touched or held on the one hand and a dangerously powerful eroticized transference on the other hand.

Erotic feelings accompanied by sexual fantasies which the patient knows are unrealistic present little problem and may even be helpful in maintaining a positive transference and constructive therapeutic alliance. Nevertheless it is important that the patient and therapist do not engage in physical contact other than, for example shaking a hand in greeting and so on. Problems arise when a borderline patient is unable to maintain either non-sexual feelings within normal limits or sexual feelings become intense, vivid, persistent, urgent, and irrational, sometimes infusing the whole of treatment so that all events are interpreted by the patient as indicating that their desires may become reality. Extensive sexualization of the relationship occurs when the patient's sense of identity is seriously threatened. Attempts may be made to seduce the therapist into a clandestine relationship. The therapist initially resists the demands but gradually can be induced to believe that a special, and eventually sexual, relationship may 'save' the patient. This is particularly likely when the patient's declaration of sexual feelings escalates and is accompanied by threats of self-harm. In contrast the patient may experience himself as being the victim of or having been abused by the therapist who has resisted seduction and a sado-masochistic interaction is set up in which the patient persistently attacks the therapist and the therapist counter-attacks verbally.

Sexual feelings of such intensity can interfere with treatment whatever the nature of the therapeutic dyad and are not confined to male–female interactions. In fact some of the more difficult therapeutic problems may result from same-sex interactions which stimulate homosexual anxieties in both patient and therapist.

Individual session

It is in the individual session that sexual feelings can become prominent. The privacy and unstructured form of the session and the fact that material is not shared with the patient's peer group allows expression of intimate feelings. Sometimes a patient may openly express love for the therapist and it is important that the therapist does not simply reject this but tries to understand it as a communication. Sometimes the expression of sexual feelings is disguised within the material, or by undue regard being given to the private life of the therapist, or even by dressing or behaving seductively or using sexual innuendo. For example, a patient may attend the individual session in sexually provocative attire and relate stories of abuse and sexual molestation in a way that distracts from other themes that are causing anxiety. The therapist may be drawn into such stories when it is more important not to focus on the sexual aspects within the session.

A patient spent many therapeutic hours trying unsuccessfully to get some token of love from her male therapist, asking him if he liked her, describing how most men found her enormously attractive, pleading with him to say something that would counteract the contempt and despair she felt she had received from her physically and sexually abusive father, and going into great detail of her romantic and sexual fantasies about the therapist. These entreaties regularly reached a crescendo just before breaks, and were steadfastly interpreted as a response to separation and as an identification with her importuning father, but to little avail. One day, weakened by a session of relentless demands, the therapist explained how if he were to respond to her advances it would completely jeopardize the therapy. During the next session it became clear that she felt that she had at last got him to admit that he really did desire her and that he was only holding back because of his professional restrictions. The patient offered to stop therapy so that they could at last start a relationship.

In the individual session the therapist should:

- be alert to countertransference. If sexual feelings are stimulated, consider whether they are induced by the patient's behaviour;
- discuss any sexual feelings within the individual session with the clinical team but not with the patient unless this is agreed by the whole teams;
- be aware of therapist contributions which encourage the situation;
- identify the process by which the patient creates a sexually-charged atmosphere;
- explore whether the sexualization is a defence against other needs which create greater anxiety;
- identify whether sexualization has been used in the same way before;
- interpret the attempt to place the relationship on a sexual basis in relation to the underlying anxieties, for example about self-esteem and identity;
- confront the patient about their fantasy that such an intimate relationship may be possible and reaffirm the boundaries of the treatment.

Group therapy

Group therapy is the most useful treatment setting in which to discuss a patient's propensity to sexualize interpersonal relationships. It is likely that a patient's propensity to sexualize relationships will be clear to other members of the group and they may be aware that the patient has a special relationship to their individual therapist. At these times the group therapists will need to capitalize on this whilst respecting the confidentiality of the individual session. In group therapy sexual feelings may be expressed safely towards the therapists or towards other patients although both interfere with treatment. Nevertheless it is important that members of the group feel safe to talk about such feelings for each other and towards the therapists, otherwise their expression is kept secret and is not available for examination. Some patients sexualize their relationship with the whole group just as they sexualize all their contacts with others in the world. This general method of relating covers anxieties about being rejected, disliked, considered unattractive, and provides a sense of identity for the patient within the group. Other members of the group may challenge this and recognize the underlying anxiety or depression that is often present. More troublesome for a group is if two patients form a 'pair' within the group and this develops into expressions of attraction for each other which leaves other members on the edge of a special relationship. Feelings of envy may be stimulated and the pair attacked within the group. On other occasions the development of a 'special' relationship between patients takes place outside the group and the therapists only hear about it through fragments of gossip within the group. The task for the therapists is to ensure that all aspects of relationships between patients are discussed in the group and that it is part of the group culture that the place to work out such relationships is within rather than without the group. Sexual feelings towards the therapists should also not be avoided since it is important that the therapists are experienced by the group as being neither less nor more involved with one patient than another although this inevitably occurs at times.

The group therapist should:

- alight on any suggestion of or allusion to a 'special' relationship between two patients or between a patient and themselves;
- take opportunities to explore a sexualized relationship that is occurring within an individual session;
- ensure that the recommendations of abstaining from intimate relationships between patients and the reasons for them are fully understood by all members of the group;
- develop a safe group culture in which intimate feelings for others and about others can be expressed and talked about including those towards the therapists;

- understand the defensive nature of sexual expressions within the group and how a patient may erroneously feel safe and cared for by another patient if they form a 'couple';
- accept that the co-therapist may recognize the developing sexual feelings of a patient towards him before he, himself, does;
- identify the distortion of the group process when patients pair together and the destructive effect on the group;
- insist on talking about a sexual relationship if it is occurring;
- interpret the sense of safety and identity that the relationship gives whilst identifying how patients use sexual feelings and their expression to avoid underlying anxieties.

Hate and contempt

Hate and contempt are affects that borderline patients use to protect their self-esteem. Rather than being simple, chronic, resistances to treatment, they may be mobilized at times when change is imminent. Therapists are summarily dismissed and sneered at. All interventions in all contexts are seen as laughable or, at best, obvious. The patient may become grandiose and arrogant but feel that they are not getting anything because everything that they are given is rendered useless. At times the patient may be extremely hurtful to a particular therapist playing on an area of weakness that they have detected.

A patient pre-occupied with sadistic impulses discovered that her therapist kept cats having seen her buy cat food in the local supermarket. The patient herself kept cats and as far as the team were aware looked after them well. However, one morning the patient left a message on the answer machine saying that she had put one of her cats in the washing machine and killed it because 'it would not behave itself and hadn't shown her proper affection'. She asked the team to ensure that her therapist knew about this. Inevitably the team were appalled and the therapist began to feel that she would be unable to see the patient in her next session. It was agreed that another member of the team would see the patient first to discuss the incident. It transpired that the patient had not committed the act of cruelty but had become so angry with her individual therapist that she wanted to taunt her.

The effect of the hate and contempt is to distance the patient from others and to protect a fragile self which has been threatened by an experience of need. The emotions cover a deep mistrust of others and inner fears of becoming dependent on others and having to recognize that others have a separate existence and their own individual motivations. The identity of the borderline patient is safe in their inner castle, contemptuously obliterating all others as unnecessary or useless to them. There is an illusory sense of control. Occasionally a patient may appear better when this state of mind is manifest since it distances them from closer interpersonal interactions and closes their mind to that of others. It is when their mind is open and they are able to experience their feelings for and the feelings from others that they become more disturbed. More subtle ways of expressing hate and contempt include 'already knowing things' when the therapist draws their attention to something or quietly leaving sessions for specious reasons. In all these circumstances, the therapists must engage with the hate and contempt and not simply try to interpret it away.

Individual session

At the most severe end of the spectrum, the individual therapist may find it difficult to help the patient attend the sessions. The hate and contempt may be so great that the patient states openly that it is not worth turning up and that the sessions are a waste of their time. Sometimes the patient will sit outside and not bother to go into the session, seemingly to express their contempt for the therapist openly and publicly. The therapist should go and talk to the patient about their not coming into the therapy room and continue the discussion for as long as possible, pointing out how difficult it is to address the problem in public. At other times the patient makes persistent derogatory remarks about the therapist and enlists support from other patients in their quest to show that the therapist is useless. This can result in a two-pronged attack on the therapist who is derided as a group therapist as well as an individual therapist. Patients may convey that the therapist is lucky to have them around, that the therapist seems to need them more than they need the therapist. It is important, initially, that the breakdown of the therapy is not seen as solely being caused by the patient. Within the session itself, the dismissal of everything the therapist says must be tolerated by the therapist who may need some support from the team to maintain their sense of therapeutic potency. Sometimes the therapist will react by offering more and more and trying harder and harder only to find that this makes things worse. As long as the therapist recognizes the function of the hate and contempt rather than reacting to the experience of it this response can be reduced.

The individual therapist should:

- accept the problem of the therapy being useless by recognizing the patient's experience of it;
- recognize that there may be some useless elements within it and identify the primary task of therapy to turn it into something that is useful;
- continue to try to engage the patient in dialogue even if the patient does not come into the therapy room;
- identify the hate and contempt as interfering with consideration about whether what the therapist says has any merit or not;
- constructively use their own feelings of revenge following a period of relentless hate from the patient or after a period during which they feel

hateful towards the patient by, for example, considering them as a reversal of transference roles that is, they are treating you as they were treated themselves in their past;

- discuss such feelings with the team and in supervision, being honest about slips that may have occurred in which the patient is attacked;
- be honest with the patient about such events, especially when challenged by the patient who may have recognized that the therapist was angry with them;
- establish with the patient the nature of the relationship before the period in which hate is expressed. Often it will have been a time when the patient has expressed a need for the therapist or appreciated something the therapist has done or helped them understand;
- interpret the purpose served by the hate and contempt for example as a way of controlling emotions, distancing the therapist, or as a need for a particular type of relationship;
- help the patient understand that they have closed their mind to the mind of others.

Group therapy

Hate and contempt may be less pronounced in group therapy because of peer pressure. It is more difficult for patients to dismiss their entire peer group than it is to disdain the staff team or individual therapists. Nevertheless, one patient may find it difficult to listen to others in the group, sneer at things that are said, and fail to attend or arrive late. Lateness as a symptom of contempt must be addressed in the group since it interferes with treatment of others. At times a whole group may round on the therapists or even attack one patient who becomes the object of 'group hate'. The group may take an anti-authoritarian stance with therapists being portrayed as setting rules and controlling what patients do and do not do. A patient can lead a revolt within the group suggesting that no one turn up or that the group meet in another venue at the time of the group therapy. At times a patient may continually draw the attention of the group to themselves and the whole group becomes dominated by their problems leaving others with no time or place to discuss themselves. Self-reference may become extreme because of the low regard in which the individual holds his peers.

The group therapists should:

- establish whether it is one individual or the whole group that are in a contemptuous state of mind;
- maintain a thoughtful dialogue within the group about the hate and contempt;
- be honest that some aspects of the group or what the therapists have said have been unhelpful;
- engage other members of the group in thinking about whether what was said had any value or not, especially after it has been dismissed;

- link the attitude and feelings to underlying anxieties which are commonly feelings of dependency, need, and loss of control as well as a threatened identity;
- pay particular attention to lateness and absences by establishing the problem as one of patients wanting to come but finding themselves unable to do so;
- beware of their own responses becoming defensive. Discuss carefully the group process within supervision including countertransference feelings;
- judiciously appeal to the group when the hate and contempt from one member becomes relentless by asking the group to focus on the problem and how the individual can be helped to find something useful within the group.

Love and attachment

It is often stated that aggression is a central problem for borderline patients but, in our view, the experience of love and positive attachment causes severe difficulty. Patients are unable to distinguish between love and other feelings such as dependency, need, and sexual desire and attraction described above. During early stages of treatment, feelings of love and positive attachment are rare and because of this the relationship may appear problem-free. As the therapist gradually activates feelings of attachment in the patient, disorganization of the attachment system becomes more evident. For example a patient may start to cling helplessly believing that physical proximity is necessary which in turn can be met with inappropriate attempts by the therapist to avoid the patient who is experienced as devouring and controlling. Alternatively attachment to the therapist can be manifest paradoxically by intensification of enactments including suicidal gestures and manifest hate of the therapist. It can be hard to remember that the root cause of increasing difficulty in the therapy is the patient's increasing awareness that the therapist and treatment matter. Commonly the patient remains unaware of the strength of their attachment. Statements early in treatment by the patient of the importance of treatment and of strong attachments are more likely to indicate eroticized or idealized feelings than a robust and secure attachment.

One patient began to sit outside the unit at nights and at weekends. It appeared that she had to be able to see the unit to know that it was still there. If the building was out of sight it was out of mind and therefore no longer existed. She talked about how she could not cope 'without the Halliwick'. The focus of treatment became helping her to manage away from the unit. First, hospital security was alerted about her presence at night so that they did not expel her from the site and second, work was done on establishing a transitional representation of the Unit.

Individual session

In general the strongest feelings about treatment are manifest within the individual session. To this extent it is the individual session that disorganizes a patient early in therapy. The therapist needs to be aware that expressions of hostility and fears of breakdown or madness may be the consequence of the mobilization of loving feelings of which the patient is unaware. Therapists may make two common errors when this occurs. First the therapist may take expressions of hostility at face value and second the therapist can react provocatively by indicating to the patient that his antagonism results from a struggle with positive feelings that are difficult to cope with. Whilst this may be partially correct, it is experienced as seductive by the patient at an early stage in treatment and will elicit an even more negative response. The principle of treatment is to explore the defences rather than to interpret the underlying loving feelings themselves. Sometimes the patient seems to need the therapist just to have someone to maltreat or to have him in close proximity, for example to hear the therapist's voice. This may put increasing pressure on the therapist to be available. It should not be confused with attachment that evokes internal feelings of security since it is more likely to represent the opposite, namely a profound sense of insecurity.

The individual therapist should:

- be aware that, as the relationship intensifies, problems within the therapeutic relationship are going to increase;
- consider that mobilization of affectionate feelings may underlie sudden hostility;
- recognize enactments within therapy as being part of transference manifestations;
- be able to retain an 'as if' stance in the face of the lack of pretence within the patient's behaviour, threats, statements of love;
- recognize the need of the patient to talk to someone during periods when the therapist is absent;
- affirm the patient's capacity to manage without the therapist, initially over weekends but later over breaks for holidays;
- interpret the underlying causes of the patient's need for the therapist. Often this may require understanding the underlying aggression and rage towards the therapist for his absence or fears in the patient that he may harm himself;
- recognize the reality of the devastating effect that apparently minor absences may have on the patient.

Group therapy

Patients become strongly attached both to the group and the group therapists. They become more and more able to use the group as treatment progresses. At later stages of treatment they express concerns about the group and particularly about absences which they find not only disruptive but also a source of sadness. Whilst challenging the therapists to do something about it they also try and do something themselves. They express the meaning of the group to them and often try to explain this to other members by considering how they were themselves when they first started and how that has changed. A narrative of their history in the group is built up which includes both good and bad aspects of the group and the group therapists. There is an assessment of its failings and its useful aspects. This can be helpful especially when it occurs in the context of a new patient joining the group or of another member expressing serious concerns about the usefulness of the group. Therapists may use the expression of opposing feelings within the group to explore the same internal conflict around good and bad found in all borderline patients.

The group therapist should:

- maintain a focus on reactions of patients to change particularly concerning absences of the therapists or other patients with whom they have been talking;
- allow a patient to explore the good and bad aspects of the group without interpretation;
- encourage patients to ask each other about their experiences within the group over time;
- interpret the external expression of positive and negative feelings about the group to the internal split within the patients themselves who need to see the group as either being all bad or all good;
- positively encourage the patients' attempts to think about what the group has meant to them over time and what their feelings have been about the therapists over time;
- link the recognition of something good in the group to the inner realization that something useful can be obtained from others and that something can also be given in return.

Establishment of stable representational systems

General principles

Rationale

Whenever borderline patients develop a relationship of personal importance, their interpersonal representational system is at risk of becoming unstable. The representation of their own internal states and those of others becomes fluid and so they are unable accurately to recognize what they are feeling and thinking in relation to the other or to know what the other is feeling or thinking in relation to them. As a consequence, they resort to rigid and crude schemas in which relationships lose their subtlety and can become exaggerated caricatures of normal ways of relating. The therapeutic task is to establish internal experiences as more robust states. This is most effectively done after affects are more stable and present less of an interference with the patients' and therapists' ability to think. This is the case both in the overall treatment programme and within the microcosm of the individual session or the group. It is usually ineffective to attempt to stabilize internal representations when there is too much 'affect noise' in the background. Affects are exaggerated because beliefs are experienced as having comparable force to physical reality. Thus emotional responses to physical events can be hard to understand without explicating the overwhelming power of the beliefs they give rise to.

General strategic recommendations

Throughout the treatment programme it is important:

- to focus on currently-experienced mental states;
- to help the patient to recognize a hierarchy of complexity of internal mental states;
- not to overestimate the patient's capacity to reflect on internal states and assume that the patient is capable of conceiving of complex internal states such as conflicting beliefs, particularly during the initial stages of treatment;
- to recognize the need to rework continually any understanding of internal mental states that may have developed.

In order to fulfil these general strategic recommendations, the therapist needs to develop and maintain a 'mentalizing therapeutic stance' (see p. 203) both in the group and individual sessions.

Individual and group sessions

The techniques required to maintain a mentalizing stance on the part of the therapist are similar within group and individual sessions. Whilst they are only effective after unstable affect states have been controlled, they are also frequently part of the technique by which those affects are stabilized. They include:

- identifying primary beliefs and linking them to affects (epistemic states);
- identifying and understanding second-order belief states (beliefs about other people's beliefs);
- exploring wishes, hopes, fears, and other motivational (or desire) states.

It is helpful to focus on each aspect in turn although in clinical practice the dynamic state of the patient determines the emphasis in any particular session. Nevertheless, it is helpful to remember that the focus for each patient changes as they progress through the programme. The order of interventions for stabilizing internal representational systems is:

1. control affect state (see above);
2. identify primary belief;
3. establish second-order belief;
4. explore underlying motivations and wishes.

Identifying primary beliefs and linking them to affects

Borderline patients hold particular beliefs about themselves and about how the world has treated them in the past and how others will treat them in the future. These beliefs are held with a tenacity that goes well beyond any present reality and govern all interpersonal interactions, especially when anxiety is aroused. Therapy will therefore stimulate them at an early stage and they are commonly manifest in the first meeting with the therapist. Primary beliefs have to be identified early in treatment. Common examples include 'the world is a malevolent place', 'anyone whom I like rejects me', 'I am the most difficult patient you have ever treated', 'people can't be trusted'. However, it is important for the therapist to understand that these are more than straightforward beliefs, that could be questioned through, for example, Socratic techniques. The beliefs form part of the way in which the borderline patient organizes his internal world through harnessing the interpersonal context. Primary beliefs are but one aspect of a complex representational system that determines how the individual understands and interprets events. Unable to experience thinking about himself internally ('from within'), the borderline patient is forced to understand himself by establishing relationship configurations, as it were from without. A situation is created in which what is normally an intrapsychic process is established through an interpersonal interaction.

For a patient to feel safe, not to feel persecuted from within, the therapist must play the assigned role in order for the patient to confirm his expectations about himself and relationships. Yet for the therapist to be effective, he must not fully engage with the patient's efforts to force him into a specific role-relationship. The therapist must go alongside the beliefs but not go along with them or argue against them. If he challenges or opposes them at an early stage the patient is either thrown into confusion and distress or disengages from therapy. Typically, the therapist feels provoked, forced to oppose an accusation, to deny a complaint, or to defend himself. If he does so the patient has no choice but to insist further on his representation of events in order to protect his fragile sense of reality and to stabilize his self-representation. Ideally, the therapist must accept the patient's need for a 'flawed' therapist without actually enacting too many of the limitations the patient imposes. As soon as rigid beliefs become apparent, the therapist must identify the triggering event, the overpowering viewpoint it gave rise to, and the affects which naturally accompany the experience.

In the individual and group sessions the therapist should:

- label belief states about the self and others and establish them as a topic for scrutiny;
- link events and belief states and affects e.g., I was late (event) so you believed that I didn't want to speak to you (belief) and so you shouted at me (affect);
- explore earlier examples of the triad of events/beliefs/affects in patients past, in the past of the group or in the past of the individual sessions and look at outcome for self and others;
- help the patient to understand alternative views of the same events in the context of the group process and individual therapy.

In the individual session the therapist should:

- help the patient reflect on his behaviour and feelings in the group therapy;
- recognize and gently challenge excessive or pathological use of mental mechanisms of projection, denial, splitting, and other powerful forms of distortion;
- focus initially on understanding 'patient–other' interactions outside the session. This will include 'patient–hospital', 'patient–day–hospital', 'patient–staff group' interactions;
- gradually move towards 'patient–therapist' interactions within session and make 'small' transference interpretations concerning relatively trivial features of the interaction between patient and therapist.

In the group session the therapists:

- link primary beliefs to the relationship with the whole team or to both therapists;
- encourage patients to question their rigidly held beliefs of others as well as those about themselves;
- continually seek alternative perspectives from others about the patient's belief about himself and others;
- encourage 'Other-centred' interactions—'explain to the group why you think that he behaved as he did';
- interpret group process to demonstrate that the group is more than each individual and that the relationship of the individual to the group influences the group process e.g. non-attendance interferes with the group process and other patients' treatment;
- sharpen the patient's views of the differences in perspective between his/her view and that of the therapist or other patients in the group.

Identifying and understanding second-order belief states

The rudimentary development of mentalization in borderline patients reduces the complexity of their representation of mental states and understanding of the motivation of others; only one version of reality is possible, there can be no false belief. A remarkable rigidity of beliefs is the consequence. Mentalization acts as a buffer: when actions of others are unexpected, this buffer function allows one to create auxiliary hypotheses about beliefs, which forestall automatic conclusions about malicious intentions. These are second-order belief states. But for the borderline patient, at times of close engagement with another person, no such process is possible.

Internal reality becomes identical with physical reality. Thus the imagination of threat is tantamount to the reality of threat. Some of these reactions can be readily understood. For example, internal working models constructed on the basis of abuse assume that malevolence is not improbable. However, being unable to generate auxiliary alternative hypotheses, particularly under stress, makes the experience of danger far more compelling. Normally, access to the mentalization buffer allows one to play with reality since understanding is known to be fallible. But the borderline patient cannot play with the ideas. No alternative realities can be envisioned, there is only one way of seeing things. This state of affairs changes only slowly. It is, therefore, important during the early part of the treatment not to try to argue patients out of their understanding. Attempts by a third party, such as a therapist, to persuade the patient that they are wrong may be experienced as an assault and an attempt to drive them crazy. Only when mentalization has been to some degree re-established can the therapist begin to challenge the patient's perspective.

The impact of these experiences is greatest in the group setting when the reality of others' putative beliefs about the self can be devastating and the individual may take extreme measures to attempt to protect themselves from the overwhelming painful reality associated with these thoughts. Shame associated with beliefs about critical views that others might hold can be experienced as devastating. Violence towards the self (or the other) might be the only way of reducing the discomfort. The problem is exaggerated by the rudimentary nature of the patient's capacity accurately to identify the belief that the other actually holds about the self. Similarly, their flawed beliefs about beliefs might lead them to experience their minds as non-opaque to the scrutiny of others. The patient comes to feel that others can read his mind and this in turn can lead to unrealistic expectations about the extent to which the other can meet the patient's need. Frequently the patient might feel distressed because the other has not acted in ways that indicates accommodation to their thoughts and feelings. This feeling is rooted in the false assumption that the other had access to the internal experience of the patient without it being communicated verbally.

In the individual session, the therapist should:

- clarify the beliefs of the patient and question them initially without challenge;
- seek alternative explanations for firmly held beliefs;
- use the transference relationship to highlight false understanding and to develop other understandings without insisting on the veracity of any one explanation;
- explore the underlying reasons for a patient's belief through transference manifestations e.g. how they organize their present understanding from their previous experience rather than consider the present situation itself;
- challenge the patient's beliefs once a robust therapeutic alliance has been established and highlight alternative accounts;
- seek to increase the patient's capacity to question and to challenge himself
- focus on differences in perspective when they occur for example when the patient reports both his own view and that of someone else.

In the group session, the therapists:

- establish a therapeutic stance of 'not knowing' by making no *a priori* assumptions;
- continually clarify beliefs with the patient and the group;
- encourage each individual and the whole group to ask questions of each other and the therapists if they do not understand something;
- focus on thinking about powerful feelings which have occurred in the group such as suicidal impulses in the group or someone walking out of the group;
- side with a patient towards whom highly critical views have been expressed;
- foster the patient's ability to ask himself why he feels something in the group at that time and who may have engendered that feeling. Then;
- encourage the expression of that experience and help the other patients react to it constructively e.g. by explaining that they had not understood something or that they did not know the other patient felt like he did.

Exploring wishes, hopes, fears, and other motivational states

The third phase of reflecting on internal states involves exploration of motivations. This involves first identifying affect states as suggested in the first section of this chapter. When this has been achieved to some degree, the underlying states need exploration within an interpersonal context. The affects are seen in terms of how they are expressed in the individual's motivations within the group, towards the individual therapist or with other people in their life.

In both the group and individual session it is important:

- to clarify with the individual their current feeling;
- to identify the other feeling which the current feeling is a reaction to;
- to explore the underlying reason for that second feeling;
- and tentatively to suggest that this was the underlying hope, fear etc. that went unrecognized or was thwarted.

Individual therapy

Individual therapy enables the patient not only to consider his own motives but to consider his understanding of others. During group therapy, patients are confronted with the motives of others directly since patients are asked to explain to each other why they have done something. In individual therapy the patient has to challenge his own understanding of others which presents considerable difficulty since it confronts his rigid, schematic representations of his own motives as well as those of others along with their teleological beliefs.

A patient invested a great deal of her time between therapy sessions drawing cartoons which she rarely showed to anyone. One day she left them in the art room. Another patient added some dialogue to the pictures in pencil and pinned them up on the wall. Some of this was marginally offensive towards and yet full of humour about the staff. The patient herself became angry saying that he had destroyed all her work. However, she believed that his motivation was to expose her as a useless cartoonist and to humiliate her by speaking for her. The fact that he had added the dialogue to each picture meant that the cartoons must have been useless when she believed them to be complete. The individual therapist explored the rigidity of this understanding of his motivation but the patient said that if he had added dialogue then he had wanted to spoil her drawings. Eventually, the patient decided to ask the other patient why he had done it when she next saw him. He explained that the pictures were so evocative and professional that they had made him think about all sorts of different aspects of the staff in relation to himself and so he had wanted to express it. He apologized if she felt that he had spoiled her work but he had done them in light pencil deliberately to ensure that his comments could be erased.

The individual therapist should:

- continually explore the patient's understanding of others' motives;
- identify the effect of the patient's understanding of others motives and wishes on the patient herself e.g. If a patient believes someone does everything for malign reasons until proved otherwise it is not surprising that they do not like them or cannot develop a closer or more constructive relationship;

- highlight evidence within the transference relationship that conflicts with the patient's own conscious motives;
- interpret why the patient experiences things in a distorted way when the evidence is clear within therapy itself e.g. you believe I don't like you and so you are avoiding me because I went away on holiday;
- consider the underlying wishes and fears of the patient as understood through the form of the sessions e.g. the patient may attend only half the session representing a wish to develop a relationship with the therapist on the one hand and a fear of sitting in the room with them for too long on the other hand which is experienced as dangerously intimate.

A patient who always left the individual session after about 20 min and returned 10 min later was eventually able to explain that after about 20 min she felt the therapist's mind was taking over hers and she had to get out of the room to get her mind back. When she had retrieved her mind she could return for the last 20 min. Her experience was that her thoughts became muddled and this was followed by a feeling that she had no thoughts other than those expressed by the therapist. This was linked to her recurrent experience that 'my mother does my head in. I can't think when I am with her'.

Group therapy

The concern in the group is to look beyond the manifest emotion and behaviour. For example, a person's anger with a group may be understood in terms of his disappointment at being overlooked. The critical elements involved may be

- identifying the anger;
- establishing the anger as a reaction to a disappointment or subjective sense of abandonment;
- understanding it in the context of the perceived motivations implicit in the disappointment.

A patient fell and twisted her knee but despite some pain she managed to attend the group the following morning. When she tried to talk about the pain in her knee, the group took little notice. However, the therapist detected the dismissive attitude of the group and asked some of the group members to consider why they were ignoring the patient's complaint of her pain. One member of the group stated that he thought that she was just attention-seeking. Shortly after this the patient became angry with the group and then fell silent and left the group as soon as it ended. The same evening she took an overdose. Exploring her overdose in relation to the group established that not only had she felt angry at the patient's disbelief of her pain but also hurt and upset that no one had appreciated her 'self-sacrifice' in coming to the group when she could 'hardly walk'. She had wished for sympathy about her knee. The therapists explored in the group her sense of abandonment and the lack of recognition of her efforts and her resulting feeling that she was not believed.

In this example the patient's desire was to be recognized by the group as having made an effort and being in need of sympathy, she felt (rightly or wrongly) that this was being overlooked and, unable to cope with the disappointment that was engendered, she became angry with the group and the group therapists.

At first the process of exploration of motivations should remain simple and easily understandable to both patient and therapist. Later the situations may become more complex and be explored in a more detailed way. For example, at the beginning of treatment, surprise may be expressed at apparently incompatible ideas but the patient is not confronted with them. Later in treatment it may be possible to work on the conflicting wishes and desires or beliefs and to explore how they affect the patient's relationships.

Formation of a coherent sense of self

General principles

Rationale

During development, borderline patients fail to find their current mental state mirrored by their caregiver. As a result they have no choice but to internalize their mother's actual state rather than their own as seen and processed within the mind of the mother and this becomes part of their own self-structure. When confronted with a frightened or frightening caregiver, the infant takes in as part of himself the mother's feeling of rage, hatred, or fear, and her image of him as frightening or unmanageable instead of a more coherent reflection of their own experience. This image fragments his self-organization and not only leads to some confusion of what is self and what is not self but also to the development of an alien self.

A stable sense of self is illusorily achieved when the alien self (see p. 89) is externalized onto the other and controlled therein. The individual then is an active agent who is in control, despite the fragility of the self. A heavy price is paid. By forcing the other to behave as if they were part of his internal representation, the potential of a 'real' relationship has been lost and the patient is actually preparing the way for abandonment. If the other is needed for self-coherence, separation or abandonment means the re-internalization of the intolerable, alien self-image, and consequent destruction of the self. Suicide represents the fantasized destruction of this alien other within the self. The impact of the threat of suicide on another appears to be aimed at forestalling the possibility of abandonment although this is not the primary motive.

Borderline patients cope by refusing to conceive of others' thoughts, and thus avoid having to think about others who they believe may wish to harm them or whose thoughts they experience as dominating their mind.

Continuing to defensively disrupt their capacity to depict mental states in themselves and in others leaves them operating on inaccurate, yet rigidly held, schematic impressions of thoughts and feelings. They are consequently immensely vulnerable in intimate relationships which undermine their sense of self whenever the other behaves in a way that suggests the alien self is out of their control. This means that the therapists have to tread a fine line between being aspects of the alien self, an unreal relationship, and placing some of it back with the patient, a real relationship in which the therapist has a mind which differs from that of the patient.

General strategic recommendations

Throughout the programme it is necessary to:

- focus on self-states and perceptions of state of mind of others;
- monitor therapist 'role-responsiveness' in self–other interactions;
- consider when self-alien self-transferences evolve;
- maintain awareness of countertransference and its effect on the therapeutic relationship;
- validate accurate perceptions of others or the therapist;
- try to understand how the actions or feelings of others were induced partly by the patient.

Once again it is necessary for the therapist to strive for a 'mentalizing stance' to help the patient establish a coherent sense of self. Only within the mentalizing stance can the therapist ensure that he becomes part of the alien self but at the same time remains partly outside it so that he can reflect the patient's state of mind. Initially this is best shown by how the therapist actually behaves with the patient rather than through interpretation. He may show through small gestures, such as seeing the patient for a brief talk outside the session time that he is fully aware that the patient is finding things difficult. In more complex circumstances, 'large' gestures may be evoked in the team. A patient may threaten such serious self-harm that the therapist or team begin to consider compulsory admission. At this point they need to consider whether they are becoming an alien self which is projected by the patient onto the team as a way of forcing them to control him. Borderline patients commonly evoke external control to stabilize their sense of self. If at all possible such large gestures are to be avoided.

Individual therapy

The task of the individual therapist is to accept becoming and being seen as the alien self but at the same time to stand alongside it. If the therapist enacts the alien self he cannot help the patient change because he becomes part of the patient's mental structure and is controlled by the patient. This may occur in extreme circumstances that engender anxiety in the therapist, for example when a patient is seriously suicidal or develops a powerful erotic transference to the therapist. In these circumstances projective systems are active leading to a confusing emotional picture which bewilders both patient and therapist. As long as the therapist is partly the alien self but also separate from it, the patient will have some stability and affect storms will be minimized but as soon as the therapist wavers or questions the patient, takes a different perspective, goes on holiday, or is unavailable, the patient becomes unstable and anxious. The therapist has to walk a fine line between the Scylla of being what the patient wants him to be and the Charybdis of being himself and challenging the patient's perspective. It is important for the therapist to recognize what he is and is not because borderline patients, especially those with some narcissistic features, have a highly-developed capacity to recognize accurately our strengths and weaknesses. Thus the sense of self of the therapist needs to be coherent and robust but alloyed with some uncertainty and flexibility. Coherence is not the same as rigidity but a recognition of what one is and is not, what one has done and not done, what one is responsible for and not responsible for, when one has made an error and not done so, and acceptance and understanding of weakness and strength without inappropriate defensiveness.

In the individual session the therapist should:

- establish a dialogue about joint responsibility for the relationship;
- monitor countertransference reactions;
- maintain an awareness of his own vulnerabilities;
- clarify when he is being perceived by the patient as something that he is not and question this and accept that the patient may also question how he is seen by the therapist;
- openly accept the patients view of him when he is seen as something that he is;
- recognize his responsibility when charged with having done something that he has done;
- move from elaboration and clarification of the individual relationship to interpretation in the 'here and now'.

Group therapy

Groups engender considerable anxiety in borderline patients leading to fragmentation of the self, a loss of embryonic mentalizing capacity, and the emergence of more extreme psychological processes. Coherence of the self can only be maintained within groups through splitting, projection, idealization and denigration and the use of other defences. Group therapists must recognize that the use of these defences is very much a two-edged phenomenon. On the one hand they are a necessity to ensure that a core sense of self is maintained without contamination with rage, disappointment, and other bad feelings. On the other hand, they rigidify the group and act as a brake on development and change. The difficulty for the therapists is when to challenge and interpret the defensive organizations within the group and when they are best left alone. If the therapists insist a group face their negative and positive transferences to each other too early, the patients may not have the resources and imagination to countenance their fears, wishes, rigid beliefs, and desires. The result will be non-attendance, dismissal of the therapists, denigration of the group, and derogation of other patients in the group. In general, it is best for the therapists to foster a group process in which individual views of others are identified and questioned by other members of the group rather than by the therapists themselves.

In the group sessions the therapists should:

- establish a group culture of self–other observation;
- identify and explore how a patient may evoke the same response from different members of the group;
- focus on splits in the group and establish how each sub-group characterizes the other;
- challenge such splits through the 'split' group as a metaphor for the individual minds of the patients;
- challenge self-states characterized by contempt and dismissal of others;
- explore aspects of self that are seen in others.

Development of a capacity to form secure relationships

General principles

Rationale

We have already emphasized the importance of consistency and reliability of the therapeutic programme if borderline patients are to form stable self-representations and develop the capacity to 'mentalize'. Mentalizing models are uniquely valuable in complex interpersonal situations, involving for instance conflict, potential deception, or irrationality. Unfortunately, non-reflective internal working models come to dominate the behaviour of borderline personality-disordered individuals especially in emotionally charged intimate relationships and in any interpersonal situation which calls forth relationship representations derived from the primary attachment relationships. Group and individual therapy stimulate internal experiences of earlier representations but borderline individuals are disadvantaged when this occurs because their caregivers did not facilitate mentalizing capacity within a secure attachment relationship (vulnerability) and they have subsequently acquired an emotional disincentive for taking the perspective of others who are seen as hostile as well as non-reflective (trauma). Subsequent relationships are jeopardized because patients divide their mentalizing resources unevenly between their external and internal worlds, becoming hypervigilant towards others but uncomprehending of their own states. All these factors distort the interpersonal life of patients with their friends and with the therapy team leaving the relationships insecure or disorganized.

The juxtaposition of need for support and understanding from others with fear of intimacy and distrust of their motives leaves the borderline patient beleaguered and insecure. Relationships become unstable and rapidly changeable and a supportive friend can suddenly be experienced as malevolent and dangerous. Therapy must therefore attempt to embody a secure base and not to repeat this pattern of interpersonal interaction. This can only be done by constant attempts to maintain mental closeness with the patient (see p. 210). But the patient is terrified of and actively fights mental closeness, even when physical proximity appears to be his overarching goal. Retaining such proximity while under persistent attack is neither comfortable nor likely to be achieved if the therapists are too sensitive. Therapists need to be robust within themselves and able to maintain their focus irrespective of provocation. The danger during treatment is that therapists will themselves react in a non-mentalizing manner and demonstrate the very thing that the patient fears, namely that no one thinks about things from their viewpoint. This leads to an insecure attachment. A secure attachment develops if interventions are always made from a 'mentalizing' standpoint and there is a continual focus on the interpersonal arena. The therapist who makes 'mind-minded' statements and continually strives to see things from the patient's perspective strengthens the security of the relationship and keeps his patient in treatment.

It is important to differentiate the work on interpersonal interactions from interventions using transference. The two are used together to complement each other and the therapist may be able to move from one to the other, often starting with the manifest interpersonal life of the patient and deepening the intervention later. Interpersonal work explores the processes between people rather than focusing on the mind itself. It is concerned with the individual's family relationships, friendship patterns, work interactions, and community relations and how they impinge on the patient's life both constructively and destructively. In some ways this is the most supportive aspect of the programme since it takes the manifest aspects of the patient's relationships and looks at how they can help or hinder the patient or be harnessed to give support in times of crisis. One problem for many borderline patients is the instability of supportive relationships which may leave them isolated and alone just at the time when they need comfort or encouragement.

General strategic recommendations

It is necessary for the therapist to consider the interpersonal life of the patient:

- during the engagement process (see p. 158)
- throughout the course of treatment
- during crises
- towards the end of treatment.

Often borderline patients have a very limited supportive network on which they can rely at the beginning of treatment. Years of distrust, emotional volatility, suspicion of others, and unstable housing take their toll leaving patients isolated and vulnerable. It is for this reason that patients may need more support early in treatment than later. During the course of treatment the staff should be alert to any development of friendships and relationships in the patient's life and help them negotiate the inevitable stresses that ensue, facilitate thinking about the emotional aspects of the relationship, and maintain expectations within reasonable bounds. Certainly supportive friendships may be of assistance during crises and the more a patient is able to use an interpersonal network to cope with mood change and anxiety the lower the level of personal risk. Towards the end of treatment the patient has to consider managing without the support of the therapist and staff team and instead invoking the interpersonal network and considering how it can be used constructively.

Individual therapy

As well as considering the patient's life outside treatment, the therapist needs to consider his own interpersonal interaction with the patient. Is it considerate, fair, moderate, concerned, and interested? The development of a secure attachment can only take place over time and each interaction during treatment needs to end with a sense for the patient that the problem has been thought about, at least to some extent, from his point of view. Whilst this is not always possible it is an important aim which therapists need to keep in mind at all times. A focus in the mind of the therapist about the interpersonal aspects of treatment will ensure that a similar process begins to develop in the mind of the patient.

The individual therapist should have gathered details about and become familiar with the patient's interpersonal world during the initial sessions of the engagement process (see p. 158). Similarly he should be aware of the problematic symptoms and behaviours. The primary interest over time is in determining which aspects of the patient's social and interpersonal function are central to the current symptoms or behaviours. Initially the patient may find little link between, for example, a suicide attempt and an interpersonal aspect of the patient's life and so it is important to understand that interpersonal interactions not only may lead to problems but also protect against them.

An emotionally-charged relationship may provoke self-harm but equally a supportive, constructive friendship may protect against it. Throughout the treatment the individual therapist should:

- focus on current and past interpersonal relationships identifying constructive and destructive elements;
- explore symptoms and behaviours in relation to the interpersonal world of the patient;
- identify relationships which are positive and evoke pleasure for the patient;
- discuss who the patient turns to when feeling troubled and explore the effect of that interaction;
- consider what may interfere with the stability of constructive relationships.

Group therapy

The task of the group therapists is to maintain a link between the processes within the group and the patients' lives outside treatment. Therapists constantly need to ask themselves 'who is there in this patient's life'? The group itself should not become a closed system—detached, encapsulated, and without links to the rest of the programme. Relationships within the group are prototypes of other relationships and as one patient said in a group – 'if you can deal with people here, you can deal with anyone'. The need for support and understanding from others and corresponding fear of intimacy and distrust of their motives means that group therapy is a useful medium in which to explore the insecurities of patients and to help them develop greater security with others.

In group therapy the therapists:

- keep in mind the interpersonal network of each patient;
- balance exploration of relationships between the members of the group with consideration of their relationships outside the treatment programme;
- stimulate discussion about external supports and how they may be used constructively to help with emotional distress;
- explore the satisfying and dissatisfying aspects of relationships within the group and outside;
- link the patients' experience in the group to their relationships outside;
- identify patterns in external relationships that are repeated within the group; and finally;
- maintain equipoise when under attack. Displays of anxiety, panic, retribution, and retaliation by therapists rapidly undermine development of a secure relationship.

Conclusions

The initial strategy in individual and group psychotherapy is to help the patient improve emotional control. In order to do this, therapists must keep in mind challenging affect states which include paranoid and passive aggression, envy, idealization, hate, sexual attraction, love and attachment and aim to give meaning to bewildering feelings. This is done by gradually linking incomprehensible emotions to events within the individual and group treatment using transference and countertransference.

The principal focus of therapy is on currently experienced mental states and recognition of the need to rework an understanding of them. This requires identification of primary beliefs and second-order belief states and meaningful links to be made to underlying affects. Inevitably this necessitates exploration of wishes, hopes and fears, and other motivational states but the sole focus should not be on the individual. Whilst a focus on self-states is essential, patient perceptions of state of mind and motivation of others are equally important.

9 Implementation pathway

A key feature of any treatment is whether mental health professionals can be trained relatively easily to implement it competently and effectively within everyday clinical practice. The evidence so far suggests that this goal is far from being realized for most treatments within psychiatric services. For example family interventions in schizophrenia remain poorly realized within clinical services despite training programmes and a robust evidence-base for effectiveness. The underlying reasons are unclear. Practitioners show competence and adherence to treatment at the end of training but when applying it to their own service find it problematic to implement, fail to obtain the support of their organization, cannot maintain their skills, and eventually give up feeling undervalued and demoralized (Baguley *et al.* 2000). These findings suggest that training should be done within an organization rather than without and that a team rather than an individual should be trained to ensure an on-going peer group. In addition, there needs to be someone with leadership skills who is more highly trained offering continued supervision and support.

Our programme was originally implemented by generically-trained mental health nurses under supervision rather than highly-trained doctoral students, analysts, therapists, or other specialist practitioners. But publication of this manual is unlikely to be enough to ensure the effective transmission of appropriate skills in treatment of personality disorder (PD) to mental health practitioners and to address the problems of translating theory into practice. A number of developers of psychotherapeutic treatments take great care in accrediting practitioners but geographical obstacles and costs associated with training create barriers to programme implementation. Our aim has been not to develop a therapy in its own right but to create an approach to treatment that orientates the thinking of the practitioner and gives a framework in which to use his or her specialist skills. This final chapter is a 'do-it-yourself' guide to implementing the treatment described in this manual and is the first step in developing a minimal cost, learner-driven package with local trainer and peer supervision and nominal direct training, support, and supervision from a centre. In this manual we have described how we have organized our programme but there is no reason to believe that the form of our implementation is either sacrosanct or optimal. In fact there is little doubt that it will need modifying to suit local circumstances, for example in secure settings, prisons, or medium-secure conditions, and consequently the aim of this chapter is to act as a blueprint outlining some of the features of treatment that have to be discussed, practised, and agreed before effective implementation can take place. It should be read with the training materials in Appendix 2 at hand.

Step 1: Consider the context in which you work, identify your skills and how you practice, and audit your resources

Context

All practitioners can use some of the techniques described in this manual irrespective of whether they work in an in-patient, day-patient, out-patient, or community setting. Patients with PD are common throughout the mental health and social systems with their prevalence steadily increasing with each level of care from general practice, through psychiatric in-patients to prison populations so there is no shortage of patients.

The specifics of his work environment will determine how the practitioner attempts to practice within the overall system so it is important to think about it in detail. It is important to consider how the practitioner/team link with the rest of the service including accident and emergency departments, how patients are referred and how other services are accessed. Are the pathways for patient care clear, or do they become confused for both patients and practitioners? What are the procedures for emergency assessment? It is helpful to draw a diagram of how patients who self-harm or attempt suicide access treatment; borderline patients make up a large proportion of this group. This diagram will immediately reveal any inadequacies in the pathways to treatment and the confusion that may exist in the minds of referrers such as Accident and Emergency practitioners.

Most mental health practitioners now work within teams rather than operating as independent individuals so the team should consider how they work together in treatment of patients. Is there a forum for discussion of how the team work together; is it possible to change the work pattern of the team?

The pathway to community mental health support is commonly via the psychiatric out-patient service with specific localities being serviced by particular teams. In order to start working with patients with PD the community team can consider identifying a named team member for initial contact for all patients with PD. This can only occur following a discussion within the team to define who has an interest in working with these patients. The identified individual may then act as the key worker whose task is to co-ordinate treatment within the team. He should make an initial assessment defining the immediate problems, identify who is involved in the care of the patient and delineate their role and responsibility. He may arrange an initial case conference to organize a treatment plan and to arrange emergency pathways to support.

Within a closed system such as a locked psychiatric ward or a prison, the whole team should attempt to define some of the characteristics of PD that create the most difficult problems for staff and agree a strategy for managing them that can be agreed and understood by all members of the team. Common examples include developing strategies for self-harm, provocative behaviour, threatened violence, and suicidal risk. First the team should examine previous episodes and review what happened both from the perspective of the patient and the staff. Alternative ways of dealing with the situation should be discussed and rehearsed within the team and tested out on the next occasion and the outcome once again subjected to the same 'autopsy' process. If possible this should be done with the patient once the 'heat' of the moment is over.

When implementing this process on a medium secure ward, the staff found that the suicidal patients with PD were unaware of why a nurse accompanied them to the eating area which was away from the ward. Further the nurses themselves, who tended to be temporary staff, thought that their only role was to prevent a patient from killing himself by restraining him if he attempted to harm himself, so they rarely bothered to talk to the patient. After discussion it was agreed that the patient would be informed about why the nurse was present. The reasons included working with the patient to develop ways of reducing suicidal impulses, controlling impulsivity, and identifying feelings and their possible consequences. These topics were agreed with the patient and focused on at pre-arranged times. This was the start of an organized mentalization process within the treatment team.

Skills

Honest appraisal of one's own professional skills as well as those of others is difficult because it involves reflection on and acceptance of weak points without showing undue diffidence as well as clarity about strengths without tripping into arrogance, or becoming overconfident. Not only is there a need to assess specific skills, for example who is competent in managing patients who become suicidal, but also a requirement to consider general attributes and it may be appropriate to discuss these with others within an appraisal system. The practitioner who finds it problematic to be on time for appointments needs to be open about it and accept that working with borderline patients may not be the right focus of his work. The practitioner should ask himself whether he is flexible enough, willing to listen, open to new perspectives, and secure in relationships.

Most practitioners have some specific psychotherapeutic skills and all have some ability to develop a therapeutic alliance with patients. Within a whole team there may be a range of skills which when packaged form a coherent synergistic intervention. Some practitioners may have cognitive or behavioural skills whilst others are able sensitively and competently to use transference and countertransference. Mentalization-based treatment within a health service setting is the frame within which these interventions are practised rather than an alternative and should not replace them leaving the practitioner feeling de-skilled and wondering what to do. Our core techniques of mentalization, retaining mental closeness, bridging the gaps, focusing on the interpersonal and current mental context are not incompatible with different models and may make their implementation more effective. One member of the team might offer individual dynamically-based psychotherapy whilst another focuses on acquisition of skills. The key element is to meet together and think about the patient within a mentalizing frame and integrate the aims of treatment in a way that is understandable to everyone whilst ensuring overall safety of treatment by arranging pathways to emergency care, facilitating advice about medication, and negotiating rapid access to in-patient care. It is crucial to have a shared perspective and if one cannot be developed treatment cannot begin. The essential point is integrating therapists rather than integration of therapies. Each individual member involved in treatment needs to know about and respect the work of the others.

Audit of resources

How many people are in the team? How many patients do they have? Which of their characteristics cause the most trouble? What is the optimal number of patients for each practitioner working in this particular context? What facilities are there in the local area?

A 'quick and dirty' survey is one way of establishing approximate numbers of patients within clinical services who have a diagnosis of borderline personality disorder. Key clinicians in the community can be asked to count the number of patients in active treatment or in contact with services who have a primary diagnosis of PD. In-patient monitoring systems will reveal the number of individuals on the wards with a primary or secondary diagnosis of PD. In addition a survey of all the resources that can be harnessed in treatment of patients and how to access them is useful. Some facilities may already have skills in treatment of PD or offer crisis care in a community setting. Resource 'mapping' should include not only mental health and social facilities but also educational and voluntary schemes.

Step 2: Apply organizational principles

Having mapped out resources, identified skills, and carefully appraised practice, organizational principles as specified in Chapter 6 should be applied to the system. The aim here is to modify the system to make room for implementation of treatment in as effective a manner as possible. There is potential for the system not only to render ineffective even those techniques applied with fidelity and care but also to undermine their initial application so first the practitioner should ensure that he has the support of management and other clinical staff. This is likely to mean development of an outline of proposals for discussion. The key aim here is to move from a 'single practitioner' approach to a coordinated 'divided functions' model or, better still, to take steps towards formation of a 'specialist team' who can increase and maintain their skills more easily.

Structure

Each element of treatment as set out in this manual should be defined by the team by specifying its aims and its boundaries. At minimum this must include the purpose of individual and/or group therapy along with any other organized contact with the service. We reproduce here an example for individual therapy used by a practitioner just starting to work with a patient with BPD.

Individual psychotherapy

Aims

- to take an individual approach to the patient's problems
- to focus on engagement in treatment programme
- to focus on self-destructive behaviour
- to develop a dynamic formulation understandable to patient and team
- to ensure support for group psychotherapy
- to increase mentalization

Boundaries

- Once per week for 50 min
- Emergency sessions offered for 15 min only
- Telephone contact allowed but patient asked to speak to key worker if problem not reduced in an initial discussion
- Patient and therapist both agree to arrive on time and to treat each other with respect and dignity

This format was used for group psychotherapy, medication, crisis responses, in-patient admission, and the case review.

The roles and responsibilities of the staff involved in the care of the patient should be clarified and the patient should be made aware of them and their limits. The practitioner should bear in mind that family or carers involved with the patient may also need to be aware of who does what and who may be contacted for advice or in an emergency. If necessary the details of treatment and the function of professionals should be written down for the patient.

Clarity

What is the best way to explain the aims of treatment to the patient? Often psychiatric interventions are not explained adequately to a patient and he is supposed to trust in the 'doctor'. This is insufficient for most patients but especially inadequate for borderline patients who are often suspicious of the motives of others and wary of treatment that they do not understand. It is important to set up treatment in a way that is understandable to both practitioner and patient. If the practitioner is confused about what he is and is not offering and why he is offering it, the patient will be too, resulting in ample room for misunderstanding, unrealized expectation, and crushing disappointment, all of which lead to chaotic treatment interactions between patient, therapist, and services. Whilst explanation of treatment is part of the structure of treatment it is also necessary to put in plain words to the patient what the practitioner is doing and why. The practitioner should talk to the patient about individual therapy, its focus, how it is believed to work, its side-effects and dangers, its emotional pain. He should also discuss with the patient how they manage in group situations in everyday life. Do they dominate social interactions or remain in the background? Are they manifestly anxious when meeting friends or do they feel supported by others? The answers to these kinds of questions will enable the practitioner to discuss with the patient how they might find group therapy, which until this point may be a mystery to them. It is important to explain the reasons for undertaking group therapy in terms of the patient's life and problems and not simply in general terms.

Consistency

The reason that structure is so important is to ensure consistency. All structures within the organization need to function consistently both across time and across contexts. This is essential given that inconsistency undermines the development of mentalization in so far as it provides incongruity in place of contingency. It is easy to understand why a mental health professional may act differently at different times given the chaotic nature of the patient group and the vicissitudes of the transference and countertransference relationship. To maintain consistency protocols should be developed which are agreed across groups and directed towards common problems.

Intrapersonal consistency is assured by three mechanisms. First is the development of clear and simple protocols which are carefully thought through and understood. Second is training in the protocols with constant monitoring to ensure that they are appropriately implemented, for example through supervision. Third is monitoring of inconsistency, recognizing when it happens and undertaking a review without recrimination.

Interpersonal consistency refers to the whole team and people within the system doing the same thing in common clinical situations. Clear leadership is necessary to ensure the agreed protocols are implemented between groups throughout the system. Leadership requires a willingness on the part of team to assign the responsibility of leadership to a member of the team as well as that member being willing to undertake the leadership role. Underlying rivalries within a team will inevitably bring with them inconsistency as members of the team attempt to develop greater influence. The natural tendency to want to make an individual contribution has to become sub-dominant to the team itself. In order to achieve this, development of an iterative process is necessary in which the team move towards a consensus that is then held by the team itself. New members of the team can then be educated by the team in the team-perspective.

Relationship focus

The opening sessions with a patient need to clarify the importance of the relationship with the therapist as a key feature of treatment. In the assessment the interpersonal aspects of the patient's problems should be the focus. These should be linked to the developing relationship with services and the therapist should suggest that similar patterns might emerge and even encroach on the experience with the therapist. Following an assessment interview, a further discussion is often necessary before a treatment plan can be agreed and so it may be helpful to tell the patient at the outset that before anything is decided it is likely that two interviews will be needed. The second interview might begin with an opening remark such as 'have you had any further thoughts about the previous discussion'? If this leads to a struggle on the part of the patient, the therapist can tell him about his own thoughts about the previous session and what he made of the assessment. This shows the patient that the therapist has been thinking about the problems and this can be used as an example of what the therapist will expect the patient to try to do—a simple example of mentalization with which the patient may then be able to identify. The point here is that the patient should not be able to leave the second session without recognizing that the manner in which he forms and negotiates his relationship to services and to the therapist is of paramount importance in understanding himself and others and has a bearing on the outcome of treatment.

The therapist should think about how he forms a therapeutic alliance with patients. A friendly, sympathetic attitude, encouraging collaboration and joint responsibility, and careful attention to the patient–therapist interaction are known to facilitate an alliance and are dependent on thoughtful consideration of the therapist's relationship with the patient, whilst a more autocratic approach is unlikely to lead to engagement in treatment. Mentalizing, working with current mental states, and addressing negative feelings expressed towards the therapist will also foster a therapeutic alliance and may relate to a positive outcome. Equally important is the negotiation of breaks in the alliance which are inevitable in treatment of BPD. Successful repair of relationship ruptures has been strongly linked to good outcome (Safran *et al.* 1990). When a collapse in trust occurs, it is necessary for the therapist to consider aspects of his current relationship with the patient so that it can be understood in terms of the patient's narrative and perception of the world. That is not to suggest the blame is placed on the patient for the broken alliance because it is just as likely that the therapist has not become what the patient needed him to be at a particular moment or that he has responded in a manner that confirms their distrust or stimulates fear of abandonment. The focus on the relationship means that the therapist first needs to consider his role in the problem and communicate that to the patient. Often this needs to be on the telephone initially and useful opening remarks are 'I am just ringing to discuss what has happened and to understand what I might have done or not done that has led to you not attending your appointment'; 'we need to work this out and understand what went wrong'. The purpose of this type of remark is to continue the emphasis on mentalization and to demonstrate willingness to consider the roles of both patient and therapist in the problem. Too often borderline patients are blamed for problems in treatment just as they were made a scapegoat and held culpable for difficulties in their family.

Intensity

Intensity of treatment of BPD is a dialectic. In the early phases of treatment the intensity of the in-put that will help the patient in the long term is also toxic. A group environment enables patients to engage in splitting, destructiveness, and to use other people as parts of themselves which decreases the stability of their self-structure rather than increasing it. But the very same situation of interpersonal interaction is necessary for them to get better. The key is to find a clinically-effective dose, which may vary over time. In a day-hospital programme it is possible to vary the amount of therapy over a day or week as well as the kind of therapy. This is its strength. Some approaches fail because they offer a sub-clinical dose of treatment whilst others offer such high levels of intervention that it either pushes the patient into pretend mode and hypermentalization or creates so much instability that the patient leaves treatment. In a day-hospital programme patients can be allowed to titrate their dose of treatment initially so that a balance is found between too much and too little. The environment can adapt to the patient rather than the patient having to fit in with his surroundings. The patient should be allowed not to attend at times without being confronted about it and the therapist should keep in mind that this may be all that he can do at one moment. To attend more becomes too intense and so is avoided. Less intensive treatment at this point can be more effective but the sensitive therapist will recognize when a patient can attend more and focus on this in the sessions. The question for the team is at what stage to tackle the issue of infrequent or erratic attendance. In order to do this the therapist has to keep in mind that the patient is not attending because of anxiety which threatens to destabilize him. Rarely is non-attendance an attack on therapy or the therapist.

Medication

The therapist should keep in mind that the use of polypharmacy is to be discouraged. Who is going to prescribe for the patient and how is it going to be co-ordinated with treatment? Unless the team are clear how this is to be done, the whole process will become fragmented and the patient denied 'best' care. The practitioner/team should remain as neutral as possible about medication in relation to psychotherapy; there is no place for emphasizing one over the other because both are necessary and medication may help the patient cope with the stress of psychotherapy. The split between a biological self and a psychological self is iatrogenic and rarely in our experience forms a concern of the borderline patient unless the therapist has been unable to integrate the two models. Prescribing cannot be left to a psychiatrist working without reference to the treatment team and he should be part of the team itself or have well-defined links. But non-medically-trained staff need to have a working knowledge of medication in BPD and be able to clarify the effects of present and past medication, understand the dose prescribed, and have a working knowledge of their negative and positive effects. Staff should be able to explain the potential benefit of medication and be fully aware of its dangers as a method for suicide. Often, the practitioner will know the patient better than the prescriber and so should be prepared to advise about the quantity of medication that should be prescribed at any one time.

It should not be assumed that the patient is taking the medication as prescribed. Exploratory questions such as 'how do you remember to take it'; 'do you ever try to do without it'; 'I suppose that sometimes you have taken more than you should have' should be utilized. Discussion of medication and the patient's relationship with it should be part of therapy. Adherence to medication is least likely when a patient has experienced an interpersonal loss or whilst experiencing strong negative, positive, or dependency feelings towards the therapist and at these times the therapist should beware of misuse of medication to suppress feelings or to dampen painful thoughts.

The simplest way to understand the use of medication in BPD is to refer to our summary in this book (see p. 199), to be able to categorize symptoms as affective, impulsive, or cognitive perceptual, and to follow the algorithms provided in the Practice Guideline for Treatment of Patients with BPD (Oldham *et al.* 2001).

Step 3: Modify the aims and techniques of your current practice

Identify iatrogenic aspects of current practice

Interview techniques and interventions in general psychiatric practice commonly focus on reducing a patient's symptoms. There is no need to dispense with this useful approach because an ability to elicit symptoms and show that they are understandable is an essential element of all treatment and will enhance the therapeutic alliance with the patient. However, its centrality in treatment should be reduced. It has to be supplemented with our core techniques (see Chapter 7) which focus on the affect and mental function of the patient and place them within an interpersonal and developmental context. Increasing these skills, adding them to the existing repertoire of interventions, and integrating them with the team's present set of skills is the most demanding part of this implementation pathway and requires a reorientation of aims from straightforward symptom reduction towards helping the patient identify and give meaning to emotions, stabilize internal representations, work towards a robust self-structure, and form increasingly secure relationships.

In order for the practitioner/team to understand the iatrogenic aspects of their current practice it is useful to review our concepts of teleological function, psychic equivalence, and pretend mode (see Chapter 3).

Borderline patients function, to some degree, by understanding actions in terms of their physical as opposed to mental outcomes—the teleological stance. Their capacity to understand mental states of self and other is enfeebled; awareness of mental states takes place either within a mode of psychic equivalence or of pretend. Psychic equivalence equates the internal with the external and there cannot be differences in perspective about the external world because it is isomorphic with the internal. In pretend mode, the mental state is decoupled from external or physical reality but is separated from the rest of the patient's mental world. The result of these two modes of function is that in psychic equivalence, experience is too real and therefore overwhelming while pretend is too unreal and therefore detached and isolating. As we have seen, the consequences of this for technique are serious if therapists assume borderline patients have cognitive capacities that they simply do not have. If a patient judges motivation and attributes meaning on outcomes, iatrogenic aspects of technique include:

- the use of metaphor
- complex interpretation
- focus on conflict
- emphasis on content

Most of these assume the ability to hold different mental representations in different forms at the same time. So their use in therapy becomes meaningless or, worse, provokes confusion in the patient. The practitioner/team should consider whether their normal therapeutic practice uses these techniques and ensure that they reduce them in their work with patients with PD and replace them. More importantly, if metaphor and conflict interpretation are used, the patient may engage with the therapist in pretend mode leading the therapist to believe erroneously that therapy is progressing well. Sadly, therapy with borderline patients too easily becomes a pretence in which change becomes impossible because the understanding in treatment is encapsulated and has no meaningful links with the patient's life. When a patient appears to be responding well to treatment, the therapist should ask himself if the patient's attitudes and activities outside therapy have altered. Patients in pretend mode will betray their lack of robust change in other areas of their life. Personal relationships may cease to exist as they organize their life around therapy which becomes ultimately the only relationship governing their existence. Supervision and case discussion should be arranged urgently.

The now rare classical psychoanalytic stance, characterized by the 'analyst as a blank screen reflecting back to the patient' will create problems in therapy, being experienced by the patient as authoritarian, cold, lacking in understanding, and unsympathetic. Further, paranoid fantasies will be stimulated resulting in angry reactions and increased anxiety. Greater activity on the part of the therapist is required with more collaboration and openness than is implied in the classical analytic imperatives of free association and rules of abstinence (Freud 1915). The therapist should bear in mind that from a mentalizing perspective neither therapist nor patient experiences the therapeutic process and interactions other than impressionistically.

Increase mentalization skill set incrementally to replace current iatrogenic techniques

Most of the techniques described in this manual are directed towards increasing mentalization. Already practitioners will be familiar with many techniques which do this. These include

- clarification
- elaboration
- empathy
- confrontation

As soon as practitioners are comfortable with these techniques they will need to add in new skills. Initial clinical tasks are commonly to reduce behavioural manifestations of distress so there must be a focus on action as avoidance of internal experience and a persistent attempt on the therapist's part to remain focused on the task of mentalizing the antecedent of action. The patient's denial of the importance of damaging behaviours should not be accepted. The dialogue should be brought back to the internal experience of the patient before, during, and after the action.

The best way to practice mentalizing techniques is by breaking down the process into constituent elements. These include:

- Thinking about feelings—what does the patient feel now and what was the feeling at the time?
- Relating the feeling to their current internal state and their present contexts, including the treatment programme, the services, their current life, and their past life;
- The therapist's exploration of his own reactions to the patient without expressing them directly to the patient;
- The therapist asking himself what is going on in the patient or himself that is making him feel this way;
- Consideration of whether the therapist's own feelings are relevant to the patient's state and whether expressing them verbally will offer an alternative perspective that the patient will understand;
- Only when the answers to these questions are clear should interpretation be considered.

Practising each component of this hierarchy of skills will enable the therapist to move around them smoothly without disrupting the flow of the patient–therapist interaction. Mentalizing in psychotherapy is a process of joint awareness in which the patient's mental states are the object of attention and optimally patient and therapist are engaged in a process of representational redescription in which implicit information in the mind subsequently becomes explicit knowledge to the mind. The therapist should reduce excessive reliance on content and be more concerned with helping the patient to generate multiple perspectives 'on the fly' and to free himself up from being stuck in the 'reality' of one view.

The therapist should draw attention to the patient's experience of an array of mental states and point them out as examples of secondary representations.

A patient was discussing how she had felt at a party and how varied her reactions had been to people, at first feeling joyous and excited but then abandoned and hurt when people had moved away to talk to others. This had led her to become faint and to collapse at the party requiring an ambulance to be called. The therapist said 'you seem to realize that you can feel different things in different circumstances. The fact that we can talk about them now and imagine you in that situation with other people means that we can consider what led you to collapse so that we can keep it in mind for next time when you feel the same'.

The experience of 'feeling felt' (mentalized affectivity) should be highlighted and recognized as progress towards development of meta-representation. This is in some respects comparable to the experience of 'exposure' in the context of a cognitive behavioural treatment. However, it also has an interpersonal dimension in that the patient becomes aware and is exposed to the feeling via the involvement of another person, normally the therapist. It is recognizing the therapist's experience of the patient's feeling that helps the patient experience all aspects of an emotional reaction to something which they avoided because of the anxiety it generated. Again, at the beginning of therapy the therapist should find ways of pointing this out and if necessary take some time to discuss the idea of how the mind works in terms of representations as a buffer to difficult feelings.

Step 4: Implement procedures for dealing with challenging behaviours

First and foremost protocols for challenging behaviour must be agreed with colleagues and everyone must be signed up to them. Practitioners should have a well-identified hierarchy for advice to ensure the most vulnerable member of the team is not left unsupported and each member of the team should be aware of the pathway to admission. The patient must be included in this and should be given clear instructions about how to access emergency help outside normal working hours. Whilst outlining the pathway to emergency care and in-patient care to the patient we also summarize the disadvantages, for example seeing people who know little about the problems, and re-emphasize our more constructive aim of helping the patient manage the problem himself until a member of the team is available.

Appendix 2 contains a 'check list' and aide-de-memoir for dealing with challenging behaviours and therapists should ensure that they are able to follow smoothly the therapist actions outlined under suicide and self-harm, crisis telephone calls, and affect storms. This outline can be used as a reminder. Some of our therapists keep it near the telephone so that they can bring some of the ideas to mind 'when under fire'. In a crisis it is easy to forget what to do and become embroiled in the anxiety of the situation, which inevitably leads to unproductive countertransference enactments.

Step 5: Constantly evaluate your practice

Therapy adherence

It is helpful to photocopy the adherence scale in Appendix 4. Whilst it is primarily for use by an independent assessor who is listening to an audio tape, watching a video tape, or supervising a verbatim report of a session, the therapist can score himself on each item by writing down some examples. If no clear instances from the session spring to mind, it should be considered whether the item was relevant to that particular session or not. If it might have been, the therapist should review what he might have said and make a note of it. He should try to use it in the next session at a relevant point and monitor its effect. The therapist can then report his session to another team member asking him to score this presentation according to the scale, and his reasons for placing an intervention in a particular category can be explored. Gradually, the therapist will be able to build up a clearer picture of his style and increase his understanding of different types of intervention.

Systemic adherence

The principles that hold at the level of the individual need to be applied at the systemic level. Just as the individual therapist is scrutinized by another individual in supervision, so the system needs an outside observer. Specialist organizations can become excessively private, make wild claims about their client group, grow to be protective of their procedures and beliefs, and become resistant to transparency and question. A closed system results in a team and organization becoming fearful of others.

It is difficult to ensure that principles are adhered to throughout an organization. An external person may be best placed to identify whether implementation of agreed procedures is being maintained to a high standard. One method of doing this is to ask others involved in similar work to visit and to look at case notes and to interview staff. Questions to be answered are (1) Are there established structures which are clear to everybody within the system; (2) Are the rules clearly formulated; (3) Do patients have a clear sense of the aims of each aspect of treatment and can these be explained by all staff; (4) Is implementation uniform across the system, across treaters, across patients, and across time. Scrutiny of medical records of a number of critical incidents helps establish if protocols are being consistently applied; (5) Is there a clear supervisory and leadership structure; (6) Is there a way in which clinical decision, making can take place. This forms part of audit and clinical governance as well as continuing professional development.

Patient experience of treatment

We assume that practitioners will normally be collecting qualitative information using formal feedback instruments but we believe that it is also helpful to have some narrative comments from patients. Formal feedback forms tend to have a ceiling effect and patients are inclined to state that things are either wonderful or dreadful. Reports from patients of their experience of treatment are helpful for the therapist as well as for future patients. Borderline patients are not shy about coming forward and pointing out your shortcomings and the failings of treatment. When they do, it is important not to become defensive but to listen carefully and consider the validity of their criticisms. This is part of the continuing mentalization process and practitioners should identify with the patient the context in which the failings occurred, the effect that they had, whether they were adequately addressed, and what suggestions the patient has for improvement. At the individual level this is part of the treatment process. At the group level it can inform the overall arrangement of treatment and if a patient makes a suggestion to staff he should be told that it will be discussed within the team.

In the day-hospital programme patients were admitted for treatment without meeting other patients and were simply introduced in their first group by staff. New patients found this provoked massive anxiety and suggested that before admission or on the morning of admission one of the present patients should be nominated to meet with them beforehand, to discuss treatment with them and to accompany them to their first group. This is now part of our admission process and is helpful in reducing the individual patient's anxiety as well as improving engagement in treatment.

Formal feedback on treatment is commonly used in mental health services nowadays, particularly following short term treatments. The question to consider in treatment of PD is when to give a feedback form and whether different feedback forms are necessary at different times. After considerable discussion, we now ask each patient to complete a form 3 months after admission and about 3 months following the end of intensive treatment and to bring it for discussion to their individual session or their follow-up appointment respectively. By now readers should recognize that this arrangement is in keeping with a focus on mentalization and, in the case of the final feedback form, the time-lag between ending treatment and completing the form may reduce the interference of countertransference phenomena and contamination from ending treatment or reducing its intensity. Outline questionnaires are to be found in Appendix 6.

So, it is to the patients who have given us written feedback that we give the last words of this chapter. The following reports, reproduced with their permission, describe their experience more accurately and vividly than we could ever do.

Patient 1

My experiences at the Halliwick Day Unit are many.

I arrived at the unit in a very volatile and chaotic state, after trying to end my life on numerous occasions.

The staff were welcoming as well as being tough, showed me that I deserved a better way of living. I found my initial period in the Unit very shaky and confrontational, both from staff and patients. However, I was so distrustful of anyone that it took a while to find my safety within the Unit. I started working hard on myself and my many disorders, the main ones were food and behaviour-related. I engaged on a more honest level with all the staff and probably the best person who helped me through the painful chaotic mess was my therapist whom I saw every week for an individual session and in other group work too. The collaborative approach by the team was the most helpful way for me in that the boundaries were set in conjunction with myself, my therapist, and the rest of the Unit team. We all knew where we were heading and any attempts at getting something from someone and saying it had been promised by someone else in the earlier stages in treatment were dealt with in a strong yet caring and very safe way. This allowed me to develop a sense of self-esteem and start looking forward to managing my urges for self-harm in less destructive ways. I learnt about developing safe healthy relationships and how to deal with 'endings' that was always so painful for me. Halliwick gave me the space to discover my real potential that was previously hidden in a life that revolved around self-destruction. The time spent in the art room for me was useful too as at times I really needed to express myself non-verbally or behaviourally. Groups were good as so many territories for me were explored. Relationships, space, silences, anger, despair and compassion. Exploring change. One senior therapist had a classic line of 'what is it about this change that makes it so so painful?'

I still come to the unit but as an out-patient to see 'The Boss' and my life is far from perfect. However, through the day unit, I allowed myself to have a life obviated from multiple health professionals and encouraged me to start looking after myself instead of professionals looking after me.

Patient 2

I'd never had experience of group therapy before and never with individual together. It was more challenging than one-to-one therapy although I liked the one-to-one sessions. I think they kept me safe. I had never thought about the effect of my behaviour on others before and the group made you do that. I hadn't had close friendships so I never realized that there were effects on others when you are destructive. You just think about yourself and never what it is about and who might it affect and what it has done to them. I never used to ask others about how they feel or listen to what they think about me. I can deal with anyone now if I can deal with people here.

The staff were different here. They are more consistent. In other places they all do something different. Here they don't change their mind and you ask one staff one thing and they say the same as someone else. They were flexible too and accept that people need different things. Someone might need something more than someone else. It is a long-term treatment as well. I have had lots of treatment before but staff just leave and then there is nothing after only a short time. I feel dropped and go back to how I was. At least there is some follow-up here. It was good that I could maintain my independence when I came here. I have been an in-patient before and it was too much for me.

My self-harm is better. My eating is OK. I have little lapses but it is better. I can interact with other people now and don't have big blow-ups because I can understand others now and get inside their heads. I know how to respond, how to talk to people, and think about how they are feeling. I can manage my emotions now and don't run away from them. But I still feel lonely when I am on my own and my moods go up and down but I think that I can manage to go to College now. I am not 100% better but better than I have ever been before. I still find very close relationships hard. People are hard to meet and then taking it a step further is even more difficult but I have more friendships than I ever had before. I don't look too far in advance. I get frightened but I want to be independent and to manage like everyone else does.

Appendix 1 Suicide and self-harm inventory

This instrument is designed to ensure accurate collection of data about attempted acts of suicide and incidents of self-harm. For the purposes of the research project the instrument is categorical. The interviewer should note that a trained rater will assess if a particular episode meets the criteria for either a suicide attempt or self-harm. **The instrument is not a measure of severity.** The aim of the interview is to assess the frequency of attempts of both suicide and self-harm over a six-month time period.

Criteria for suicidal acts

The criteria for suicidal acts are:

(1) **deliberate**
This means that the act could not be construed as an accident and there was planning involved. The subject accepts ownership of the act e.g. claiming not to have read the indications on a bottle of medications before taking it in excess would not be considered as a suicidal act.

(2) **life-threatening**
The subject's life was seriously at risk as a consequence of the act. Even if the subject considered, at the time of the attempt, that their life was at risk as a consequence of the act, but in reality it was not, the gesture would not be considered suicidal but as an act of self-harm (if other criteria were met).

(3) **have resulted in medical intervention**
The subject must have either sought medical intervention or medical intervention was sought on their behalf. Medical intervention need not be treatment but

at the minimum a physical examination is implied. If a doctor is not able to confirm the attempt you should not consider it under this heading. Confirmation consists of a note in the medical records, a letter to the RMO or some other service. It requires more than the patient's claim of medical intervention for this criterion to be met.

(4) **medical assessment was consistent with a suicide attempt**
The medical record must provide evidence that medical opinion was consistent with the patient's act being deliberate, potentially lethal, and requiring medical attention. Please ensure that the records are carefully searched. A positive finding is necessary if an act is to be coded as suicidal.

Attempted suicide

Over the past 6 months have you attempted to kill yourself? (The interviewer should describe to the patient the definition of an attempt at suicide given above).

On how many occasions can you recall trying to kill yourself?

List in chronological order: Date/Method

The interviewer should assess the accuracy of this statement at the end of the interview
Accurate/reasonably accurate/questionable/inaccurate

The interviewer should then elicit the following information for each act commencing with the earliest attempt over the last 6 months:

Suicidal act 1

Date of the event:

Overdose/Self-laceration/Burning/Head banging/Swallowing razor blades/ Hanging/Shooting/Jumping from height or under train/Other—please specify

(Only include life threatening self-induced injury here e.g. overdose necessitating hospital assessment or admission, self-laceration leading to severe loss of blood requiring transfusion, head banging resulting in sub-dural haematoma, razor blade ingestion leading to surgical intervention, etc)

How long before the act did the patient know that he was going to harm himself?

Were plans made? If so, what were those plans

Did the patient contact anyone about the possible attempt? Mother/Father/ Partner/ Other patient/Mental health worker/General practitioner

Did the patient leave a note indicating that the act was suicidal?

Did anyone try and help the patient? i.e. friend, carer, professional, patient

Was anyone present at the time of the attempt?

Did the patient expect anyone to visit?

Was the attempt associated with alcohol or illicit drugs? Yes/No Alone or with other?

If so, with whom was the patient drinking or taking drugs prior to the act and where?

What were those drugs or alcohol and in what quantity?

If found, how was the patient found and by whom?

Who arranged for the patient to go to hospital?

How did the patient get to hospital?

Which hospital was the patient admitted to?

Is there evidence for admission? If so, are there medical notes?

Please enter here the details of those medical notes e.g. Patient Identification Number

Do they confirm the stated act?

Is there a note to state that the act was potentially life-threatening? Please copy verbatim the statement suggesting that the act was a suicide attempt.

What medical and nursing action was taken?

How long was the patient in hospital?

To whose care was the patient discharged and was follow-up given?

Criteria for acts of self-harm

(1) **deliberate**

This means that the act could not be construed as an accident and that the subject accepts ownership of the act. Planning may have been involved. Common examples include the purchase of razor blades, carrying them around in a bag, and, in an organized fashion, cutting the wrists or other areas of the body; lighting a cigarette and burning oneself. In other instances, planning may not occur. The individual may harm himself in an emotional crisis. Often head-banging occurs under these circumstances but self-laceration may also happen at these times and frenzied cutting results. Under these circumstances the frenzied self-harm only counts as one act as long as other criteria are met. Similarly, if a patient reports events that occur within hours of each other, these are to be considered as one event. ONLY when 48 h has passed between events are they to be considered as separate acts.

(2) **resulting in visible tissue damage**

Clear tissue damage should be present. Common examples are recent scars, bruises, and burns. The interviewer should make a note of where the tissue damage is so that an interviewer in 6 months time can ask for evidence of new damage. Please note that it may be impossible to ask the patient to show the tissue damage either because of sensitivity in the interview or because of the site of the damage. In this case it is adequate to make a note of the type, site, and time of the self-harm BUT in all cases there must be evidence under criterion 3.

(3) **nursing or medical intervention required**

It is important that the information is collected as accurately as possible. The rater will decide whether or not a patient scores positively based on the information that you collect. The subject must have either sought medical or nursing intervention or medical/nursing intervention was sought on their behalf. For example the arms may have required bandaging following self-laceration. Medical/nursing intervention need not be treatment but at the minimum a physical examination is implied. If a doctor or nurse is not able to confirm the attempt you should not consider it under this heading. Confirmation consists of a note in the medical records, a letter to the RMO or some other service. It requires more than the patient's claim of medical intervention for this criterion to be met.

Acts of self-harm

Have you harmed yourself in any other way over the last 6 months? For example by cutting or burning yourself, banging your head?

(The interviewer should describe to the patient the definition of self-harm given above).

Yes/No

How many times have you harmed yourself in any of these ways over the last 6 months? (Interviewer should assess the accuracy of this statement at the end of the interview).

Date/Method

Accurate/reasonably accurate/questionable/inaccurate

Date/Method

Accurate/reasonably accurate/questionable/inaccurate

Date/Method

Accurate/reasonably accurate/questionable/inaccurate

The interviewer should then elicit the following information for each act commencing with the earliest attempt over the last 6 months:

Date of act:
Self laceration, head banging, burning, Other-specify

If possible and clinically appropriate please ask the patient to show the results of the act of self-harm e.g. is there clear tissue damage of self-laceration/burns to the wrists and arms. Is there bruising to the face? Describe the evidence. (Do not embarrass or shame the patient. If in doubt DO NOT ASK)

Please document the site of self-harm in such a way that an interviewer will be clear in 6 months time where the previous acts were sited e.g. upper arm, breasts, face, genitals. Draw picture if necessary.

Was the act part of a frenzied process or a single act e.g. some patients cut themselves many times over a short period of time or head bang for a period of hours.

Is the patient clear that all the acts were part of the same incident?

If multiple acts were committed please indicate over what period of time

Was there a period of over 48 h between the multiple acts (acts occurring within 48 h of each other are counted as one incident)

How long before the act did the patient know that he was going to harm himself?

If so what were the warning signs as described by the patient?

Were plans made? If so what were those plans e.g. did the patient go out and buy razor blades, did he lay them out before hand?

Did the patient contact anyone prior to the act?

Did anyone try and help the patient? i.e. friend, carer, professional

Was anyone present at the time of the act?

Was the attempt associated with alcohol or illicit drugs?

Was the patient with someone? If so with whom was the patient drinking or taking drugs prior to the act and where?

Estimate the quantity and list the substances used

Did the result of self-harm require medical or nursing intervention?

If so, by whom and where?

Notes ID number:

What intervention was given? e.g. cleaning, dressing, observation on medical in-patient ward

Is there evidence in the medical notes of the medical or nursing intervention? Yes/No

Copy verbatim the entry made by the nurse or doctor.

If no evidence in the notes, do you have corroboration of the self-harm from an independent witness, for example a health care worker.

Please confirm that you have reviewed the medical notes. Yes/No

Appendix 2 Training materials

Framework of treatment

The therapist needs to organize a robust framework for treatment, ensure that treatment is safe and co-ordinated, and be able to explain the frame to the patient. He has to negotiate sensitively the joint role of therapist and key worker.

As a key worker the therapist needs to:

- structure treatment
  - arrange a timetable with the patient
  - clarify roles and responsibilities
  - organize a crisis plan
  - provide access to in-patient care
  - explain and maintain boundaries
  - explain broad contract of treatment
  - arrange review of medication
- identify the initial hierarchy of therapeutic goals with the patient. In descending order of importance these are commonly:
  - engagement in therapy/begin to develop therapeutic alliance in first session
  - ensure safety, by structural change if necessary, to reduce suicidal acts
  - consider appropriate use of emergency services
  - stabilize accommodation
  - rationalize medication
  - start development of a psychodynamic formulation
- develop consistency and coherence to minimize splitting
  - rationalize the number of people involved in the patient's care
  - organize an admission case conference
  - provide adequate notice of absences and breaks
  - ensure the patient accepts and agrees the limits of confidentiality

- explain the rationale of treatment
  - clarify the purpose of individual and group therapy
  - personalize the treatment—give examples of problems and how they will be addressed
  - discuss the common anxieties associated with treatment
  - identify factors that might lead to drop-out
- work flexibly whilst maintaining boundaries
  - avoid becoming increasingly rigid in response to chaotic behaviour
  - address missed appointments by considering the underlying anxiety
  - use the individual session to consider the anxieties of group therapy and the group to challenge antitherapeutic attitudes in individual session
- recognize the importance of supervision and team work
  - commit to regular supervision times
  - attend team meetings regularly
  - consider colleagues' viewpoint even when different from one's own
  - report countertransference responses honestly and without modification

Mentalization

The aim of this module is (1) for the therapist to recognize that the borderline patient deviates from the normal intentional stance in which an individual is assumed to be a rational agent with understandable desires and predictable beliefs who will act to further his goals in light of those beliefs and (2) to learn ways of increasing a patient's level of mentalization through questioning and exploration. Mentalization is the process by which an individual implicitly and explicitly interprets his own actions and those of others as meaningful on the basis of intentional mental states (e.g. desires, needs, feelings, beliefs, and reasons). It acts as a buffer between feeling and action helping the individual to form a deeper understanding of others, to recognize his own and others' misunderstandings, to consider if others or his own motivation or reaction is deceitful and manipulative, or honest and true, and to modulate interpersonal and emotional distance. For training purposes and patient information leaflets this has been characterized as helping the patient 'PUSH THE PAUSE BUTTON' (Jon Allen–personal communication).

The therapist needs to learn to recognize the different clinical manifestations of mentalization. Signs of mentalization include:

- distinguishing between appearance and reality
- reflecting on mental states

- monitoring thoughts, feelings, and language to give meaning
- reasoning, using an appropriate knowledge base
- attending to primary themes without distraction from sub-dominant themes or emotional states

The task of the therapist is to increase the patient's capacities in all these areas.

Therapist techniques

The therapist needs to maintain a genuine stance of not-knowing and to PUSH THE PAUSE BUTTON by:

- asking questions or using questioning comments to promote exploration
  - what do you make of what has happened?
  - why do you think that he said that?
  - I wonder if that was related to the group yesterday?
  - perhaps you felt that I was judging you?
  - what do you make of her suicidal feeling (in the group)?
  - why do you think that he behaved towards you as he did?
- using the therapeutic relationship (transference manifestations) to highlight alternative perspectives
  - I saw it as a way to control yourself rather than to attack me (patient explanation), can you think about that for a moment
  - you seem to think that I don't like you and yet I am not sure what makes you think that.
  - just as you distrusted everyone around you because you couldn't predict how they would respond, you now are suspicious of me
  - you have to see me as critical so that you can feel vindicated in your dismissal of what I say
- within the day-hospital programme encouraging use of expressive therapy
  - art therapy
  - journaling
  - psychodrama

These expressive therapies, only done in group form, allow the internal to be placed outside in a different form and considered from a distance. The therapist technique is not only to get the patient to verbalize what he has written or painted, but to consider what others are trying to express in their work.

Working with current mental states

The therapist should not get lost in the past. Borderline patients are pulled into the past because of its powerful influence on the present and they become imprisoned by it, suffering understandable bitterness and desire for retribution and reparation which only serve to anchor the patient more firmly in the trauma. The therapist needs to ensure that the past does not become a retreat and must concentrate on the emotional present.

Therapist techniques

The therapist always works within the moment until the influence of the past on the present is clearly distorting the therapeutic relationship.
The therapist needs to:

- attend to current emotions
  - what is the feeling
  - towards whom is it directed
  - is there an underlying feeling covered by the manifest feeling
- focus on expression of emotions
  - keep talking to patient if he is in an emotional crisis
  - state what the patient is expressing to you and help them to consider other ways of expressing it
  - confront patient with negative effects of their expression
  - formulate the problem (if possible) in simple terms—you are doing this because …
- identify immediate or recent interpersonal contexts especially within group and individual therapy
  - detail time since last session, including outside events
  - ask about group or individual therapy and feelings evoked
  - interpret the current mental state in terms of the interpersonal interactions including the here and now
  - understand the situation in terms of the patient's instability of the self and the need to restabilize
  - consider the repetition of the present mental state in different guises in other situations in current life–isn't this how you were with…? Wasn't this what happened when … ?
  - predict future episodes and outline their likely context as an early warning system

- relate current events to the 'explored' past only when the 'explored' current has been understood and affect expression controlled
  - is this a repetition and if so what stimulates it
  - is the patient dealing with the present in a way that has developed from his treatment in the past
  - identify and interpret the unconscious need to stabilize the self

Bridging the gaps

The gap between affective experience and its representation has to be bridged in therapy and a major aim of therapy is to strengthen the secondary representational system.
In order to do this the therapist needs to:

- reflect the patient's expression in a modified form
  - empathize with patient's internal state
  - accept what is real for the patient
  - break down the experience into small components keeping to the interpersonal focus
  - explore alternative understanding of the verbalized events and internal experience
  - validate correct experience and representation but explore its continuing interference in functioning
  - focus on translation of behaviour into verbal expression
- focus the patient's attention on therapist experience when it offers an opportunity to clarify misunderstandings and to develop prototypical representations
  - highlight the patient's experience of therapist
  - use transference to emphasize different experiences and perspectives
  - negotiate negative reactions and ruptures in therapeutic alliance by identifying patient and therapist roles in the problem
- develop a transitional area in sessions in which to play with ideas
  - help the patient use ideas as representations rather than as 'real' things
  - judiciously use humour to heighten meaning
  - explore different meanings in one idea
  - later in therapy move from the concrete to some abstraction

Transference

Transference is used to demonstrate alternative perspectives and not as a tool to reconstruct the past. Transference is the medium through which patients' past experience influences their perception of the present and represents the interactions of their internal object representations.

The therapist needs to:

- ensure that the patient does not experience transference as a mystery
  - explain the concept of transference at the beginning of treatment
  - identify transference features in the patient–therapist relationship to example the explanation
  - highlight the usefulness of considering the patient–therapist relationship as a focus of treatment
- join together aspects of patients' interpersonal life with transference tracers
  - link the patient–therapist relationship to affiliations outside
  - understand the relevance of external relationships to the therapy relationship
  - demonstrate that the pattern of interaction with the treatment system reflects the form of relationships outside
- contrast his own perception with that of patient
  - do not insist on one view being correct but identify underlying reasons for alternative explanation
  - be sensitive to the reality of the patient's experience even if different from yours
  - recognize there is a shared reality but no absolute reality
- consider the present in terms of the past but only later in therapy
  - focus on current problems but build up a narrative linking them with the past
  - identify the role that the patient places you in now and consider reversal of roles
  - reflect on forced role responsiveness as a method to maintain stability or make sense of the incomprehensible

Suicide and self-harm

The therapist needs to

- remain calm—anxiety in the therapist reduces his ability to mentalize
  - what can I do to help the patient not do this?

 - I am not responsible for the patient's life but I am here to help them reduce risk
 - I have the team to discuss the problem with and I can tell the patient that I would like to do that

- sensitively monitor countertransference and other responses
 - am I anxious because the patient is anxious or is it because I am worried about being blamed
 - do I feel angry because I am being portrayed as something I don't believe that I am or is it so that the patient can feel more stable.
 - if the patient is at lower risk by experiencing me in a specific manner then it is my task to accept that role until the crisis passes, Therefore I must:
 - beware of forcefully returning projections

- assess the immediacy of the threat and consider it in terms of previous acts of self-harm or suicide attempts
 - at least the patient has spoken about it rather than just doing it
 - what was the previous pattern
 - did anything calm the situation last time
 - is the patient so angry, dismissive, hopeless, anxious that they find it impossible to listen to me
 - would it help if both of us had 'time-out' from the meeting for a few minutes
 - place previous acts within a context, commonly a context of problematic emotional relationships, and link to the present situation

- be aware of the well-known risk factors for suicide
 - previous attempts
 - hopelessness
 - severe anxiety
 - alcohol and drug misuse
 - isolation, loneliness, and lack of supportive relationships
 - notes and written final wishes

- keep talking to the patient about the feeling and its immediate precipitants
 - who was the patient with when the feeling started
 - what was being talked about
 - was there a fear of abandonment which includes apparently small issues such as someone close showing independence of mind
 - has the patient discussed it with others in the group and did anything help

  - link recent acts within the relationship of the patient to the partial hospital, intensive out-patient programme or to the therapist
  - show the patient that their actions are understandable given their feelings immediately prior to the act of self-harm, inability to deal with these feelings, and their past experiences, and instability of self

- engage the patient in discussing his action to establish communication about it and to maintain this communication for as long as possible
  - what are the likely experiences or reactions of others to the action
  - consider confronting the patient with the destructive nature of the acts
  - explore the affective changes since the previous individual session linking them with events within treatment
  - help the patient to modify their responses to their multiply-determined feelings

- make a systematic attempt to place some of the responsibility for the patient's actions back with the patient with an aim of re-establishing self-control.
  - I cannot stop you harming yourself but we can work together to reduce the need to do it
  - positively state the importance of bringing the risk to the attention of therapist as being the first step in helping themselves not act dangerously
  - state that the patient will be the judge of whether hospital admission is necessary

- make clear that the staff are able and willing to respond to the emergency.
  - we will see you, if only for a short time, if you believe that will help you reduce your risk
  - we will help you negotiate hospital admission even if it is just for one night

- refrain from interpreting the patient's actions in terms of their personal history and the putative unconscious motivations or their current possible manipulative intent at the time of crisis
  - rarely are suicide threats and anxiety of self-harm motivated by manipulation
  - the patient cannot think in this way during a crisis and experiences the therapist as failing to understand the current emergency

- be clear about his role whilst the suicide risk remains high
  - keep to what has been agreed—if a meeting is arranged ensure that it happens

  - do not increase contact because of anxiety but only if it is obvious that risk is escalating
  - contact the patient judiciously to show that he is still being thought about
  - inform the patient that the level of risk will be discussed in the team and will be considered in all the therapeutic contexts e.g. group and individual, expressive therapy

- following the episode ensure a thorough review in a number of contexts including individual and group therapy
  - the episode is discussed actively by the group and individual therapist
  - link to current problems within the therapy
  - explore the interpersonal context and the group process before development of the risk of suicide and self-harm
  - identify the effect of the event or threatened event on the individual session and the group therapy
  - interpret the unconscious meaning later when the patient has retrieved some capacity to mentalize. Consider it in terms of maintenance of stability of the self and organisation of meaning predicated on past experience

Crisis telephone calls

At the beginning of treatment patients are given the unit telephone numbers and informed that a member of staff will discuss a problem with them over the telephone if it is urgent. The unit numbers have an answering machine and if messages are left overnight a member of the team will return the call by 10 am the next working day. Telephone calls are not therapy and should not be used in this way by either patient or therapist. Interpretation is not used as a technique in telephone calls although empathy, elaboration, clarification, and confrontation are. Telephone calls can be deliberately brief if a patient has not been attending and continues to contact by phone only. Under these circumstances, the content of any telephone conversation must be related to non-attendance. Use of telephone contact varies from the rare to the excessive and both may be a problem. The patient who fails to contact but acts out may need help to use the service more effectively whilst the patient who contacts compulsively will need support to reduce the need. In our experience the frequent contact patients find separation difficult and if they are to remain stable require confirmation that staff continue 'have them in mind'. Sometimes the answer machine is an adequate substitute and one patient only ever called out-of-hours stating that no reply was needed although we made it clear in the following treatment session that the call had been received and listened to.

Therapist strategies for dealing with telephone calls are:

- clarify the purpose of the call
  - listen
  - ask the patient why he is calling at this particular time
  - identify any interpersonal circumstances outside that are contributing to the problem
  - consider factors from group and individual therapy that might have provoked the crisis and mention them to the patient
  - if the crisis is life-threatening, follow suggestions in dealing with self-harm and suicide threats and ask the patient to attend for further discussion
- make the call as brief as possible and try to complete the conversation with clear agreement about what is being done about the problem
  - decide how long the conversation can last and explain why, for example another appointment
  - ensure that the patient recognizes the need to explore the problem further in treatment
  - confirm that information will be passed on to the treatment team
  - be specific about the next appointment time in group or individual therapy
- do nothing that encourages telephone calls in place of therapy or promotes the use of urgent telephone conversations to resolve crises
  - ask about what the patient has done to address the problem and, if constructive, build on that
  - who else has the patient talked to about the problem and what was their suggestion
  - insist that the patient thinks about solutions
  - identify the patients' use of you in the conversation. Is it as a transference figure? Is it to show that nothing can help?

Therapist reasons for contacting the patient are:

- administrative
- part of the engagement process
- repair or enhance therapeutic alliance
- reduce risk by demonstrating continuing mentalization
- agreed part of treatment plan e.g. scheduled phone call
  - ≺ do not contact the patient to reduce therapist anxiety unless discussed with at least one other team member

Affect storms

Failure of affect control leads to irrational behaviour and inappropriate responses from others. It is important that therapists are confident in dealing with outbursts of emotion and do not retaliate or react impulsively themselves. Appropriate intervention reduces the risk of enactments.
The therapist should:

- maintain a dialogue throughout the emotional crisis:
  - keep talking calmly and confidently to the patient
  - remember that the emotion will recede over time and remind the patient of this
  - if the patient is agitated do not insist he sits down. Allow them to walk around the room if necessary
  - continue thinking about why the patient is like this now and if in a group ask other patients if they can understand the reasons
- clarify the feeling
  - do not insist on what the feeling is but try to get the patient to describe it
  - label the feeling if possible
  - identify likely consequences if the feeling is not controlled e.g. self-harm
  - what effect is the emotional expression likely to have on others
- address possible underlying causes for the affect storm
  - identify any interpersonal precursors in the patient's current life
  - consider group and individual therapy as a cause of the outburst
  - explore feelings beneath the manifest emotion e.g. hurt behind anger, love behind aggression
  - identify previous outbursts and mention how they were understood within the treatment
  - link to previous or current relationships

Appendix 3 Crisis plan

This plan is to be agreed by all members of treatment team.

Mr Anthony Challenge experiences regular episodes of .... (Insert self-harm, suicide attempt, dangerous behaviour, etc). This is a result of his personality difficulties.
He has been assessed by (Insert Name) and the following crisis plan developed with him:

1. He will report indicators of forthcoming crisis by contacting (Insert Name and Telephone Number).
2. If (Insert name) is unavailable Mr A Challenge will contact (insert office administrator Name and number) who will inform another member of team.
3. The team aim to respond within X hours during normal working hours or before 10 am on the next working day.
4. Known factors include: (Insert List e.g. alcohol, increase in drug use, feelings of rejection, and interpersonal difficulties).
5. If contact is made during normal working hours (Insert Name) the crisis will be discussed over the phone initially.
6. If resolution is problematic or risk considered high, a brief appointment will be made to decide on further action including in-patient admission, referral to medical services.
7. The crisis, once resolved, will be discussed in detail in the next clinical sessions.
8. No change in overall treatment plan will be made during a crisis and there will be no change in medication without discussion with the team.
9. **Out of hours** Mr Anthony Challenge will contact (Insert Emergency Details). They will listen to the problems, assess risk but not alter or prescribe

medication, and offer appropriate intervention until a member of treatment team can be contacted on the following working day.

Signed:

Patient:

Key worker:

Agreed by team : Yes ❑ No ❑

Appendix 4 Rating of MBT adherence and competence

Patient:______________________ **Rater:**______________________

Therapist:______________________ **Today's date:**____________________

Group session No:_________________ **Individual session No**:____________

Form of presentation (circle one) Verbal Audiotape Videotape

Type of rating (circle one) Peer group Supervisor Research staff

Please rate the extent to which the therapist's interventions reflect optimal MBT procedures, *in light of this patient's presentation in this session*. Make your ratings using the following scale:

1. does not use MBT procedures
2. attempts to use MBT procedures but strays from routine; clearly needs supervisory assistance
3. utilizes MBT procedures adequately but may need some supervisory assistance
4. utilizes MBT procedures adequately
5. excellent use of MBT procedures

0. does not apply

Framework of treatment

1 2 3 4 5 0 Treatment is offered in a clearly structured context that is transparent to patients and treaters?

1 2 3 4 5 0 Clear hierarchy of therapeutic goals agreed with patient?

1 2 3 4 5 0	Crisis plan identified?
1 2 3 4 5 0	Admission case conference been organized where roles of staff have been identified, and the limits of confidentiality agreed?
1 2 3 4 5 0	Patient appears to understand the rationale of treatment and the purpose of group and individual therapy?
1 2 3 4 5 0	Boundaries of therapy have been explained?
1 2 3 4 5 0	Therapist committed to supervision either in peer group or with senior practitioner?

Overall score for framework of treatment 1 2 3 4 5 0

Mentalization

1 2 3 4 5 0	Taking a genuine stance of 'not–knowing' but attempting to 'find out'
1 2 3 4 5 0	Therapist asks appropriate questions to promote exploration
1 2 3 4 5 0	Adequate consideration of patient's understanding of motives of others
1 2 3 4 5 0	Use of transference tracers at beginning of therapy
1 2 3 4 5 0	Using transference interpretation to highlight alternative perspectives
1 2 3 4 5 0	Appropriate confrontation and challenge of unwarranted beliefs about self and other
1 2 3 4 5 0	Avoidance of presenting the patient with complex mental states
1 2 3 4 5 0	Avoidance of simplified historical accounts
1 2 3 4 5 0	Avoiding confrontation with patient when in psychic equivalence mode
1 2 3 4 5 0	Identifying and addressing pretend mode of mentalization in the patient
1 2 3 4 5 0	Addresses reversibility of mental states and challenges psychic equivalence

Overall score for mentalization 1 2 3 4 5 0

Working with current mental states

1 2 3 4 5 0 Attending to current emotions

1 2 3 4 5 0 Focus on appropriate expression of emotions

1 2 3 4 5 0 Linking affect with immediate or recent interpersonal contexts

1 2 3 4 5 0 Relates understanding in current interpersonal context to appropriate past experiences

Overall score for working with mental states 1 2 3 4 5 0

Bridging the gaps

1 2 3 4 5 0 Reflects the patient's internal state in a modified form

1 2 3 4 5 0 Recognizes patient's experience of psychic equivalence

1 2 3 4 5 0 Focuses attention of patient on therapist experience without being persistently self-referent

1 2 3 4 5 0 Negotiates ruptures in alliance by clarifying patient and therapist roles

1 2 3 4 5 0 Develops a transitional 'as if' playful way of linking internal and external reality in sessions

1 2 3 4 5 0 Judiciously uses humour

Overall score for bridging the gaps 1 2 3 4 5 0

Affect storms

1 2 3 4 5 0 Maintains a dialogue throughout the emotional outburst

1 2 3 4 5 0 Initially attempts to clarify the feeling and any underlying emotion without interpretation

1 2 3 4 5 0 Addresses possible underlying causes within patient's current life

1 2 3 4 5 0 Identifies triggers for the storm in patient's construal of their interpersonal experience immediately prior to it

1 2 3 4 5 0 Links affect storm to therapy only after storm has receded

Overall score for affect storms 1 2 3 4 5 0

Use of transference

1 2 3 4 5 0	Shows clear build up over time to transference interpretation
1 2 3 4 5 0	Only uses transference interpretation when therapeutic alliance is established
1 2 3 4 5 0	Transference not used as simple repetition of the past
1 2 3 4 5 0	Transference is used to demonstrate alternative perspectives between self and other
1 2 3 4 5 0	Avoids interpreting the therapeutic relationship as part of another relationship that the patient currently has or has had in the past
1 2 3 4 5 0	Transference interpretations brief and to the point
1 2 3 4 5 0	Refrains from use of metaphor
1 2 3 4 5 0	Does not focus on conflict

Overall score for transference 1 2 3 4 5 0

How much overall competence does the therapist exhibit in this session?

1	**2**	**3**	**4**	**5**
Very little				**A great deal**

What difficulties are present in the therapist's current approach? Use the space below to record your comments.

Appendix 5 Text of intensive out-patient programme (IOP) leaflet

Who is the service for?

This service is tailored to those individuals who

- have difficulties in forming and maintaining relationships
- have problems in controlling their impulses
- have frequently experienced difficult emotions
- may engage in self-harming activity.

The aim of the programme is:

- to explore how your difficulties have come about, particularly in relation to past experiences
- to identify factors that maintain your problems
- to help find ways of dealing with the problems as they are affecting you now.

What form does the treatment take?

The treatment takes the form of both individual and group psychotherapy.

Individual therapy

One individual session is offered on a weekly basis. This session lasts 50 min. You will see the same therapist each week.

Exploratory group

This group will have a maximum of 6–8 people and last for 1½ hours. The group will help you explore your relationships with others, what past experiences influence them, and how these experiences affect your relationships now.

Psychiatric review

You will be offered a regular psychiatric review to discuss medication and to discuss how your treatment is progressing. Other mental health professionals may be present at this meeting, particularly if you have housing or other social needs.

When are these groups and individual sessions?

The exploratory groups take place at a pre-arranged time and this will be discussed with you when you start treatment. The individual session will be arranged at a time that is mutually convenient for you and your therapist.

What is expected from me and what can I expect from the service?

In order to participate in the treatment you will

- try and attend all meetings
- stay in treatment for one year
- not abuse alcohol or drugs
- listen thoughtfully to other group members
- try to complete any homework assignments
- try to limit any self-damaging behaviour.

We will

- listen to you with respect
- organize the programme professionally and competently
- maintain confidentiality as discussed below
- continually try to understand your problem and not be judgmental.

Is the service confidential?

The service is provided within the confines of medical confidentiality. Information will only be shared with other mental health professionals outside the service after it has been discussed with you.

The therapists running IOPP share information. This information is kept confidential within the team.

Why do I have to keep filling forms in?

The IOPP is a research-based service. The service has been set up as part of a research project. It is, therefore, necessary for us to ask you to complete some questionnaires at regular intervals. Hopefully, these do not take too much of your time and it will allow us to develop the programme according to the feedback that you give us.

The answers you give on your forms are confidential and not used by the therapists. Only the researcher will know your answers. If, at any time, you want feedback from the questionnaires, this will be available.

Appendix 6 Admission feedback questionnaire

Name :

Date :

Please summarize your main problems before you entered treatment.

Was your referral handled in an efficient and helpful manner?

Yes ❑ No ❑ To some extent ❑

Please describe your experience of the assessment.

Following the assessment, was it clear what was going to happen next?

Yes ❑ No ❑ To some extent ❑

Were you given an understandable outline of treatment?

Yes ❑ No ❑ To some extent ❑

Was a crisis plan given to you?

Yes ❑ No ❑ To some extent ❑

Did you have a reasonable idea of the aims of treatment as discussed before admission?

Yes ❑ No ❑ To some extent ❑

Was a patient available to meet with you before you started treatment?

Yes ❑ No ❑

Please describe your experience of starting treatment.

Was there anything you think that could have been done to improve the process of assessment and admission for treatment?

Thank you for your comments. To ensure that they are discussed it would be helpful if you could bring this form to your next meeting with a member of staff.

References

Ad-Dab'bagh, Y. and Greenfield, B. (2001). Multiple complex developmental disorder: the "multiple and complex" evolution of the "childhood borderline syndrome" construct. *Journal of the American Academy of Child and Adolescent Psychiatry*, **40**: 954–64.

Adler, G. and Buie, D. (1979). Aloneness and borderline psychopathology: The possible relevance of some child developmental issues. *International Journal of Psycho-Analysis*, **60**: 83–96.

Adolphs, R. (2003). Cognitive neuroscience of human social behaviour. *Nature Reviews*, **4**: 165–78.

Aggleton, J. P. and Young, A. W. (2000). The enigma of the amygdala: On its contribution to human emotion. In: *Cognitive Neuroscience of Emotion* (ed. R. D. Lane and L. Nadel), pp. 106–28. New York: Oxford University Press.

Ainsworth, M. D. S., Blehar, M. C., Waters, E., and Wall, S. (1978). *Patterns of Attachment: A Psychological Study of the Strange Situation.* Hillsdale, NJ: Erlbaum.

Akiskal, H. S. (1983). Dysthymic disorder: psychopathology of proposed chronic depressive subtypes. *The American Journal of Psychiatry*, **140**: 11–20.

Akiskal, H. S., Hirschfeld, R. M., and Yerevanian, B. I. (1983). The relationship of personality to affective disorders. *Archives of General Psychiatry*, **40**: 801–10.

Akiskal, H. S., Chen, S. E., Davis, G. C., Puzantian, V. R., Kashgarian, M., and Bolinger, J. M. (1985). Borderline: An adjective in search of a noun. *The Journal of Clinical Psychiatry*, **46**: 41–8.

Alford, B. and Beck, A. (1997). *The Integrative Power of Cogntive Therapy.* New York: Guilford.

Allen, J. G. (2001). *Interpersonal Trauma and Serious Mental Disorder.* Wiley: Chichester.

Allen, J. G. and Fonagy, P. (2002). The development of mentalizing and its role in psychopathology and psychotherapy. (Technical Report No. 02–0048). The Menninger Clinic, Research Department, Topeka, KS.

Allen, J. G. (2003). Mentalizing. *Bulletin of the Menninger Clinic*, **67**: 91–112.

Allen, J. P., Moore, C., Kuperminc, G., and Bell, K. (1998). Attachment and adolescent psychosocial functioning. *Child Development*, **69**: 1406–19.

Amen, D. G., Stubblefield, M., Carmicheal, B., and Thisted, R. (1996). Brain SPECT findings and aggressiveness. *Annals of Clinical Psychiatry*, **8**: 129–37.

American Psychiatric Association (1980). *Diagnostic and Statistical Manual of Mental Disorders (3rd Ed., DSM-III).* Washington, DC: American Psychiatric Press.

American Psychiatric Association (1994). *Diagnostic and Statistical Manual of Mental Disorders (DSM-IV).* Washington, DC: American Psychiatric Association.

American Psychiatric Association (2001). Practice guideline for the treatment of patients with borderline personality disorder. *American Journal of Psychiatry* **158**: 1–52.

Anderson, S. W., Bechara, A., Damasio, H., Tranel, D., and Damasio, A. R. (1999). Impairment of social and moral behavior related to early damage in human prefrontal cortex. *Nature Neuroscience*, **2**: 1032–7.

Andrews, J. (1990). Interpersonal self-confirmation and challenge in psychotherapy. *Psychotherapy*, **27**: 485–504.

Andrulonis, P., Glueck, B., Stroebel, C., Vogel, N., Shapiro, A., and Aldridge, D. (1980). Organic brain dysfunction and the borderline syndrome. *Psychiatric Clinics of North America*, **4**: 47–66.

Antikainen, R., Hintikka, J., Lehtonen, J., Koponen, H., and Arstila, A. (1995). A prospective three-year follow-up study of borderline personality disorder inpatients. *Acta Psychiatrica Scandinavica*, **92**: 327–35.

Arnsten, A. F. and Goldman-Rakic, P. S. (1998). Noise stress impairs prefrontal cortical cognitive function in monkeys: evidence for a hyperdopaminergic mechanism. *Archives of General Psychiatry*, **55**: 362–8.

Arnsten, A. F. T. (1998). The biology of being frazzled. *Science*, **280**: 1711–2.

Arnsten, A. F. T. Mathew, R. Ubriani, R. Taylor, J. R., and Li, B.-M. (1999). Alpha-1 noradrenergic receptor stimulation impairs prefrontal cortical cognitive function. *Biological Psychiatry*, **45**: 26–31.

Arntz, A., Appels, C., and Sieswerda, S. (2000). Hypervigilance in borderline disorder: a test with the emotional Stroop paradigm. *Journal of Personality Disorders*, **14**: 366–73.

Arntz, A. and Veen, G. (2001). Evaluations of others by borderline patients. *The Journal of Nervons and Mental Disease*, **189**: 513–21.

Asberg, M., Traskman, L., and Thoren, P. (1976). 5-HIAA in the cerebrospinal fluid: A biochemical suicide predictor? *Archives of General Psychiatry*, **33**: 1193–7.

Astington, J., Harris, P., and Olson, D. (1988). *Developing Theories of Mind.* New York: Cambridge University Press.

Astington, J. W. and Jenkins, J. M. (1995). Theory of mind development and social understanding. *Cognition and Emotion*, **9**: 151–65.

Baddeley, A. (2002). The concept of episodic memory. In: *Episodic Memory: New Directions in Research.* (pp. 1–10) (ed. Baddeley, A., Aggleton, A., and Conway, M. (2002)). London: Oxford University Press.

Baguley, I., Butterworth, A., Fahy, K., Haddock, G., Lancashire, S., and Tarrier, N. (2000). Bringing into clinical practice skills shown to be effective in research settings: a follow-up of 'Thorn Training' in psychosocial family interventions for psychosis. In *Psychosis: Psychological Approaches and their Effectiveness* (ed. Martindale, B., Bateman, A., Crowe, M., and Margison, F.). London: Gaskell.

Bahrick, L. R. and Watson, J. S. (1985). Detection of intermodal proprioceptive-visual contingency as a potential basis of self-perception in infancy. *Developmental Psychology*, **21**: 963–73.

Balint, M. (1968). *The Basic Fault.* London: Tavistock.

Barkham, M., Rees, A., Shapiro, D. A. *et al* (1996). Outcome of time-limited psychotherapy in applied settings: replication of the Second Sheffield Psychotherapy Project. *Journal of Consulting and Clinical Psychology*, **64**: 1079–85.

Barkley, R. A. (1997). *ADHD and the Nature of Self-Control.* New York: Guilford Press.

Barley, W. D., Buie, S. E., Peterson, E. W., *et al.* (1993). The development of an inpatient cognitive-behavioural treatment programme for borderline personality disorder. *Journal of Personality Disorders*, **7**: 232–41.

Barnett, D., Ganiban, J., and Cicchetti, D. (1999). Maltreatment, emotional reactivity and the development of Type D attachments from 12 to 24 months of age. *Monographs of the Society for Research in Child Development.*

Baron-Cohen, S., Tager-Flusberg, H., and Cohen, D. J. (1993). *Understanding Other Minds: Perspectives from Autism.* Oxford: Oxford University Press.

Baron-Cohen, S. (1995). *Mindblindness: An Essay on Autism and Theory of Mind.* Cambridge, MA: MIT Press.

Baron-Cohen, S. and Swettenham, J. (1996). The relationship between SAM and ToMM: Two hypotheses. In: *Theories of Theories of Mind* (ed. P. Carruthers and P. K. Smith), pp. 158–68. Cambridge: Cambridge University Press.

Baron-Cohen, S. (1999). Does the study of autism justify minimalist innate modularity? *Learning and Individual Differences*, **10**: 179–91.

Baron-Cohen, S., Tager-Flusberg, H., and Cohen, D. J. (eds.) (2000). *Understanding Other Minds: Perspectives from Developmental Cognitive Neuroscience.* Oxford: Oxford University Press.

Bartholomew, K. and Horowitz, L. M. (1991). Attachment styles among young adults: A test of a four-category model. *Journal of Personality and Social Psychology*, **61**: 226–44.

Bartholomew, K., Kwong, M. J., and Hart, S. D. (2001). Attachment. In: *Handbook of Personality Disorders: Theory, Research and Treatment* (ed. W. J. Livesley), pp. 196–230. New York: Guilford Press.

Bassarath, L. (2001). Neuroimaging studies of antisocial behaviour. *Canadian Journal of Psychiatry*, **46**: 728–32.

Bateman, A. W. and Holmes, J. (1995). *Introduction to Psychoanalysis: Contemporary Theory and Practice.* London: Routledge.

Bateman, A. W. and Fonagy, P. (1999). The effectiveness of partial hospitalization in the treatment of borderline personality disorder—A randomised controlled trial. *The American Journal of Psychiatry*, **156**: 1563–69.

Bateman, A. W. (2000). Integration in psychotherapy: an evolving reality in personality disorder. *British Journal of Psychotherapy*, **17**: 147–56.

Bateman, A. W. and Fonagy, P. (2000). Effectiveness of psychotherapeutic treatment of personality disorder. *British Journal of Psychiatry*, **177**: 138–43.

Bateman, A. W. and Fonagy, P. (2001). Treatment of borderline personality disorder with psychoanalytically oriented partial hospitalisation: an 18-month follow-up. *The American Journal of Psychiatry*, **158**: 36–42.

Bateman, A. W. and Fonagy, P. (2003). Health service utilisation costs for borderline personality disorder patients treated with psychoanalytically oriented partial hospitalisation versus general psychiatric care. *The American Journal of Psychiatry*, **160**: 169–71.

Bateman, A. W. and Tyrer, P. (2003). Effective management of personality disorder. *www.doh.gov.uk/mentalhealth/batemantyrer.pdf.*

Beck, A. T. and Freeman, A. (1990). *Cognitive Therapy of Personality Disorders.* New York: Guilford Press.

Beebe, B., Jaffe, J., Feldstein, S., Mays, K., and Alson, D. (1985). Interpersonal timing: The application of an adult dialogue model to mother-infant vocal and kinesic interactions. In: *Social Perception in Infants* (ed. T. M. Field and N. A. Fox), pp. 217–47. Norwood, NJ: Ablex.

Beeghly, M. and Cicchetti, D. (1994). Child maltreatment, attachment, and the self system: Emergence of an internal state lexicon in toddlers at high social risk. *Development and Psychopathology*, **6**: 5–30.

Bell, K. and Calkins, S. (2000). Relationships as inputs and outputs of emotion regulation. *Psychological Inquiry*, **11**: 160–3.

Benjamin, L. S. (1993). *Interpersonal Diagnosis and Treatment of Personality Disorder.* New York: Guilford Press.

Bergvall, A. H., Wessely, H., Forsman, A., and Hansen, S. (2001). A deficit in attentional set-shifting of violent offenders. *Psychological Medicine*, **31**: 1095–105.

Bernstein, A. (1990). The impact of incest trauma on ego development. In: *Adult Analysis and Child Sexual Abuse* (ed. H. Levine), pp. 65–91. Hillsdale, NJ: Analytic Press.

Bernstein, D. P., Cohen, P., Velez, C. N., Schwab-Stone, M., Siever, L. J., and Shinsato, L. (1993). Prevalence and stability of the DSM-III-R personality disorders in a community-based survey of adolescents. *The American Journal of Psychiatry*, **150**: 1237–43.

Bernstein, G. A., Garfinkel, B. D., and Borchardt, C. M. (1990). Comparative studies of pharmacotherapy for school refusal. *Journal of the American Academy of Child and Adolescent Psychiatry*, **29**: 773–81.

Beutler, L. E. Machado, P. P. P., and Neufeldt, S. A. (1994). Therapist variables. In: *Handbook of Psychotherapy and Behavior Change* (ed. A. E. Bergin and S. L. Garfield). New York: Wiley.

Bifulco, A., Brown, G. W., Lillie, A., and Jarvis, J. (1997). Memories of childhood neglect and abuse: corroboration in a series of sisters. *Journal of Child Psychology and Psychiatry*, **38**: 365–74.

Bion, W. R. (1957). Differentiation of the psychotic from the non-psychotic personalities. *International Journal of Psychoanalysis*, **38**: 266–75.

Bion, W. R. (1962*a*). *Learning from Experience.* London: Heinemann.

Bion, W. R. (1962*b*). A theory of thinking. *International Journal of Psychoanalysis*, **43**: 306–10.

Bion, W. R. (1963). *Elements of Psycho-Analysis.* London: Heinemann.

Bion, W. R. (1965). *Transformations.* London: Heinemann.

Bion, W. R. (1970). *Attention and Interpretation.* London: Tavistock.

Bizot, J., Le Bihan, C., Puech, A. J., Hamon, M., and Thiebot, M. (1999). Serotonin and tolerance to delay of reward in rats. *Psychopharmacology (Berl)*, **146**: 400–12.

Blackburn, R., Crellin, M., Morgan, E., and Tulloch, R. (1990). Prevalence of personality disorders in a special hospital population. *Journal of Forensic Psychiatry*, **1**: 43–52.

Blair, R. J. and Cipolotti, L. (2000). Impaired social response reversal. A case of 'acquired sociopathy'. *Brain*, **123**: 1122–41.

Blair, R. J. (2001). Neurocognitive models of aggression, the antisocial personality disorders, and psychopathy. *Journal of Neurology, Neurosurgery and Psychiatry*, **71**: 727–31.

Blair, R. J., Colledge, E., and Mitchell, D. G. (2001). Somatic markers and response reversal: is there orbitofrontal cortex dysfunction in boys with psychopathic tendencies? *Journal of Abnormal Child Psychology*, **29**: 499–511.

Blais, M. A. (1997). Clinician ratings of the five-factor model of personality and the DSM-IV personality disorders. *Journal of Nervous and Mental Disease*, **185**: 388–93.

Blatt, S. J., Stayner, D., Auerbach, J. S., and Behrends, R. S. (1996). Change in object and self representations in long-term, intensive, inpatient treatment of seriously disturbed adolescents and young adults. *Psychiatry: Interpersonal and Biological Processes*, **59**: 82–107.

Bleiberg, E. (1994). Borderline disorders in children and adolescents: The concept, the diagnosis, and the controversies. *Bulletin of the Menninger Clinic*, **58**: 169–96.

Block, J. (1996). Some jangly remarks on Baumeister and Heatherton. *Psychological Inquiry*, **7**: 28–32.

Blum, H. P. (2003). Repression, transference and reconstruction. *International Journal of Psychoanalysis*, **84**: 497–503.

Blume, E. S. (1990). *Secret Survivors: Uncovering Incest and its After-Effects in Women.* New York: Ballantine.

Bogdan, R. J. (1997). *Interpreting Minds.* Cambridge, MA: MIT Press.

Bogdan, R. J. (2001). *Minding Minds.* Cambridge, MA: MIT Press.

Bohus, M., Haaf, B., Simms, T. C, S., Unckel, C., and Linehan, M. (2002). Effectiveness of inpatient Dialectical Behavioural Therapy for Borderline Personality Disorder: A controlled trial. Paper presented at the 5th ISSPD European Congress on Personality Disorders. Germany: Munich.

Bolton, D. and Hill, J. (1996). *Mind, Meaning and Mental Disorder.* Oxford: Oxford University Press.

Bond, M. P., Paris, J., and Zweig-Frank, H. (1994). Defense styles and borderline personality disorder. *Journal of Personal Disorders*, **8**: 28–31.

Bonda, E., Petrides, M., Ostry, D., and Evans, A. (1996). Specific involvement of human parietal systems and the amygdala in the perception of biological motion. *Journal of Neuroscience*, **16**: 3737–44.

Bouchard, M.-A., Target, M., Lecours, S., Fonagy, P., and Tremblay L-M (submitted). Mentalization in Adult Attachment: Reflective Functioning, Mental States and Affect Elaboration Compared.

Bowlby, J. (1969). *Attachment and Loss, Vol. 1: Attachment.* London: Hogarth Press and the Institute of Psycho-Analysis.

Bowlby, J. (1973). *Attachment and Loss, Vol. 2: Separation: Anxiety and Anger.* London: Hogarth Press and Institute of Psycho-Analysis.

Bowlby, J. (1980). *Attachment and Loss, Vol. 3: Loss: Sadness and Depression.* London: Hogarth Press and Institute of Psycho-Analysis.

Bowlby, J. (1988). *A Secure Base: Clinical Applications of Attachment Theory.* London: Routledge.

Bowlby, J. (1991). *Charles Darwin: A New Life.* New York: Norton.

Bradley, S. J. (1979). The relationship of early maternal separation to borderline personality in children and adolescents. *The American Journal of Psychiatry*, **136**: 424–26.

Bram, A. D. and Gabbard, G. O. (2001). Potential space and reflective functioning. Towards conceptual clarification and preliminary clinical implications. *The International Journal of Psychoanalysis*, **82**: 685–99.

Brazelton, T., Kowslowski, B., and Main, M. (1974). The origins of reciprocity: The early mother-infant interaction. In: *The Effect of the Infant on Its Caregiver* (ed. M. Lewis and L. Rosenblum), pp. 49–76. New York: John Wiley.

Brazelton, T. B. and Tronick, E. (1980). Preverbal communication between mothers and infants. In: *The Social Foundations of Language and Thought* (ed. D. R. Olson), pp. 299–315. New York: Norton.

Bremner, J., Southwick, S., Brett, E., Fontana, A., Rosenheck, R., and Charney, D. (1992). Dissociation and posttraumatic stress disorder in Vietnam combat veterans. *The American Journal of Psychiatry*, **149**: 328–32.

Bremner, J. D., Davis, M., Southwick, S. M., Krystal, J. H., and Charney, D. S. (1993*a*). *Neurobiology of Posttraumatic Stress Disorder.* Washington, DC: American Psychiatric Press.

Bremner, J. D., Scott, T. M., Delaney, R. C. *et al.* (1993*b*). Deficits in short-term memory in posttraumatic stress disorder. *The American Journal of Psychiatry*, **150**:1015–9.

Bremner, J. D., Southwick, S. M., Yehuda, R., and Charney, D. F. (1993*c*). Childhood physical abuse and combat-related post-traumatic stress disorder in Vietnam veterans. *The American Journal of Psychiatry*, **150**: 235–9.

Bremner, J. D., Licinio, J., Darnell, A. *et al.* (1997). Elevated CSF corticotropin-releasing factor concentrations in posttraumatic stress disorder. *American Journal of Psychiatry*, **154**: 624–9.

Bremner, J. D., Narayan, M., Staib, L. H., Southwick, S. M., McGlashan, T., and Charney, D. S. (1999*a*). Neural correlates of memories of childhood sexual abuse in women with and without posttraumatic stress disorder. *The American Journal of Psychiatry*, **156**: 1787–95.

Bremner, J. D., Staib, L. H., Kaloupek, D., Southwick, S. M., Soufer, R., and Charney, D. S. (1999*b*). Neural correlates of exposure to traumatic pictures and sound in Vietnam combat veterans with and without posttraumatic stress disorder: a positron emission tomography study. *Biological Psychiatry*, **45**: 806–16.

Brennan, K. A. and Shaver, P. R. (1998). Attachment styles and personality disorders: their connections to each other and to parental divorce, parental death, and perceptions of parental caregiving. *Journal of Personality*, **66**: 835–78.

Breslau, N., Davis, G. C., Peterson, E. L., and Schultz, L. R. (2000). A second look at comorbidity in victims of trauma: the posttraumatic stress disorder-major depression connection. *Biological Psychiatry*, **48**: 902–9.

Bretherton, I. (1991). Pouring new wine into old bottles: the social self as internal working model. In: *Self Processes and Development: Minnesota Symposia on Child Psychology* (ed. M. R. Gunnar and L. A. Sroufe), pp. 1–41. Hillsdale, NJ: Lawrence Erlbaum Associates.

Bretherton, K. and Munholland, K. A. (1999). Internal working models in attachment relationships: A construct revisited. In: *Handbook of Attachment: Theory, Research and Clinical Applications* (ed. J. Cassidy and P. R. Shaver), pp. 89–114. New York: Guilford.

Brewin, C. R., Andrews, B., and Gotlib, I. H. (1993). Psychopathology and early experience: A reappraisal of retrospective reports. *Psychological Bulletin*, **113**: 82–98.

Briere, J. and Runtz, M. (1987). Post-sexual abuse trauma: data and implications for clinical practice. *Journal of Interpersonal Violence*, **2**: 367–97.

Britton, R. (1992). The Oedipus situation and the depressive position. In: *Clinical Lectures on Klein and Bion* (ed. R. Anderson), pp. 34–45. London: Routledge.

Brothers, L. (1997). *Friday's Footprint: How Society Shapes the Human Mind.* New York: Oxford University Press.

Broussard, E. R. (1995). Infant attachment in a sample of adolescent mothers. *Child Psychiatry and Human Development*, **25**: 211–9.

Brower, M. C. and Price, B. H. (2001). Neuropsychiatry of frontal lobe dysfunction in violent and criminal behaviour: a critical review. *Journal of Neurology, Neurosurgery and Psychiatry*, **71**: 720–6.

Brown, J. R., Donelan-McCall, N., and Dunn, J. (1996). Why talk about mental states? The significance of children's conversations with friends, siblings, and mothers. *Child Development*, **67**: 836–49.

Brownell, H., Griffin, R., Winner, E., Friedman, O., and Happe, F. (2000). Cerebral lateralization and theory of mind. In: *Understanding Other Minds: Perspectives from Developmental Cognitive Neuroscience.* 4th ed. (ed. S. Baron-Cohen, H. Tager-Flusberg, and D. J. Cohen), pp. 306–33. New York: Oxford University Press.

Byford, S., Knapp, M., Greenshields, J., *et al.* (2003). Cost-effectiveness of brief cognitive behaviour therapy versus treatment as usual in recurrent deliberate self-harm: a decision-making approach. *Psychological Medicine*, **33**(6): 977–86.

Camras, L. A., Sachs-Alter, E., and Ribordy, S. C. (1996). Emotion understanding in maltreated children: Recognition of facial expressions and integration with other emotion cues. In: *Emotional Development in Atypical Children* (ed. M. D. Lewis and M. Sullivan), pp. 203–25. Mahwah, NJ: Erlbaum.

Cardasis, W., Hochman, J. A., and Silk, K. R. (1997). Transitional objects and borderline personality disorder. *The American Journal of Psychiatry*, **154**: 250–5.

Carlson, S. M. and Moses, L. J. (2001). Individual differences in inhibitory control and children's theory of mind. *Child Development*, **72**: 1032–53.

Carpendale, J. I. M. and Lewis, C. (in press). Constructing an understanding of mind: The development of children's social understanding within social interaction. *Behavioral and Brain Sciences.*

Carpenter, P. A. Just, M. A., and Reichle, E. D. (2000). Working memory and executive function: Evidence from neuro-imaging. *Current Opinion in Neurobiology*, **10**: 195–9.

Caspi, A., McClay, J., Moffitt, T. E., *et al.* (2002). Role of genotype in the cycle of violence in maltreated children. *Science*, **297**(5582): 851–4.

Caspi, A., Sugden, K., Moffitt, T. E., *et al.* (2003). Influence of life stress on depression: moderation by a polymorphism in the 5-HTT gene. *Science*, **301**(5631): 386–9.

Cassam, Q. (ed.) (1994). *Self-knowledge.* Oxford: Oxford University Press.

Champion, L. A., Goodall, G. M., and Rutter, M. (1995). Behavioural problems in childhood and stressors in early adult life: A 20 year follow-up of London school children. *Psychological Medicine*, **25**: 231–46.

Chengappa, K., Ebeling, T., Kang, J., Levine, J., and Parepally, H. (1999). Clozapine reduces severe self-mutilation and aggression in psychotic patients with borderline personality disorder. *The Journal of Clinical Psychiatry*, **60**: 477–84.

Chiesa, M. and Fonagy, P. (2000). The Cassel personality disorder study: methodology and treatment effects. *British Journal of Psychiatry*, **176**: 485–91.

Chiesa, M., Bateman, A., Wilberg, T., and Friis, S. (2002*a*). Patients' characteristics, outcome and cost-benefit of hospital-based treatment for patients with personality disorder: A comparison of three different programmes. *Psychology and Psychotherapy: Theory, Research and Practice*, **75**: 381–92.

Chiesa, M., Fonagy, P., Holmes, J., Drahorad, C., and Harrison-Hall, A. (2002*b*). Health Service use costs by personality disorder following specialist and non-specialist treatment: a comparative study. *Journal of Personality Disorders*, **16**: 160–73.

Chiesa, M., Fonagy, P., Holmes, J., and Drahorad, C. (in press). Residential versus community treatment of personality disorder: a comparative study of three treatment programmes. *American Journal of Psychiatry*.

Christianson, S. and Nilsson, L. (1989). Hysterical amnesia: A case of aversively motivated isolation of memory. In: *Aversion, Avoidance, and Anxiety: Perspectives on Aversively Motivated Behaviour* (ed. T. Archer and L. Nilsson), pp. 289–310. Hillsdale, NH: Erlbaum.

Christianson, S. (1992). Remembering emotional events: Potential mechanisms. In: *The Handbook of Emotion and Memory: Research and Theory* (ed. S. Christianson), pp. 307–40. Hillsdale, NJ: Erlbaum.

Chugani, H. T., Behen, M. E., Muzik, O., Juhasz, C., Nagy, F., and Chugani, D. C. (2001). Local brain functional activity following early deprivation: a study of postinstitutionalized Romanian orphans. *Neuroimage*, **14**: 1290–301.

Cicchetti, D. and Beeghly, M. (1987). Symbolic development in maltreated youngsters: An organizational perspective. In: *Atypical Symbolic Development. New Directions for Child Development* (ed. D. Cicchetti and M. Beeghly), pp. 5–29. San Francisco: Jossey-Bass.

Cicchetti, D. and Lynch, M. (1995). Failures in the expectable environment and their impact on individual development: The case of child maltreatment. In: *Developmental Psychopathology (vol. 2)* (ed. D. Cicchetti and D. J. Cohen), pp. 32–71. New York: Wiley.

Clark, L. A., Livesley, W. J., and Morey, L. (1997). Personality disorder assessment: The challenge of construct validity. *Journal of Personality Disorders*, **11**: 205–31.

Clarkin, J., Hull, J., Cantor, J. *et al.* (1993*a*). Borderline personality disorder and personality traits: A comparison of SCID-II BPD and NEO-PI. *Psychological Assessment*, **5**: 472–6.

Clarkin, J. F., Hull, J. W., and Hurt, S. W. (1993*b*). Factor structure of borderline personality disorder criteria. *Journal of Personality Disorders*, **7**: 137–43.

Clarkin, J., Foelsch, P. A., and Kernberg, O. F. (1996). Manual for the Inventory of Personality Organization (IPO). In: *The Personality Disorder Institute, Department of Psychiatry.* Cornell University Medical College.

Clarkin, J. F. and Lenzenweger, M. F. (1996). *Major Theories of Personality Disorder.* New York: Guilford.

Clarkin, J. F., Yeomans, F., and Kernberg, O. F. (1998). *Psychodynamic Psychotherapy of Borderline Personality Organisation: A Treatment Manual.* New York: Wiley.

Clarkin, J. F., Kernberg, O. F., and Yeomans, F. (1999). *Transference-Focused Psychotherapy for Borderline Personality Disorder Patients.* New York, NY: Guilford Press.

Clarkin, J. F., Foelsch, P., Levy, K., Hull, J., Delaney, J., and Kernberg, O. (2001). The development of a psychodynamic treatment for patients with borderline personality disorder: a preliminary study of behavioural change. *Journal of Personality Disorders*, **15**: 487–95.

Claussen, A. H., Mundy, P. C., Mallik, S. A., and Willoughby, J. C. (2002). Joint attention and disorganised attachment status in infants at risk. *Development and Psychopathology*, **14**: 279–91.

Cleare, A. J., Murray, R. M., and O'Keane, V. (1996). Reduced prolactin and cortisol responses to d-fenfluramine in depressed compared to healthy matched control subjects. *Neuropsychopharmacology*, **14**: 349–54.

Cloitre, M., Scarvalone, P., and Difede, J. (1997). Posttraumatic stress disorder self-and interpersonal dysfunction among sexually retraumatized women. *Journal of Traumatic Stress*, **10**: 437–52.

Cloninger, C. R., Svrakic, D. M., and Przybeck, T. R. (1993). A psychobiological model of temperament and character. *Archives of General Psychiatry*, **50**: 975–90.

Clyman, R. B. (1991). The procedural organization of emotions: A contribution from cognitive science to the psychoanalytic theory of therapeutic action. *Journal of the American Psychoanalytic Association*, **39**: 349–82.

Coccaro, E. F., Berman, M. E., Kavoussi, R. J., and Hauger, R. L. (1996). Relationship of prolactin response to d-fenfluramine to behavioral and questionnaire assessments of aggression in personality-disordered men. *Biological Psychiatry*, **40**: 157–64.

Coccaro, E. F., Bergman, C. S., Kavoussi, R. J., and Seroczynski, A. D. (1997). Heritability of aggression and irritability: A twin study of the Buss-Durkee Aggression Scales in adult male subjects. *Biological Psychiatry*, **41**: 273–84.

Coccaro, E. F. (1998). Neurotransmitter function in personality disorders. In: *Biology of Personality Disorders* (ed. K. R. Silk), pp. 1–25. Washington, DC: American Psychiatric Press.

Cohen, P., Brown, J., and Smaile, E. (2001). Child abuse and neglect and the development of mental disorders in the general population. *Development and Psychopathology*, **13**: 981–99.

Cohen, T. (1995). Motherhood among incest survivors. *Child Abuse and Neglect*, **19**: 1423–9.

Cole, K. and Mitchell, P. (2000). Siblings in the development of executive control and a theory of mind. *British Journal of Developmental Psychology*, **18**: 279–95.

Cooke, T. and Campbell, D. (1979). *Quasi-Experimentation*. Boston: Houghton-Mifflin.

Coolidge, F. L., Thede, L. L., and Jang, K. L. (2001). Heritability of personality disorders in childhood: a preliminary investigation. *Journal of Personality Disorders*, **15**: 33–40.

Corkum, V. and Moore, C. (1995). Development of joint visual attention in infants. In: *Joint Attention: Its Origins and Role in Development* (ed. C. Moore and P. Dunham), pp. 61–83. New York: Erlbaum.

Courtois, C. A. (1992). The memory retrieval process in incest survivor therapy. *Journal of Child Sexual Abuse*, **1**: 15–32.

Cousens, P. and Nunn, K. (1997). Is "self-regulation" a more helpful construct than "attention"? *Clinical Child Psychology and Psychiatry*, **2**: 27–43.

Cowdry, R. W., Gardner, D. L,. O'Leary, K. M., Leibenluft, E., and Rubinow, D. R. (1991). Mood variability: a study of four groups. *The American Journal of Psychiatry*, **148**: 1505–11.

Crawford, T. N., Cohen, P., and Brook, J. S. (2001*a*). Dramatic-erratic personality disorder symptoms: I. Continuity from early adolescence into adulthood. *Journal of Personality Disorders*, **15**: 319–35.

Crawford, T. N., Cohen, P., and Brook, J. S. (2001*b*). Dramatic-erratic personality disorder symptoms: II. Developmental pathways from early adolescence to adulthood. *Journal of Personality Disorders*, **15**: 336–50.

Crittenden, P. M. (1981). Abusing, neglecting, problematic, and adequate dyads: Differentiating by patterns of interaction. *Merrill-Palmer Quarterly*, **27**: 201–18.

Crittenden, P. M. (1990). Internal representational models of attachment relationships. *Infant Mental Health Journal*, **11**: 259–77.

Crittenden, P. M. (1994). Peering into the black box: An exploratory treatise on the development of self in young children. In: *Disorders and Dysfunctions of the Self. Rochester Symposium on Developmental Psychopathology, Vol 5* (ed. D. Cicchetti and S. L. Toth), pp. 79–148. Rochester, NY: University of Rochester Press.

Crittenden, P. M. (1997). Toward an integrative theory of trauma: A dynamic-maturation approach. In: *Rochester Symposium on Developmental Psychopathology: Developmental Perspectives on Trauma* (ed. D. Cicchetti and S. L. Toth), pp. 33–84. Rochester, NY: University of Rochester Press.

Csibra, G. and Gergely, G. (1998). The teleological origins of mentalistic action explanations: A developmental hypothesis. *Developmental Science*, **1**: 255–9.

Csibra, G., Gergely, G., Brockbank, M., Biro, S., and Koós, O. (1999). Twelve-month-olds can infer a goal for an incomplete action. In: *11th Biennial Conference on Infant Studies (ICIS).* Georgia: Atlanta.

Cutting, A. L. and Dunn, J. (1999). Theory of mind, emotion understanding, language, and family background: Individual differences and interrelations. *Child Development*, **70**: 853–65.

Daley, S. E., Hammen, C., Burge, D. *et al.* (1999). Depression and Axis II symptomatology in an adolescent community sample: concurrent and longitudinal associations. *Journal of Personality Disorders*, **13**: 47–59.

Damasio, A. R. (1994). Descartes' error and the future of human life. *Scientific American*, **271**: 144.

Damasio, A. R. (1999). *The Feeling of What Happens: Body and Emotion in the Making of Consciousness.* New York: Harcourt Brace.

Damasio, A. R. (2000). A neural basis for sociopathy. *Archives of General Psychiatry*, **57**: 128–9.

Damasio, A. R. (2003). *Looking for Spinoza: Joy, Sorrow, and the Feeling Brain.* New York: Harvest Books.

Davidson, K. and Tyrer, P. (1996). Cognitive therapy for antisocial and borderline personality disorders: Single case study series. *British Journal of Clinical Psychology*, **35**: 413–29.

Davidson, K. (2000). *Cognitive Therapy for Personality Disorders: A Guide for Clinicians.* Oxford: Butterworth–Heinemann.

Davidson, R. J., Putnam, K. M., and Larson, C. L. (2000). Dysfunction in the neural circuitry of emotion regulation—A possible prelude to violence. *Science*, **289**: 591–4.

Davies, J. and Frawley, M. (1991). Dissociative processes and transference-countertransference paradigms in the psychoanalytically oriented treatment of adult survivors of childhood sexual abuse. *Psychoanalytic Dialogues*, **2**: 5–36.

Davies, S., Campling, P., and Ryan, K. (1998). Therapeutic community provision at regional and district levels. *Psychiatric Bulletin*, **23**: 79–83.

Dawson, D. (1988). Treatment of the borderline patient: Relationship management. *Canadian Journal of Psychiatry*, **33**: 370–4.

De Bellis, M. D., Lefter, L., Trickett, P. K., and Putnam, F. W. Jr. (1994). Urinary catecholamine excretion in sexually abused girls. *Journal of the American Academy of Child and Adolescent Psychiatry*, **33**: 320–7.

De Bellis, M. D., Baum, A. S., Birmaher, B. *et al.* (1999*a*). A. E. Bennett research award. Developmental traumatology. Part I: Biological stress systems. *Biological Psychiatry*, **45**: 1259–70.

De Bellis, M. D., Keshavan, M. S., Clark, D. B. *et al.* (1999*b*). A.E. Bennett Research Award. Developmental traumatology. Part II: Brain development. *Biological Psychiatry*, **45**: 1271–84.

De Bellis, M. D., Keshavan, M. S., Spencer, S., and Hall, J. (2000). N-Acetylaspartate concentration in the anterior cingulate of maltreated children and adolescents with PTSD. *The American Journal of Psychiatry*, **157**: 1175–7.

De Bellis, M. D. (2001). Developmental traumatology: The psychobiological development of maltreated children and its implications for research, treatment, and policy. *Development and Psychopathology*, **13**: 539–64.

de Villiers, J. (2000). Language and theory of mind: What are the developmental relationships? In: *Understanding of Minds: Perspectives from Developmental Cognitive Neuroscience* (ed. S. Baron-Cohen, H. Tager-Flusberg, and D. J. Cohen). Oxford: Oxford University Press.

DeCasper, A. J. and Fifer, W. P. (1980). Of human bonding: Newborns prefer their mothers' voices. *Science*, **208**: 1174–6.

Denham, S. A., Zoller, D., and Couchoud, E. A. (1994). Socialization of preschoolers' emotion understanding. *Developmental Psychology*, **30**: 928–36.

Denman, C. (2002). Integrative developments in cognitive analytic therapy. In: *Integration in Psychotherapy: Models and Methods* (ed. J. Holmes and A. Bateman). Oxford: Oxford University Press.

Dennett, D. (1987). *The Intentional Stance.* Cambridge, Mass: MIT Press.

Dewald, P. (1989). Effects on an adult of incest in childhood: A case report. *Journal of the American Psychoanalytic Association*, **37**: 997–1014.

Dick, B. M. and Woof, K. (1986). An evaluation of a time-limited programme of dynamic group psychotherapy. *British Journal of Psychiatry*, **148**: 159–64.

Diefendorff, J., Lord, R., Hepburn, E., Quickle, J., Hall, R., and Sanders, R. (1998). Perceived self-regulation and individual differences in selective attention. *Journal of Experimental Psychology: Applied*, **4**: 228–47.

DiLillo, D. (2001). Interpersonal functioning among women reporting a history of childhood sexual abuse: empirical findings and methodological issues. *Clinical Psychology Review*, **21**: 553–76.

Dinn, W. M. and Harris, C. L. (2000). Neurocognitive function in antisocial personality disorder. *Psychiatry Research*, **97**: 173–90.

DoH (2003). Personality Disorder: No longer a diagnosis of exclusion. *Department of Health Publications, www.nimhe.org*.

Dolan, B. M. and Coid, J. (1993). *Psychopathic and Antisocial Personality Disorders: Treatment and Research Issues*. London: Gaskell.

Dozier, M., Cue, K., and Barnett, L. (1994). Clinicians as care givers: Role of attachment organisation in treatment. *Journal of Consulting and Clinical Psychology*, **62**: 793–800.

Dozier, M., Stovall, K. C., and Albus, K. E. (1999). Attachment and psychopathology in adulthood. In: *Handbook of Attachment: Theory, Research and Clinical Applications* (ed. J. Cassidy and P. R. Shaver), pp. 497–519. New York: Guilford.

Drake, R. E., Adler, D. A., and Vaillant, G. E. (1988). Antecedents of personality disorders in a community sample of men. *Journal of Personality Disorders*, **2**: 60–8.

Driessen, M., Herrmann, J., Stahl, K. *et al.* (2000). Magnetic resonance imaging volumes of the hippocampus and the amygdala in women with borderline personality disorder and early traumatization. *Archives of General Psychiatry*, **57**: 1115–22.

Dubner, A. E. and Motta, R. W. (1999). Sexually and physically abused foster care children and posttraumatic stress disorder. *Journal of Consulting and Clinical Psychology*, **67**: 367–73.

Dulit, R. A., Fyer, M. R., Leon, A. C., Brodsky, B. S., and Frances, A. J. (1994). Clinical correlates of self-mutilation in borderline personality disorder. *The American Journal of Psychiatry*, **151**: 1305–11.

Dunkle, J. and Friedlander, M. (1996). Contribution of therapists' experience and personal characteristics to the working alliance. *Journal of Consulting and Clinical Psychology*, **43**: 456–60.

Dunlop, S. A., Archer, M. A., Quinlivan, J. A., Beazley, L. D., and Newnham, J. P. (1997). Repeated prenatal corticosteroids delay myelination in the ovine central nervous system. *Journal of Maternal-Fetal Medicine*, **6**: 309–13.

Dunn, J., Brown, J., and Beardsall, L. (1991*a*). Family talk about feeling states and children's later understanding of others' emotions. *Developmental Psychology*, **27**: 448–55.

Dunn, J., Brown, J., Somkowski, C., Telsa, C., and Youngblade, L. (1991*b*). Young children's understanding of other people's feelings and beliefs: Individual differences and their antecedents. *Child Development*, **62**: 1352–66.

Dunn, J. (1996). The Emanuel Miller Memorial Lecture 1995. Children's relationships: Bridging the divide between cognitive and social development. *Journal of Child Psychology and Psychiatry*, **37**: 507–18.

Dunn, J. Deater-Deckard, K. Pickering, K., and Golding, J. (1999). Siblings, parents, and partners: family relationships within a longitudinal community study. ALSPAC study team. Avon Longitudinal Study of Pregnancy and Childhood. *Journal of Child Psychology and Psychiatry*, **40**: 1025–37.

Dunn, J., Davies, L. C., O'Connor, T. G., and Sturgess, W. (2000). Parents' and partners' life course and family experiences: links with parent–child relationships in different family settings. *Journal of Child Psychology and Psychiatry*, **41**: 955–68.

Dutton, D. G., Saunders, K., Starzomski, A., and Bartholomew, K. (1994*a*). Intimacy-anger and insecure attachment as precursors of abuse in intimate relationships. *Journal of Applied Social Psychology*, **24**: 1367–86.

Dutton, D. G., Saunders, K., Starzomski, A., and Bartholomew, K. (1994*b*). Intimacy–anger and insecure attachments as precursors of abuse in intimate relationships. *Journal of Applied Social Psychology*, **24**: 1367–86.

Dutton, D. G. (1995). Male abusiveness in intimate relationships. *Clinical Psychology Review*, **15**: 567–81.

Eagle, M. (1996). Attachment research and psychoanalytic theory. In: *Psychoanalytic Perspectives on Developmental Psychology: Empirical Studies of Psychoanalytic Theories* (ed. J. M. Masling, R. F., Bornstein et al.), pp. 105–49. Washington DC: American Psychological Association.

Early, L. F. and Lifschutz, J. E. (1974). A case of stigmata. *Archives of General Psychiatry*, **30**: 197–200.

Egeland, B. and Susman-Stillman, A. (1996). Dissociation as a mediator of child abuse across generations. *Child Abuse and Neglect*, **20**: 1123–32.

Ekselius, L. and von Knorring, L. (1998). Personality disorder comorbidity with major depression and response to treatment with sertraline or citalopram. *International Clinical Psychopharmacology*, **13**: 205–11.

Eley, T. C., Lichtenstein, P., and Stevenson, J. (1999). Sex differences in the etiology of aggressive and nonaggressive antisocial behavior: results from two twin studies. *Child Development*, **70**: 155–68.

Elliott, R., Dolan, R. J., and Frith, C. D. (2000). Dissociable functions in the medial and lateral orbitofrontal cortex: Evidence from human neuroimaging studies. *Cerebral Cortex*, **10**: 308–17.

Emde, R., Kubicek, L., and Oppenheim, D. (1997). Imaginative reality observed during early language development. *International Journal of Psychoanalysis*, **78**: 115–33.

Emery, N. J. and Perrett, D. I. (2000). How can studies of the monkey brain help us understand "theory of mind" and autism in humans? In: *Understanding Other Minds: Perspectives from Developmental Cognitive Neuroscience* (ed. S. Baron-Cohen, H. Tager-Flusberg, and D. J. Cohen), pp. 274–305. New York: Oxford University Press.

Eppright, T. D. Kashani, J. H. Robison, B. D., and Reid, J. C. (1993). Comorbidity of conduct disorder and personality disorders in an incarcerated juvenile population. *The American Journal of Psychiatry*, **150**: 1233–6.

Erikson, E. H. (1959). *Identity and the Life Cycle.* New York: International Universities Press.

Evans, K., Tyrer, P., Catalan, J. *et al.* (1999). Manual–assisted cognitive–behaviour therapy (MACT): a randomised controlled trial of a brief intervention with bibliotherapy in the treatment of recurrent deliberate self–harm. *Psychological Medicine*, **29**: 19–25.

Fantz, R. (1963). Pattern vision in newborn infants. *Science*, **140**: 296–7.

Favazza, A. R. (1992). Repetitive self–mutilation. *Psychiatric Annals*, **22**: 60–3.

Feeney, J. A. and Noller, P. (1990). Attachment style as a predictor of adult romantic relationships. *Journal of Personality and Social Psychology*, **58**: 281–91.

Field, T. (1979). Differential behavioral and cardiac responses of 3–month–old infants to a mirror and peer. *Infant Behaviour and Development*, **2**: 179–84.

Field, T. (1985). Attachment as psychobiological attunement: Being on the same wavelength. In: *The Psychobiology of Attachment and Separation* (ed. M. Reite and T. Fields), pp. 415–54. New York: Academic Press.

First, M. B., Spitzer, R. L., Gibbon, M., and Williams, J. B. W. (1995*a*). The structured clinical interview for DSM–III–R personality disorders (SCID–II) Part I: Description. *Journal of Personality Disorders*, **9**: 83–91.

First, M. B., Spitzer, R. L., Gibbon, M., Williams, J. B., W. Davies, M., and Borus, J. (1995*b*). The structured clinical interview for DSM–III–R personality disorders (SCID–II) Part II: Multi-site test-retest reliability study. *Journal of Personality Disorders*, **9**: 92–104.

Fisher, C. (1945). Amnesic states in war neurosis: The psychogenesis of fugues. *Psychoanalytic Quarterly*, **14**: 437–58.

Fletcher, P. C., Happe, F., Frith, U. *et al.* (1995). Other minds in the brain: a functional imaging study of "theory of mind" in story comprehension. *Cognition*, **57**: 109–28.

Fodor, J. (1987). *Psychosemantics*. Cambridge, Mass: MIT Press.

Fodor, J. A. (1992). A theory of the child's theory of mind. *Cognition*, **44**: 283–96.

Fonagy, P. (1991). Thinking about thinking: Some clinical and theoretical considerations in the treatment of a borderline patient. *International Journal of Psychoanalysis*, **72**: 1–18.

Fonagy, P., Steele, H., Moran, G., Steele, M., and Higgitt, A. (1991). The capacity for understanding mental states: The reflective self in parent and child and its significance for security of attachment. *Infant Mental Health Journal*, **13**: 200–17.

Fonagy, P., Steele, M., Moran, G. S., Steele, H., and Higgitt, A. (1993). Measuring the ghost in the nursery: An empirical study of the relation between parents' mental representations of childhood experiences and their infants' security of attachment. *Journal of the American Psychoanalytic Association*, **41**: 957–89.

Fonagy, P,. Steele, M., Steele, H., Higgitt, A., and Target, M. (1994). Theory and practice of resilience. *Journal of Child Psychology and Psychiatry*, **35**: 231–57.

Fonagy, P., Leigh, T., Kennedy, R. *et al.* (1995*a*). Attachment, borderline states and the representation of emotions and cognitions in self and other. In: *Rochester Symposium on Developmental Psychopathology: Cognition and emotion* (ed. D. Cicchetti and S. S. Toth), pp. 371–414. Rochester, NY: University of Rochester Press.

Fonagy, P., Steele, M., Steele, H. *et al.* (1995*b*). The predictive validity of Mary Main's Adult Attachment Interview: A psychoanalytic and developmental perspective on the transgenerational transmission of attachment and borderline states. In: *Attachment Theory: Social, Developmental and Clinical Perspectives* (ed. S. Goldberg, R. Muir, and J. Kerr), pp. 233–78. Hillsdale, NJ: The Analytic Press.

Fonagy, P., Leigh, T., Steele, M. *et al.* (1996). The relation of attachment status, psychiatric classification, and response to psychotherapy. *Journal of Consulting and Clinical Psychology*, **64**: 22–31.

Fonagy, P. and Target, M. (1996). Playing with reality: I. Theory of mind and the normal development of psychic reality. *International Journal of Psychoanalysis,* **77**: 217–33.

Fonagy, P. (1997). Attachment and theory of mind: Overlapping constructs? *Association for Child Psychology and Psychiatry Occasional Papers*, **14**: 31–40.

Fonagy, P. and Target, M. (1997). Attachment and reflective function: Their role in self-organization. *Development and Psychopathology*, **9**: 679–700.

Fonagy, P,. Redfern, S., and Charman, T. (1997*a*). The relationship between belief-desire reasoning and a projective measure of attachment security (SAT). *British Journal of Developmental Psychology*, **15**: 51–61.

Fonagy, P., Steele, H., Steele, M., and Holder, J. (1997*b*). Attachment and theory of mind: Overlapping constructs? *Association for Child Psychology and Psychiatry Occasional Papers*, **14**: 31–40.

Fonagy, P., Target, M., Steele, M., and Steele, H. (1997*c*). The development of violence and crime as it relates to security of attachment. In: *Children in a Violent Society* (ed. J. D. Osofsky), pp. 150–77. New York: Guilford Press.

Fonagy, P., Target, M., Steele, H., and Steele, M. (1998). Reflective-Functioning Manual, version 5.0, for Application to Adult Attachment Interviews. London: University College London.

Fonagy, P. (1999*a*). Male perpetrators of violence against women: An attachment theory perspective. *Journal of Applied Psychoanalytic Studies*, **1**: 7–27.

Fonagy, P. (1999*b*). The transgenerational transmission of holocaust trauma. Lessons learned from the analysis of an adolescent with obsessive-compulsive disorder. *Attachment and Human Development*, **1**: 92–114.

Fonagy, P. (2000). Attachment and borderline personality disorder. *Journal of the American Psychoanalytic Association*, **48**: 1129–46.

Fonagy, P. and Target, M. (2000). Playing with reality III: The persistence of dual psychic reality in borderline patients. *International Journal of Psychoanalysis*, **81**: 853–74.

Fonagy, P., Target, M., and Gergely, G. (2000). Attachment and borderline personality disorder: A theory and some evidence. *Psychiatric Clinics of North America*, **23**: 103–22.

Fonagy, P., Stein, H., and White, R. (2001). Dopamine receptor polymorphism and susceptibility to sexual, physical and psychological abuse: Preliminary results of a longitudinal study of maltreatment. Paper presented at the symposium on the Consequences of Sexual Abuse: Issues of Measurement and Mechanisms at the *10th Biannual Meeting of the Society for Research in Child Development*, Mineapolis.

Fonagy, P. and Target, M. (2002). Early intervention and the development of self-regulation. *Psychoanalytic Inquiry*, **22**: 307–35.

Fonagy, P., Gergely, G., Jurist, E., and Target, M. (2002). *Affect Regulation, Mentalization and the Development of the Self.* New York: Other Press.

Fonagy, P. (2003). The development of psychopathology from infancy to adulthood: the mysterious unfolding of disturbance in time. *Infant Mental Health Journal*, **24**: 212–39.

Fonagy, P., Stein, H., Allen, J., and Fultz, J. (2003). The relationship of mentalization and childhood and adolescent adversity to adult functioning. Paper presented at the *Biennial Meeting of the Society for Research in Child Development.* Tampa, FL.

Fossati, A., Madeddu, F., and Maffei, C. (1999*a*). Borderline personality disorder and childhood sexual abuse: a meta-analytic study. *Journal of Personality Disorders*, **13**: 268–80.

Fossati, A., Maffei, C., Bagnato, M., Donati, D., Namia, C., and Novella, L. (1999*b*). Latent structure analysis of DSM-IV borderline personality disorder criteria. *Comprehensive Psychiatry*, **40**: 72–9.

Fossati, A., Donati, D., Donini, M., Novella, L., Bagnato, M., and Maffei, C. (2001). Temperament, character, and attachment patterns in borderline personality disorder. *Journal of Personality Disorders*, **15**: 390–402.

Frank, H. and Paris, J. (1981). Recollections of family experience in borderline patients. *Archives of General Psychiatry*, **38**: 1031–4.

Frederickson, R. (1992). *Repressed Memories: A Journey to Recovery from Sexual Abuse.* New York: Simon and Schuster.

Freud, A. (1936). *The Ego and the Mechanisms of Defence*, 1946. New York: International Universities Press.

Freud, S. (1899). Screen memories. In: *The Standard Edition of the Complete Psychological Works of Sigmund Freud* (ed. J. Strachey), Vol. 3 pp. 301–22. London: Hogarth Press.

Freud, S. (1900). The interpretation of dreams. In: *The Standard Edition of the Complete Psychological Works of Sigmund Freud* (ed. J. Strachey), Vols. 4, 5 pp. 1–715. London: Hogarth Press.

Freud, S. (1914). On narcissism: An introduction. In: *The Standard Edition of the Complete Psychological Works of Sigmund Freud* (ed. J. Strachey), Vol. 14 pp. 67–104. London: Hogarth Press.

Freud, S. (1915). Observations on transference love. In: *The Standard Edition of the Complete Psychological Works of Sigmund Freud*, (ed. J. Strachey), Vol. 12 pp. 157–71. London: Hogarth Press.

Freud, S. (1924). The loss of reality in neurosis and psychosis. In: *The Standard Edition of the Complete Psychological Works of Sigmund Freud* (ed. J. Strachey), Vol. 19 pp. 183–90. London: Hogarth Press.

Frith, C. and Frith, U. (2000). The physiological basis of theory of mind: Functional neuroimaging studies. In: *Understanding Other Minds: Perspectives from Developmental Cognitive Neuroscience* (ed. S. Baron-Cohen, H. Tager-Flusberg, and D. J. Cohen), pp. 334–56. New York: Oxford University Press.

Frith, C. D. and Frith, U. (1999). Interacting minds—A biological basis. *Science*, **286**: 1692–5.

Frodi, A., Dernevik, M., Sepa, A., Philipson, J., and Bragesjo, M. (2001). Current attachment representations of incarcerated offenders varying in degree of psychopathy. *Attachment & Human Development*, **3**: 269–83.

Fyer, M. R., Frances, A. J., Sullivan, T., Hurt, S. W., and Clarkin, J. (1988). Suicide attempts in patients with borderline personality disorder. *The American Journal of Psychiatry*, **145**: 737–9.

Gabbard, G. O. (1991). Technical approaches to transference hate in the analysis of borderline patients. *The International Journal of Psychoanalysis*, **72**: 625–37.

Gabbard, G. O., Horwitz, L., Allen, J. G. *et al.* (1994). Transference interpretation in the psychotherapy of borderline patients: A high-risk, high-gain phenomenon. *Harvard Review of Psychiatry*, **2**: 59–69.

Gabbard, G. O. (1995). Countertransference: The emerging common ground. *The International Journal of Psychoanalysis*, **76**: 475–85.

Gabbard, G. O. and Lester, E. P. (1995). *Boundaries and Boundary Violations in Psychoanalysis.* New York: Basic Books.

Gabbard, G. O. (1996). *Love and Hate in the Analytic Setting.* New York: Jason Aronson.

Gabbard, G. O. (1997). Challenges in the analysis of adult patients with histories of childhood sexual abuse. *Canadian Journal of Psychoanalysis*, **5**: 1–25.

Gabbard, G. O. (2000*a*). *Psychodynamic Psychiatry in Clinical Practice,* 3rd ed. American Psychiatric Press, Arlington, VA.

Gabbard, G. O. (2000*b*). *Psychotherapy for Personality Disorders,* American Psychiatric Press, Washington DC.

Gabbard, G. O. (2000*c*). Psychotherapy of personality disorders. *Journal of Psychotherapy Practice and Research*, **9**: 1–6.

Gabbard, G. O. (2001). Psychodynamic psychotherapy of borderline personality disorder: a contemporary approach. *Bulletin of the Menninger Clinic*, **65**: 41–57.

Gabbard, G. O. (2003). Miscarriages of psychoanalytic treatment with suicidal patients. *International Journal of Psychoanalysis*, **84**: 249–61.

Gallagher, H. L., Happe, F., Brunswick, N., Fletcher, P. C., Frith, U., and Frith, C. D. (2000). Reading the mind in cartoons and stories: an fMRI study of 'theory of mind' in verbal and nonverbal tasks. *Neuropsychologia*, **38**: 11–21.

Gallese, V. (2000). The acting subject: Toward the neural basis of social cognition. In: *Neural Correlates of Consciousness* (ed. T. Metzinger), pp. 325–33. Cambridge, MA: MIT Press.

Gallese, V. (2001). The "shared manifold" hypothesis: From mirror neurons to empathy. *Journal of Consciousness Studies*, **8**: 33–50.

Gaston, L. (1990). The concept of the alliance and its role in psychotherapy: Theoretical and empirical considerations. *Psychotherapy*, **27**: 143–53.

Gazzaniga, M. S. (1985). *The Social Brain: Discovering the Networks of the Mind.* New York: Basic Books.

Gergely, G. and Csibra, G. (1996). Understanding rational actions in infancy: teleological interpretations without mental attribution. Paper presented at the Symposium on 'Early Perception of Social Contingencies', *10th Biennial International Conference on Infant Studies (ICIS).* RI, USA: Providence.

Gergely, G. and Watson, J. (1996). The social biofeedback model of parental affect-mirroring. *International Journal of Psychoanalysis*, **77**: 1181–212.

Gergely, G. and Csibra, G. (1997). Teleological reasoning in infancy: The infant's naive theory of rational action. A reply to Premack and Premack. *Cognition*, **63**: 227–233.

Gergely, G. and Csibra, G. (1998). La interpretacion teleologica de la conducta: La teoria infantil de la accion racional [The teleological interpretation of behaviour: the infant's theory of rational action]. *Infancia y Aprendizaje*, **84**: 45–65.

Gergely, G. and Watson, J. (1999). Early social-emotional development: Contingency perception and the social biofeedback model. In: *Early Social Cognition: Understanding Others in the First Months of Life* (ed. P. Rochat), pp. 101–37. Hillsdale, NJ: Erlbaum.

Gergely, G. and Csibra, G. (2000). The teleological origins of naive theory of mind in infancy. Paper presented at the Symposium on 'Origins of theory of mind: studies with human infants and primates'. *12th Biennial International Conference on Infant Studies (ICIS).* Brighton, England.

Gergely, G. (2001). The development of understanding of self and agency. In: *Handbook of Childhood Cognitive Development* (ed. U. Goshwami), pp. 26–46. Oxford: Blackwell.

Gergely, G., Koós, O., and Watson, J. S. (2002). Contingency perception and the role of contingent parental reactivity in early socio-emotional development. In: *Imiter pour découvrir l'human: Psychologie, neurobioligie, robotique et philosophie de l'ésprit* (ed. J. Nadel and J. Decety), pp. 59–82. Paris: Presses Universitaires de France.

Gergely, G. and Csibra, G. (2003). Teleological reasoning in infancy: The naive theory of rational action. *Trends in Cognitive Sciences*, **7**: 287–92.

Gerlsma, C., Emmelkamp, P. M. G., and Arrindell, W. A. (1990). Anxiety, depression and perception of early parenting: A meta-analysis. *Clinical Psychology Review*, **10**: 251–77.

Gidycz, C. A., Hanson, K., and Layman, M. J. (1995). A prospective analysis of the relationships among sexual assault experiences: an extension of previous findings. *Psychology of Women Quarterly*, **19**: 5–29.

Giedd, J. N., Blumenthal, J., Jeffries, N. O. *et al.* (1999). Brain development during childhood and adolescence: a longitudinal MRI study. *Nature Neuroscience*, **2**: 861–3.

Gilligan, J. (1997). *Violence: Our Deadliest Epidemic and Its Causes.* New York: Grosset/Putnam.

Glaser, D. (2000). Child abuse and neglect and the brain—A review. *Journal of Child Psychology and Psychiatry*, **41**: 97–116.

Goel, V., Grafman, N., Sadato, M., and Hallett, M. (1995). Modeling other minds. *Neuroreport*, **6**: 1741–6.

Goldberg, E. (2001). *The Executive Brain: Frontal Lobes and the Civilized Mind.* New York: Oxford University Press.

Goldberg, R. L., Mann, L., Wise, T. *et al.* (1985). Parental qualities as perceived by borderline personality disorders. *Hillside Journal of Clinical Psychiatry*, **7**: 134–40.

Goldfried, M. R. (1995). *From Cognitive-Behavior Therapy to Psychotherapy Integration.* New York: Springer.

Goldman Rakic, P. S., O Scalaidhe, S. P., Chafee, M. V. *et al.* (2000). Memory. In: *The New Cognitive Neurosciences* (ed. M. S. Gazzaniga). pp. 733–840. Cambridge, MA, US: The MIT Press.

Goldman, S. J., D'Angelo, E. J., and Demaso, D. R. (1993). Psychopathology in the families of children and adolescents with borderline personality disorder. *American Journal of Psychiatry*, **150**: 1832–5.

Goodman, G., Hull, J. W., Clarkin, J. F., and Yeomans, F. E. (1999). Childhood antisocial behaviors as predictors of psychotic symptoms and DSM-IIIR borderline personality disorder. *Journal of Personality Disorders*, **13**: 35–46.

Goodman, M. and New, A. (2000). Impulsive aggression in borderline personality disorder. *Current Psychiatry Reports*, **2**: 56–61.

Gopnik, A. and Slaughter, V. (1991). Young children's understanding of changes in their mental states. *Child Development*, **62**: 98–110.

Gorenstein, E. E. (1982). Frontal lobe functions in psychopaths. *Journal of Abnormal Psychology*, **91**: 368–79.

Gould, E., McEwen, B. S., Tanapat, P., Galea, L. A., and Fuchs, E. (1997). Neurogenesis in the dentate gyrus of the adult tree shrew is regulated by psychosocial stress and NMDA receptor activation. *Journal of Neuroscience*, **17**: 2492–98.

Goyer, P. F., Andreasen, P. J., Semple, W. E. *et al.* (1994). Positron-emission tomography and personality disorders. *Neuropsychopharmacology*, **10**: 21–8.

Green, A. (1975). The analyst, symbolization, and absence in the analytic setting. *International Journal of Psychoanalysis*, **56**: 1–22.

Green, A. (1977). The borderline concept. A conceptual framework for the understanding of borderline patients: Suggested hypotheses. In: *Borderline Personality Disorders* (ed. P. Hartcollis), pp. 15–46. New York: International Universities Press.

Greene, J. and Haidt, J. (2002). How (and where) does moral judgment work? *Trends in Cognitive Sciences*, **6**: 517–23.

Grienenberger, J., Kelly, K., and Slade, A. (2001). Maternal reflective functioning and the caregiving relationship: The link between mental states and mother-infant affective communication. Paper presented at the *Biennial Meetings of the Society for Research in Child Development,* Minneapolis, MN.

Griffin, D. W. and Bartholomew, K. (1994). The metaphysics of measurement: The case of adult attachment. In: *Advances in Personal Relationships: Vol 5. Attachment Processes in Adulthood* (ed. K. Bartholomew and D. Perlman), pp. 17–52. London: Jessica Kingsley.

Griffiths, P. and Leach, G. (1998). Face to Face with Distress: The Professional Use of Self in Psychosocial Care. In: *Psychosocial Nursing: A Model Learned from Experience* (ed. E. Barnes, P. Griffith, J. Ord, and D. Wells). Oxford: Butterworth Heinemann.

Grilo, C. M., McGlashan, T. H., and Skodol, A. E. (2000). Stability and course of personality disorders: the need to consider comorbidities and continuities between axis I psychiatric disorders and axis II personality disorders. *The Psychiatric Quarterly*, **71**: 291–307.

Grinker, R., Werble, B., and Drye, R. C. (1968). *The Borderline Syndrome: A Behavioral Study of Ego Functions.* New York: Basic Books.

Gunderson, J., Carpenter, W., and Strauss, J. (1975). Borderline and schizophrenic patients: a comparative study. *The American Journal of Psychiatry*, **132**: 1257–64.

Gunderson, J. G. and Singer, M. T. (1975). Defining borderline patients: An overview. *The American Journal of Psychiatry*, **132**: 1–10.

Gunderson, J., Kerr, J., and Englund, D. (1980). The families of borderlines: A comparative study. *Archives of General Psychiatry*, **37**: 27–33.

Gunderson, J. G., Kolb, J. E., and Austin, V. (1981). The diagnostic interview for borderline patients. *The American Journal of Psychiatry*, **138**: 896–903.

Gunderson, J. G. (1984). *Borderline Personality Disorder.* Washington, DC: American Psychiatric Press.

Gunderson, J. G. and Elliott, G. R. (1985). The interface between borderline personality disorder and affective disorder. *The American Journal of Psychiatry*, **142**: 277–88.

Gunderson, J. G., Frank, A. F., Ronningstam, E. F., Wachter, S., Lynch, V. J., and Wolf, P. J. (1989). Early discontinuance of borderline patients from psychotherapy. *Journal of Nervous and Mental Disease*, **177**: 38–42.

Gunderson, J. G. (1996). The borderline patient's intolerance of aloneness: Insecure attachments and therapist availability. *The American Journal of Psychiatry*, **153**: 752–8.

Gunderson, J. G., Najavits, L.M., Leonhard, C. *et al.* (1997). Ontogeny of the therapeutic alliance in borderline patients. *Journal of Psychotherapy Research*, **7**: 301–9.

Gunderson, J. G. (2001). *Borderline Personality Disorder: A Clinical Guide.* Washington DC: American Psychiatric Publishing.

Gurvits, I. G., Koenigsberg, H. W., and Siever, L. J. (2000). Neurotransmitter dysfunction in patients with borderline personality disorder. *The Psychiatric Clinics of North America*, **23**: 27–40, vi.

Guthrie, E., Creed, F., Dawson, D. *et al.* (1991). A controlled trial of psychological treatment for the irritable bowel syndrome. *Gastroenterology*, **100**: 450–7.

Guthrie, E. (1999*a*). Psychodynamic interpersonal therapy. *Advances in Psychiatric Treatment*, **5**: 135–145.

Guthrie, E., Moorey, J., Margison, F. *et al.* (1999*b*). Cost-effectiveness of brief psychodynamic-interpersonal therapy in high utilizers of psychiatric services. *Archives of General Psychiatry*, **56**: 519–26.

Guthrie, E., Kapur, N., Mackway-Jones, K., Chew-Graham, C., Moorey, J., Mendel, E. *et al.* (2001). Randomised controlled trial of brief psychological intervention after deliberate self-poisoning. *British Medical Journal*, **323**: 135–7.

Haaken, J. and Schlaps, A. (1991). Incest resolution therapy and the objectification of sexual abuse. *Psychotherapy*, **28**: 39–47.

Haigh, R. (1999). *The Quintessence of a Therapeutic Environment—Five Essential Qualities.* London: Jessica Kingsley.

Happe, F., Ehlers, S., Fletcher, P. *et al.* (1996). "Theory of mind" in the brain: Evidence from a PET scan study of Asperger syndrome. *NeuroReport*, **8**: 197–201.

Happé FGE (1995). The role of age and verbal ability in the theory of mind task performance of subjects with autism. *Child Development*, **66**: 843–55.

Harman, C. Rothbart, M. K., and Posner, M. I. (1997). Distress and intention interactions in early infancy. *Motivation and Emotion*, **21**: 27–43.

Harter, S. (1999). *The Construction of the Self: A Developmental Perspective.* New York: Guilford Press.

Hartmann, E. (1984). *The Nightmare: The Psychology and Biology of Terrifying Dreams.* New York: Basic Books.

Hazan, C. and Shaver, P. (1987). Romantic love conceptualized as an attachment process. *Journal of Personality and Social Psychology*, **52**: 511–24.

Hegel, G. (1807). *The Phenomenology of Spirit.* Oxford: Oxford University Press.

Henry, W. P., Schact, T., and Strupp, H. H. (1990). Patient and therapist introject, interpersonal process, and differential psychotherapy outcome. *Journal of Consulting and Clinical Psychology*, **58**: 768–74.

Herman, J. and van der Kolk, B. (1987). Traumatic antecedents of borderline personality disorder. In: *Psychological Trauma* (ed. B. van der Kolk), pp. 23–51. Washington, DC: American Psychiatric Press.

Herman, J. L., Perry, C., and van der Kolk, B. A. (1989). Childhood trauma in borderline personality disorder. *The American Journal of Psychiatry*, **146**: 490–5.

Herpertz, S. C. (1995). Self-injurious behaviour. Psychopathological and nosological characteristics in subtypes of self-injurers. *Acta Psychiatrica Scandinavica*, **91**: 57–68.

Herpertz, S. C., Steinmeyer, S. M., Marx, D., Oidtmann, A., and Sass, H. (1995). The significance of aggression and impulsivity for self-mutilative behavior. *Pharmacopsychiatry*, **28 Suppl 2**: 64–72.

Herpertz, S., Hanns, H., Schwenger, U., Eng, M., and Sass, H. (1999). Affective responsiveness in borderline personality disorder: a psychophysiological approach. *The American Journal of Psychiatry*, **156**: 1550–6.

Herpertz, S., Werth, U., Lukas, G. *et al.* (2001*a*). Emotion in criminal offenders with psychopathy and borderline personality disorder. *Archives of General Psychiatry*, **58**: 737–45.

Herpertz, S. C., Dietrich, T. M., Wenning, B. *et al.* (2001*b*). Evidence of abnormal amygdala functioning in borderline personality disorder: a functional MRI study. *Biological Psychiatry*, **50**: 292–8.

Heuer, F. and Reisberg, D. (1992). Emotion, arousal, and memory for detail. In: *The Handbook of Emotion and Memory: Research and Theory* (ed. S. Christianson), pp. 151–80. Hillsdale, NH: Erlbaum.

Higgitt, A. and Fonagy, P. (1992). The psychotherapeutic treatment of borderline and narcissistic personality disorder. *British Journal of Psychiatry*, **161**: 23–43.

Hirono, N., Mega, M., Dinov, I., Mishkin, F., and Cummings, J. L. (2000). Left frontotemporal hypoperfusion is associated with aggression in patients with dementia. *Archives of Neurology*, **57**: 861–6.

Hirschfeld, L. and Gelman, S. (1994). *Mapping the Mind: Domain Specificity in Cognition and Culture.* New York: Cambridge University Press.

Hoagwood, K., Hibbs, E., Brent, D., and Jensen, P. (1995). Introduction to the special section: Efficacy and effectiveness in studies of child and adolescent psychotherapy. *Journal of Consulting and Clinical Psychology*, **63**: 683–7.

Hobson, R. F. (1985). *Forms of Feeling: The Heart of Psychotherapy.* New York: Basic Books.

Hobson, R. P. (1993). *Autism and the Development of Mind.* London: Lawrence Erlbaum.

Hoffman, M. L. (1978). *Toward a Theory of Empathic Arousal and Development.* New York: Plenum Press.

Hofstra, M. B., van der Ende, J., and Verhulst, F. C. (2002). Child and adolescent problems predict DSM-IV disorders in adulthood: A 14-year follow-up of a Dutch epidemiological sample. *Journal of the American Academy of Child and Adolescent Psychiatry*, **41**: 182–9.

Høglend, P. (1993). Personality disorders and long-term outcome after brief psychodynamic therapy. *Journal of Personality Disorders*, **7**: 168–81.

Hollander, E., Grossman, R., Stein, D., and Kwon, J. (1996). Borderline personality disorder and impulsive-aggression: the role of Divalproex Sodium treatment. *Psychiatric Annals*, **26**: 464–9.

Holmes, H. A., Black, C., and Miller, S. A. (1996). A cross-task comparison of false-belief understanding in a Head Start population. *Journal of Experimental Child Psychology*, **63**: 263–85.

Holmes, J. (1998). Defensive and creative uses of narrative in psychotherapy: An attachment perspective. In: *Narrative and Psychotherapy and Psychiatry* (ed. G. Roberts and J. Holmes), pp. 49–68. Oxford: Oxford University Press.

Hooven, C., Gottman, J. M., and Katz, L. F. (1995). Parental meta-emotion structure predicts family and child outcomes. *Cognition and Emotion*, **9**: 229–64.

Horne, J. (1988). *Why We Sleep: The Functions of Sleep in Humans and Other Mammals.* Oxford: Oxford University Press.

Horwitz, A. V., Widom, C. S., McLaughlin, J., and White, H. R. (2001). The impact of childhood abuse and neglect on adult mental health: a prospective study. *Journal of Health and Social Behaviour*, **42**: 184–201.

Horwitz, L. (1974). *Clinical Prediction in Psychotherapy.* New York: Jason Aronson.

Horwitz, L., Gabbard, G. O., Allen, J. G. *et al.* (1996). *Borderline Personality Disorder: Tailoring the Psychotherapy to the Patient.* Washington, DC: American Psychiatric Press.

Horowitz, L. M., Rosenberg, S. E., Baer, B. A., Ureno, G., and Villasenor, G. (1988). Inventory of interpersonal problems: Psychometric properties and clinical applications. *Journal of Consulting and Clinical Psychology*, **56**: 885–92.

Horowitz, L. M., Rosenberg, S. E., and Bartholomew, K. (1993). Interpersonal problems, attachment styles and outcome in brief dynamic therapy. *Journal of Consulting and Clinical Psychology*, **61**: 549–60.

Hughes, C., Deater-Deckard, K., and Cutting, A. (1999). 'Speak roughly to your little boy?' Sex differences in the relations between parenting and preschoolers' understanding of mind. *Social Development*, **8**: 143–60.

Hyman, S. E. (2002). The new begining of research on borderline personality disorder. *Biological Psychiatry*, **51**: 933–5.

Ilardi, S. S., Craighead, W. E., and Evans, D. D. (1997). Modeling relapse in unipolar depression: The effects of dysfunctional cognitions and personality disorders. *Journal of Consulting and Clinical Psychology*, **65**: 381–91.

Ingram, R. E. and Ritter, J. (2000). Vulnerability to depression: cognitive reactivity and parental bonding in high-risk individuals. *Journal of Abnormal Psychology*, **109**: 588–96.

Intrator, J., Hare, R., Stritzke, P. *et al.* (1997). A brain-imaging (Single Photon Emission Computerized Tomography) study of semantic and affective processing in psychopaths. *Biological Psychiatry*, **42**: 96–103.

Jacobsen, T., Huss, M., Fendrich, M., Kruesi, M. J. P., and Ziegenhain, U. (1997). Children's ability to delay gratification: Longitudinal relations to mother-child attachment. *Journal of Genetic Psychology*, **158**: 411–26.

Jaffe, J., Beebe, B., Feldstein, S., Crown, C. L., and Jasnow, M. D. (2001). Rhythms of Dialogue in Infancy. *Monographs of the Society for Research in Child Development*, **66**.

James, W. (1890). *Principles of Psychology*. New York: Henry Holt & Co.

Jang, K. L., Livesley, W. J., Vernon, P. A., and Jackson, D. N. (1996). Heritability of personality disorder traits: a twin study. *Acta Psychiatrica Scandinavica*, **94**: 438–44.

Jeannerod, M. (1997). *The Cognitive Neuroscience of Action*. Oxford: Blackwell.

Jenkins, J. and Astington, J. W. (1996). Cognitive factors and family structure associated with theory of mind development in young children. *Developmental Psychology*, **32**: 70–8.

Jensen, P. S., Hibbs, E. D., and Pilkonis, P. A. (1996). From ivory tower to clinical practice: Future directions for child and adolescent psychotherapy research. In: *Psychosocial Treatments for Child and Adolescent Disorders Empirically Based Strategies for Clinical Practice* (ed. E. D. Hibbs and P. S. Jensen), pp. 701–11. Washington, DC: American Psychological Association.

Johnson, J. G., Cohen, P., Brown, J., Smailes, E. M., and Bernstein, D. P. (1999). Childhood maltreatment increases risk for personality disorders during early adulthood. *Archives of General Psychiatry*, **56**: 600–5.

Johnson, J. G., Smailes, E. M., Cohen, P., Brown, J., and Bernstein, D. P. (2000). Associations between four types of childhood neglect and personality disorder symptoms during adolescence and early adulthood: findings of a community-based longitudinal study. *Journal of Personality Disorders*, **14**: 171–87.

Kantrowitz, J. (1995). Outcome research in psychoanalysis: review and reconsiderations. In: *Research in Psychoanalysis: Process, Development, Outcome* (ed. T. Shapiro and R. Emde), pp. 313–28. Madison WI: International Universities Press Inc.

Karmiloff-Smith, A. (1992). *Beyond Modularity: A Developmental Perspective on Cognitive Science*. Cambridge, MA: MIT Press.

Karterud, S., Vaglum, S., Friis, S., Irion, T., Johns, S., and Vaglum, P. (1992). Day hospital therapeutic community treatment for patients with personality disorder: An empirical evaluation of the containment function. *The Journal of Nervous and Mental Disease*, **180**: 238–43.

Karterud, S., Pedersen, G., Friis, S., *et al.* (1998). The Norwegian network of psychotherapeutic day hospitals. *Therapeutic Communities*, **19**: 15–28.

Karterud, S., Pedersen, G., Bjordal, E., Brabrand, J., Friis, S., Haaseth, Ø., Haavaldsen, G., Irion, T., Leirvåg, H., Tørum, E., and Urnes, Ø. (2003). Day treatment of patients with personality disorders: Experiences from a Norwegian treatment research network. *Journal of Personality Disorders*, **17**: 243–62.

Kasen, S., Cohen, P., Skodol, A. E., Johnson, J. G., Smailes, E., and Brook, J. S. (2001). Childhood depression and adult personality disorder: alternative pathways of continuity. *Archives of General Psychiatry*, **58**: 231–6.

Kaye, A. L. and Shea, M. T. (2000). Personality disorders, personality traits, and defense mechanisms. In: *Handbook of Psychiatric Measures* (ed. Task Force for the Handbook of Psychiatric Measures), pp. 713–49. Washington, DC: American Psychiatric Association.

Kazniak, A. W., Nussbaum, P. D., Berren, M. R., and Santiago, J. (1988). Amnesia as a consequence of male rape: A case report. *Journal of Abnormal Psychology*, **97**: 100–4.

Keller, M. B., Lavori, P. W., Friedman, B. *et al.* (1987). The longitudinal interval follow-up evaluation. A comprehensive method for assessing outcome in prospective longitudinal studies. *Archives of General Psychiatry*, **44**: 540–8.

Kelley, W. M., Macrae, C. N., Wyland, C. L., Caglar, S., Inati, S., and Heatherton, T. F. (2002). Finding the self? An event-related fMRI study. *Journal of Cognitive Neuroscience*, **14**: 785–94.

Kemperman, I., Russ, M. J., and Shearin, E. (1997). Self-injurious behavior and mood regulation in borderline patients. *Journal of Personality Disorders*, **11**: 146–57.

Kernberg, O. F. (1967). Borderline personality organisation. *Journal of the American Psychoanalytic Association*, **15**: 641–85.

Kernberg, O. F. (1972). Final report of the Menninger Foundation's psychotherapy research project: summary and conclusions. *Bulletin of the Menninger Clinic*, **36**: 181–95.

Kernberg, O. F., *et al.* (1972). Psychotherapy and psychoanalysis: final report of the Menninger Foundation Psychotherapy Research Project. *Bulletin of the Menninger Clinic*, **36**: 3–275.

Kernberg, O. F. (1975). *Borderline Conditions and Pathological Narcissism.* New York: Jason Aronson.

Kernberg, O. F. (1976). *Object Relations Theory and Clinical Psychoanalysis.* New York: Aronson.

Kernberg, O. F. (1977). The structural diagnosis of borderline personality organization. In: *Borderline Personality Disorders: The Concept, the Syndrome, the Patient* (ed. P. Hartocollis), pp. 87–121. New York: International Universities Press.

Kernberg, O. F. (1980). *Internal World and External Reality: Object Relations Theory Applied.* New York: Aronson.

Kernberg, O. F. (1982). Self, ego, affects and drives. *Journal of the American Psychoanalytic Association*, **30**: 893–917.

Kernberg, O. F. (1983). Object relations theory and character analysis. *Journal of the American Psychoanalytic Association*, **31**: 247–71.

Kernberg, O. F. (1984*a*). *Severe Personality Disorders: Psychotherapeutic Strategies.* New Haven, CT: Yale University Press.

Kernberg, O. F. (1984*b*). *Reflections in the Mirror: Mother-Child Interactions, Self-Awareness, and Self-Recognition.* New York: Basic Books, Inc.

Kernberg, O. F., Selzer, M. A., Koenigsberg, H. W., Carr, A. C., and Appelbaum, A. H. (1989). *Psychodynamic Psychotherapy of Borderline Patients.* New York: Basic Books.

Kernberg, O. F. (1992). *Aggression in Personality Disorders and Perversions.* New Haven and London: Yale University Press.

Kernberg, O. F. and Clarkin, J. (1995). *The Inventory of Personality Organization.* White Plains, NY: The New York Hospital—Cornell Medical Center.

Kernberg, O. F., Clarkin, J. F., and Yeomans, F. E. (2002*a*). *A Primer of Transference Focused Psychotherapy for the Borderline Patient.* New York: Jason Aronson.

Kernberg, O. F., Clarkin, J. F., and Yeomans, F. E. (2002*b*). *A Primer of Transference Focused Psychotherapy for the Borderline Patient.* New York, NY: Jason Aronson.

Kiehl, K. A., Smith, A. M., Hare, R. D. *et al.* (2001). Limbic abnormalities in affective processing by criminal psychopaths as revealed by functional magnetic resonance imaging. *Biological Psychiatry*, **50**: 677–84.

Kimble, C., Oepen, G., Weinberg, E., Williams, A., and Zanarini, M. C. (1996). Neurobiological vulnerability and trauma in borderline personality disorder. In: *Role of Sexual Abuse in the Etiology of Borderline Personality Disorder* (ed. M. C. Zanarini), pp. 165–80. Washington, DC: American Psychiatric Press.

Klein, M. (1937). Love, guilt and reparation. In: *Love, Guilt and Reparation: The Writings of Melanie Klein Volume I*, pp. 306–43. New York: Macmillan, 1984.

Klein, M. (1946*a*). *Envy and Gratitude and Other Works, 1946–1962*, New York: Delta, 1975.

Klein, M. (1946*b*). Notes on some schizoid mechanisms. In: *Developments in Psychoanalysis* (ed. M. Klein, P. Heimann, S. Isaacs, and J. Riviere), pp. 292–320. London: Hogarth Press.

Klin, A., Schultz, R., and Cohen, D. J. (2000). Theory of mind in action: Developmental perspectives on social neuroscience. In: *Understanding Other Minds: Perspectives from Developmental Cognitive Neuroscience* 2nd ed. (ed. S. Baron-Cohen, H. Tager-Flusberg, and D. J. Cohen), pp. 357–88. New York: Oxford University Press.

Knight, R. (1953). Borderline states. *Bulletin of the Menninger Clinic*, **17**: 1–12.

Kochanska, G., Murray, K., Jacques, T., Koenig, A. L., and Vandegeest, K. (1996). Inhibitory control in young children and its role in emerging internalization. *Child Development*, **67**: 490–507.

Kochanska, G. (1997). Multiple pathways to conscience for children with different temperaments: from toddlerhood to age 5. *Developmental Psychology*, **33**: 228–40.

Kochanska, G., Murray, K., and Harlan, E. (2000). Effortful control in early childhood: Continuity and change, antecedents, and implications for social development. *Developmental Psychology*, **36**: 220–32.

Kochanska, G. (2001). Emotional development in children with different attachment histories: The first three years. *Child Development*, **72**: 474–90.

Kochanska, G., Coy, K. C., and Murray, K. T. (2001). The development of self-regulation in the first four years of life. *Child Development*, **72**: 1091–111.

Koenigsberg, H. W., Harvey, P. D., Mitropoulou, V. *et al.* (2001). Are the interpersonal and identity disturbances in the borderline personality disorder criteria linked to the traits of affective instability and impulsivity? *Journal of Personality Disorders*, **15**: 358–70.

Koenigsberg, H. W., Harvey, P. D., Mitropoulou, V. *et al.* (2002). Characterizing affective instability in borderline personality disorder. *The American Journal of Psychiatry*, **159**: 784–8.

Koerner, K. and Dimeff, L. A. (2000). Further data on Dialectical Behaviour Therapy. *Clinical Psychology Science and Practice*, **7**: 104–112.

Koerner, K. and Linehan, M. M. (2000). Research on Dialectical Behavior Therapy for patients with borderline personality disorder. *Psychiatric Clinics of North America*, **23**: 151–67.

Kohut, H. (1971). *The Analysis of the Self.* New York: International Universities Press.

Kohut, H. (1977). *The Restoration of the Self.* New York: International Universities Press.

Koren-Karie, N., Oppenheim, D., Dolev, S., Sher, S., and Etzion-Carasso, A. (2002). Mothers' insightfulness regarding their infants' internal experience: Relations with maternal sensitivity and infant attachment. *Developmental Psychology*, **38**: 534–42.

Korfine, L. and Hooley, J. M. (2000). Directed forgetting of emotional stimuli in borderline personality disorder. *Journal of Abnormal Psychology*, **109**: 214–21.

Kosslyn, S. M. (1994). *Image and Brain: The Resolution of the Imagery Debate.* Cambridge, MA: MIT Press.

Kraemer, G. W. (1999). Psychobiology of early social attachment in Rhesus monkeys: Clinical applications. In: *The Integrative Neurobiology of Affiliation* (ed. C. S. Carter, II Lederhendler and B. Kirkpatrick), pp. 373–90. Cambridge, MA: MIT Press.

Kramer, S. (1990). Residues of incest. In: *Adult Analysis and Childhood Sexual Abuse* (ed. H Levine), pp. 149–70. Hillsdale, NJ: Analytic Press.

Krawitz, R. (1997). A prospective psychotherapy outcome study. *Australian and New Zealand Journal of Psychiatry*, **31**: 465–73.

Kreppner, J. M., O'Connor, T. G., and Rutter, M. (2001). Can inattention/overactivity be an institutional deprivation syndrome? *Journal of Abnormal Child Psychology*, **29**: 513–28.

Kroll, J. (2000). Use of no-suicide contracts by psychiatrists in Minnesota. *The American Journal of Psychiatry*, **157**: 1684–6.

Kuebli, J., Butler, S., and Fivush, R. (1995). Mother-child talk about past emotions: Relations of maternal language and child gender over time. *Cognition and Emotion*, **9**: 265–83.

Laakso, M. P., Vaurio, O., Koivisto, E. *et al.* (2001). Psychopathy and the posterior hippocampus. *Behavioural Brain Research*, **118**: 187–93.

Lane, R. D., Ahern, G. L., Schwartz, G. E., and Kaszniak, A. W. (1997). Is alexithymia the emotional equivalent of blindsight? *Biological Psychiatry*, **42**: 834–44.

Lane, R. D., Reiman, E. M., Axelrod, B., Yun, L.-S., Holmes, A., and Schwartz, G. E. (1998). Neural correlates of levels of emotional awareness: Evidence of an interaction between emotion and attention in the anterior cingulate cortex. *Journal of Cognitive Neuroscience*, **10**: 525–35.

Lane, R. D. (2000). Neural correlates of conscious emotional experience. In: *Cognitive Neuroscience of Emotion* (ed. R. D. Lane and L. Nadel), pp. 345–70. New York: Oxford University Press.

Langeland, W. and Dijkstra, S. (1995). Breaking the intergenerational transmission of child abuse: Beyond the mother-child relationship. *Child Abuse Review*, **4**: 4–13.

Lanius, R. A., Williamson, P. C., Densmore, M. *et al.* (2001). Neural correlates of traumatic memories in posttraumatic stress disorder: a functional MRI investigation. *The American Journal of Psychiatry*, **158**: 1920–2.

Lapierre, D., Braun, C. M., and Hodgins, S. (1995). Ventral frontal deficits in psychopathy: neuropsychological test findings. *Neuropsychologia*, **33**: 139–51.

Lecours, S. and Bouchard M.-A. (1997). Dimensions of mentalisation: Outlining levels of psychic transformation. *International Journal of Psychoanalysis*, **78**: 855–75.

Lees, J., Manning, N., and Rawlings, B. (1999). *Therapeutic Community Effectiveness. A Systematic International Review of Therapeutic Community Treatment for People with Personality Disorders and Mentally Disordered Offenders*, University of York (CRD Report 17), NHS Centre for Reviews and Dissemination.

Legerstee, M. and Varghese, J. (2001). The role of maternal affect mirroring on social expectancies in 2-3 month-old infants. *Child Development*, **72**: 1301–13.

Leichsenring, F. and Leibing, E. (2003). The effectiveness of psychodynamic therapy and cognitive behavior therapy in the treatment of personality disorders: a meta-analysis. *The American Journal of Psychiatry*, **160**: 1223–32.

Lemieux, A. and Coe, C. L. (1995). Abuse-related posttraumatic stress disorder: Evidence for chronic neuroendocrine activation in women. *Psychosomatic Medicine*, **57**: 105–15.

Lenzenweger, M. F., Clarkin, J. F., Kernberg, O. F., and Foelsch, P. A. (2001). The Inventory of Personality Organization: psychometric properties, factorial composition, and criterion relations with affect, aggressive dyscontrol, psychosis proneness, and self-domains in a nonclinical sample. *Psychological Assessment*, **13**: 577–91.

Lesch, K. P., Bengel, D., Heils, A., Sabol, S. Z., Greenberg, B. D., and Petri, S. (1996). Association of anxiety-related traits with a polymorphism in the serotonin transporter gene regulatory region. *Science*, **274**: 1527–31.

Leslie, A. M. (1994). TOMM, ToBy, and agency: core architecture and domain specificity. In: *Mapping the Mind: Domain Specificity in Cognition and Culture* (ed. L. Hirschfeld and S. Gelman), pp. 119–48. New York: Cambridge University Press.

Leslie, A. M. (2000). "Theory of Mind" as a mechanism of selective attention. In: *The New Cognitive Neurosciences* (ed. M. S. Gazzaniga), pp. 1235–47. Cambridge, Massachusetts: The MIT Press.

Lewis, C., Freeman, N. H., Kyriakidou, C., Maridaki-Kassotaki, K., and Berridge, D. (1996). Social influences on false belief access: Specific sibling influences or general apprenticeship? *Child Development*, **67**: 2930–47.

Lewis, G. and Appleby, L. (1988). Personality Disorder: the patients psychiatrists dislike. *British Journal of Psychiatry*, **153**: 44–9.

Lewis, J. (2000). Repairing the bond in important relationships: a dynamic for personality maturation. *The American Journal of Psychiatry*, **157**: 1375–8.

Lewis, M. and Brooks-Gunn, J. (1979). *Social Cognition and the Acquisition of Self.* New York: Plenum Press.

Lewis, M., Allessandri, S. M., and Sullivan, M. W. (1990). Violation of expectancy, loss of control and anger expressions in young infants. *Developmental Psychology*, **26**: 745–51.

Leyton, M., Okazawa, H., Diksic, M. *et al.* (2001). Brain Regional alpha–[11C]methyl-L-tryptophan trapping in impulsive subjects with borderline personality disorder. *The American Journal of Psychiatry*, **158**: 775–82.

Linehan, M. M. (1986). Suicidal people: one population or two? *Annals of the New York Academy of Sciences*, **487**: 16–33.

Linehan, M. M. (1987). Dialectical behavioural therapy: A cognitive behavioural approach to parasuicide. *Journal of Personality Disorders*, **1**: 328–33.

Linehan, M. M., Armstrong, H. E., Suarez, A., Allmon, D., and Heard, H. (1991). Cognitive-behavioural treatment of chronically parasuicidal borderline patients. *Archives of General Psychiatry*, **48**: 1060–4.

Linehan, M. M. (1993*a*). *Cognitive-Behavioural Treatment of Borderline Personality Disorder.* New York: Guilford Press.

Linehan, M. M. (1993*b*). *The Skills Training Manual for Treating Borderline Personality Disorder.* New York: Guilford Press.

Linehan, M. M., Heard, H. L., and Armstrong, H. E. (1993). Naturalistic follow-up of a behavioral treatment for chronically parasuicidal borderline patients. *Archives of General Psychiatry*, **50**: 971–4.

Links, P. S. Steiner, M., and Huxley, G. (1988). The occurrence of borderline personality disorder in the families of borderline patients. *Journal of Personality Disorders*, **2**: 14–20.

Links, P. S., Mitton, J. E., and Steiner, M. (1993). Stability of borderline personality disorder. *Canadian Journal of Psychiatry*, **38**: 255–9.

Links, P. S., Heslegrave, R., and van Reekum, R. (1998). Prospective follow-up study of borderline personality disorder: prognosis, prediction of outcome, and Axis II comorbidity. *Canadian Journal of Psychiatry*, **43**: 265–70.

Links, P. S., Heslegrave, R., and van Reekum, R. (1999). Impulsivity: Core aspect of borderline personality disorder. *Journal of Personality Disorders*, **13**: 1–9.

Linnoila, V. M. and Virkkunen, M. (1992). Aggression, suicidality, and serotonin. *The Journal of Clinical Psychiatry*, **53 Suppl**: 46–51.

Lipschitz, D. S. Winegar, R. K. Hartnick, E. Foote, B., and Southwick, S. M. (1999). Posttraumatic stress disorder in hospitalized adolescents: psychiatric comorbidity and clinical correlates. *Journal of the American Academy of Child and Adolescent Psychiatry*, **38**: 385–92.

Livesley, W. J., Jackson, D. N., and Schroeder, M. L. (1992). Factorial structure of traits delineating personality disorders in clinical and general population samples. *Journal of Abnormal Psychology*, **101**: 432–40.

Livesley, W. J., Jang, K. L., and Vernon, P. A. (1998). Phenotypic and genetic structure of traits delineating personality disorder. *Archives of General Psychiatry*, **55**: 941–8.

Livesley, W. J. (2001). Conceptual and Taxonomic Issues. In: *Handbook of Personality Disorders Theory, Research, and Treatment* (ed. W. Livesley). New York: Guilford.

Loftus, E. F. (1993). The reality of repressed memories. *American Psychologist*, **48**: 518–37.

Logue, A. (1995). *Self-Control: Waiting Until Tomorrow for What You Want Today.* Englewood Cliffs, NJ: Prentice-Hall.

Loranger, A. W., Sartorius, N., Andreoli, A., Berger, P., Buckheim, P., and Channabasavanna, S. M. (1994). The International Personality Disorder Examination: The World Health Organization/Alcohol, Drug Abuse and Mental Health Administration International Pilot Study of Personality Disorders. *Archives of General Psychiatry*, **51**: 215–24.

Loranger, A. W. (1999). *International Personality Disorder Examination (IPDE): DSM-IV and ICD-10 Modules.* Odessa, FL: Psychological Assessment Resources.

Luntz, B. K. and Widom, C. S. (1994). Antisocial personality disorder in abused and neglected children grown up. *The American Journal of Psychiatry*, **151**: 670–4.

Luquet, P. (1988). Langage, pensee et structure psychique. *Revue Francais de Psychoanalyse*, **52**: 267–302.

Luria, A. R. (1966). *Higher Cortical Functions in Man*. New York: Plenum Press.

Lyons-Ruth, K. (1991). Rapprochement or approchement: Mahler's theory reconsidered from the vantage point of recent research in early attachment relationships. *Psychoanalytic Psychology*, **8**: 1–23.

Lyons-Ruth, K. (1996). Attachment relationships among children with aggressive behavior problems: The role of disorganized early attachment patterns. *Journal of Consulting and Clinical Psychology*, **64**: 64–73.

Lyons-Ruth, K. and Jacobovitz, D. (1999). Attachment disorganization: Unresolved loss, relational violence and lapses in behavioral and attentional strategies. In: *Handbook of Attachment Theory and Research* (ed. J. Cassidy and P. R. Shaver), pp. 520–54. New York: Guilford.

Lyons-Ruth, K., Bronfman, E., and Atwood, G. (1999*a*). A relational diathesis model of hostile–helpless states of mind: Expressions in mother-infant interaction. In: *Attachment Disorganization* (ed. J. Solomon and C. George), pp. 33–70. New York: Guilford Press.

Lyons-Ruth, K., Bronfman, E., and Parsons, E. (1999*b*). Atypical attachment in infancy and early childhood among children at developmental risk. IV. Maternal frightened, frightening, or atypical behavior and disorganized infant attachment patterns. In: *Typical Patterns of Infant Attachment: Theory, Research and Current Directions* (ed. J. Vondra and D. Barnett), pp. 67–96. Monographs of the Society for Research in Child Development.

Mahler, M. S. (1971). A study of separation-individuation process and its possible application to borderline phenomena in the psychoanalytic situation. *The Psychoanalytic Study of the Child*, **26**: 403–24.

Main, M., Kaplan, N., and Cassidy, J. (1985). Security in infancy, childhood, and adulthood: A move to the level of representation. *Monographs of the Society for Research in Child Development*, **50**: 66–104.

Main, M. and Solomon, J. (1986). Discovery of an insecure-disorganized/disoriented attachment pattern. In: *Affective Development in Infancy* (ed. T. B. Brazelton and M. W. Yogman), pp. 95–124. Norwood, NJ: Ablex.

Main, M. and Hesse, E. (1990). Parents' unresolved traumatic experiences are related to infant disorganized attachment status: Is frightened and/or frightening parental behavior the linking mechanism? In: *Attachment in the Preschool Years: Theory, Research and Intervention* (ed. M. Greenberg, D. Cicchetti, and E. M. Cummings), pp. 161–82. Chicago: University of Chicago Press.

Main, M. (1991). Metacognitive knowledge, metacognitive monitoring, and singular (coherent) vs. multiple (incoherent) model of attachment: Findings and directions for future research. In: *Attachment Across the Life Cycle* (ed. C. M. Parkes, J. Stevenson-Hinde, and P. Marris), pp. 127–59. London: Tavistock/Routledge.

Main, M. and Hesse, E. (1992). Disorganized/disoriented infant behaviour in the Strange Situation, lapses in the monitoring of reasoning and discourse during the parent's Adult Attachment Interview, and dissociative states. In: *Attachment and Psychoanalysis* (ed. M. Ammaniti and D. Stern), pp. 86–140. Rome: Gius, Latereza and Figli.

Main, M. and Hesse, E. (2001). Attachment narratives and attachment across the lifespan. *Journal of the American Psychoanalytic Association*, **48**.

Main, T. (1989). *The Ailment and Other Psychoanalytic Essays*. London: Free Association Press.

Malatesta, C. Z. and Izard, C. E. (1984). The ontogenesis of human social signals: From biological imperative to symbol utilization. In: *The Psychobiology of Affective Development* (ed. N. A. Fox and R. J. Davison), pp. 161–206. Hillsdale, NJ: Erlbaum.

Malatesta, C. Z., Culver, C., Tesman, J. R., and Shepard, B. (1989). The development of emotion expression during the first two years of life. *Monographs of the Society for Research in Child Development*, **54**: 1–104.

Margison, F. (2000). Editorial cognitive analytic therapy: A case study in treatment development. *British Journal of Medical Psychology*, **73**: 145–9.

Markovitz, P. J., Calabrese, J. R., Schulz, S. C., and Meltzer, H. Y. (1991). Fluoxetine in the treatment of borderline and schizotypal personality disorders. *The American Journal of Psychiatry*, **148**: 1064–7.

Markovitz, P. J. and Wagner, C. (1995). Venlafaxine in the treatment of borderline personality disorder. *Psychopharmacology Bulletin*, **31**: 773–7.

Marty, P. (1991). *Mentalisation et Psychosomatique*. Paris: Laboratoire Delagrange.

Marvin, R. S. and Britner, P. A. (1999). Normative development: The ontogeny of attachment. In: *Handbook of Attachment: Theory, Research and Clinical Applications* (ed. J. Cassidy and P. R. Shaver), pp. 44–67. New York: Guilford.

Marziali, E., Newman, T., Munroe-Blum, H., and Dawson, D. (1989). Manual and training materials for relationship management psychotherapy. *Unpublished Manuscript*.

Masterson, J. F. and Rinsley, D. (1975). The borderline syndrome: the role of the mother in the genesis and psychic structure of the borderline personality. *International Journal of Psychoanalysis*, **56**: 163–77.

Mauro, C. F. and Harris, Y. R. (2000). The influence of maternal child-rearing attitudes and teaching behaviors on preschoolers' delay of gratification. *The Journal of Genetic Psychology* , **161**: 292–306.

Mayes, A. R. (2000*a*). The neuropsychology of memory. In: *Memory Disorders in Psychiatric Practice* (ed. G. E. Berrios and J. R. Hodges), pp. 58–74. New York, NY, US: Cambridge University Press.

Mayes, L. C. (2000*b*). A developmental perspective on the regulation of arousal states. *Seminars in Perinatology*, **24**: 267–79.

Mayes, L. C. (2002). A behavioral teratogenic model of the impact of prenatal cocaine exposure on arousal regulatory systems. *Neurotoxicology and Teratology*, **24**: 385–95.

McDavid, J. D. and Pilkonis, P. A. (1996). The stability of personality disorder diagnosis. *Journal of Personality Disorders*, **10**: 1–15.

McEwen, B. (1999). Development of the cerebral cortex: XIII. Stress and brain development: II. *Journal of the American Academy of Child and Adolescent Psychiatry*, **38**: 101–3.

McGlashan, T. H. (1983). The borderline syndrome. I. Testing three diagnostic systems. *Archives of General Psychiatry*, **40**: 1311–8.

McGlashan, T. (1986). The Chestnut Lodge follow-up Study III: Long-term outcome of borderline personalities. *Archives of General Psychiatry*, **43**: 20–30.

McGlashan, T. (1987). Borderline personality disorder and unipolar affective disorder: Longterm effects of co-morbidity. *Journal of Nervous and Mental Disease*, **175**: 467–73.

McGlashan, T. H. (1992). The longitudinal profile of BPD: Contributions from The Chestnut Lodge Follow-Up Study. In: *Handbook of the Borderline Diagnosis* (ed. D. Silver and M. Rosenbluth). Madison, CT: International Universities Press.

McGlashan, T. H. (2002). The borderline personality disorder practice guidelines: the good, the bad, and the realistic. *Journal of Personality Disorders*, **16**: 119–21.

McLeer, S. V., Callaghan, M., Henry, D., and Wallen, J. (1994). Psychiatric disorders in sexually abused children. *Journal of the American Academy of Child and Adolescent Psychiatry*, **33**: 313–9.

McLeer, S. V., Dixon, J. F., Henry, D. *et al.* (1998). Psychopathology in non–clinically referred sexually abused children. *Journal of the American Academy of Child and Adolescent Psychiatry*, **37**: 1326–33.

Meares, R., Stevenson, J., and Comerford, A. (1999). Psychotherapy with borderline patients: A comparison between treated and untreated cohorts. *Australian and New Zealand Journal of Psychiatry*, **33**: 467–72.

Meijer, M., Goedhart, A. W., and Treffers, P. D. A. (1998). The persistence of bordeline personality disorder in adolescence. *Journal of Personality Disorders*, **12**: 13–22.

Meins, E. (1997). *Security of Attachment and the Social Development of Cognition*. London: Psychology Press.

Meins, E., Fernyhough, C., Russel, J., and Clark-Carter, D. (1998). Security of attachment as a predictor of symbolic and mentalising abilities: a longitudinal study. *Social Development*, **7**: 1–24.

Meins, E. and Fernyhough, C. (1999). Linguistic acquisitional style and mentalising development: The role of maternal mind-mindedness. *Cognitive Development*, **14**: 363–80.

Meins, E., Fernyhough, C., Fradley, E., and Tuckey, M. (2001). Rethinking maternal sensitivity: Mothers' comments on infants mental processes predict security of attachment at 12 months. *Journal of Child Psychology and Psychiatry*, **42**: 637–48.

Meloy, R. J. (1992). *Violent Attachments*. New Jersey: Jason Aronson.

Meloy, R. J. (2001). *The Mark of Cain: Psychoanalytic Insight and the Psychopath*. New York: Analytic Press.

Meltzoff, A. N. and Moore, M. K. (1977). Imitation of facial and manual gestures by human neonates. *Science*, **198**: 75–8.

Meltzoff, A. N. and Moore, M. K. (1989). Imitation in newborn infants: Exploring the range of gestures imitated and the underlying mechanisms. *Developmental Psychology*, **25**: 954–62.

Meltzoff, A. N. (1990). Foundations for developing a concept of self: The role of imitation in relating self to other and the value of social mirroring, social modeling and self practice in infancy. In: *The Self in Transition: Infancy to Childhood* (ed. D. Cicchetti and M. Beeghly). Chicago: University of Chicago Press.

Metcalfe, J. and Mischel, W. (1999). A hot/cool-system analysis of delay of gratification: dynamics of willpower. *Psychological Review*, **106**: 3–19.

Meyer, B., Pilkonis, P. A., Proietti, J. M., Heape, C. L., and Egan, M. (2001). Attachment styles and personality disorders as predictors of symptom course. *Journal of Personality Disorders*, **15**: 371–89.

Meyer, D. J. and Simon, R.I. (1999*a*). Split treatment: clarity between psychiatrists and psychotherapists. Part 1. *Psychiatric Annals*, **29**: 241–5.

Meyer, D. J. and Simon, R.I. (1999*b*). Split treatment: clarity between psychiatrists and psychotherapists. Part 2. *Psychiatric Annals*, **29**: 327–32.

Miller, A. L., McDonough, S. C., Rosenblum, K. L., and Sameroff, A. J. (2002). Emotion regulation in context: Situational effects on infant and caregiver behavior. *Infancy*, **3**: 403–33.

Milligan, K., Atkinson, L., Trhub, S. E., Benoit, D., and Poulton, L. (2003). Maternal attachment and the comunication of emotion through song. *Infant Behavior and Development*, **26**: 1–13.

Mitchell, R. W. (1993). Mental models of mirror self-recognition: Two theories. *New Ideas in Psychology*, **11**: 295–325.

Modell, A. (1963). Primitive object relationships and the predisposition to schizophrenia. *International Journal of Psychoanalysis*, **44**: 282–92.

Modestin, J. and Villiger, C. (1989). Follow-up study on borderline versus nonborderline personality disorders. *Comprehensive Psychiatry*, **30**: 236–44.

Moffitt, T. E., Caspi, A., Harrington, H., and Milne, B. J. (2002). Males on the life-course-persistent and adolescence-limited antisocial pathways: Follow-up at age 26 years. *Development and Psychopathology*, **14**: 179–207.

Mollon, P. (2002). *Remembering Trauma: A Psychotherapist's Guide to Memory and Illusion*. London: Whurr Publications.

Monroe-Blum, H. and Marziali, E. (1995). A controlled trial of short-term group treatment for borderline personality disorder. *Journal of Personality Disorders*, **9**: 190–8.

Monsen, J., Odland, T., Faugli, A., Daae, E., and Eilersten, D. E. (1995). Personality disorders: Changes and stability after intensive psychotherapy focussing on affect consciousness. *Psychotherapy Research*, **5**: 33–48.

Moore, C., Furrow, D., Chiasson, L., and Patriquin, M. (1994). Developmental relationships between production and comprehension of mental terms. *First Language*, **14**: 1–17.

Morgan, A. B. and Lilienfeld, S. O. (2000). A meta-analytic review of the relation between antisocial behavior and neuropsychological measures of executive function. *Clinical Psychology Review*, **20**: 113–36.

Morris, H., Gunderson, J. G., and Zanarini, M. C. (1986). Transitional object use and borderline psychopathology. *The American Journal of Psychiatry*, **143**: 1534–8.

Morton, J. and Johnson, M. H. (1991). CONSPEC and CONLEARN: a two-process theory of infant face recognition. *Psychological Review*, **98**: 164–81.

Mosheim, R., Zachhuber, U., Scharf, L. *et al.* (2000). Bindung und Psychotherapie: Bindungsqualitaet und interpersonale Probleme von Patienten als moegliche Einflussfaktoren auf das Ergebnis stationaerer Psychotherapie [Quality of attachment and interpersonal problems as possible predictors of inpatient therapy outcome]. *Psychotherapeut*, **45**: 223–9.

Mullen, P. E., Martin, J. L., Anderson, J. C., Romans, S. E., and Herbison, G. P. (1996). The long-term impact of the physical, emotional, and sexual abuse of children: a community study. *Child Abuse and Neglect*, **20**: 7–21.

Mundy, P. and Neal, R. (2001). Neural plasticity, joint attention, and a transactional social-orienting model of autism. In: *International Review of Mental Retardation: Autism (Vol 23)* (ed. L. Masters Glidden), pp. 139–68. San Diego, CA: Academic Press.

Munir, K. M. and Beardslee, W. R. (1999). Developmental psychiatry: is there any other kind? *Harvard Review of Psychiatry*, **6**: 250–62.

Muzik, M. and Rosenblum, K. (2003). Maternal reflective capacity: associations with sensitivity and mental state comments during interaction. In: *Biannual Meeting of the Society for Research in Child Development.* Tampa, Fl.

Neisser, U. (1988). Five kinds of self-knowledge. *Philosophical Psychology*, **1**: 35–59.

New, A. S., Gelenter, J., Yovel, Y., Trestman, R. L., Nielsen, D. A., and Silverman, J. (1998). Tryptophan hydroxylase genotype is associated with impulsive-aggression measures: a preliminary study. *American Journal of Medical Genetics*, **81**: 13–7.

New, A. S., Gelernter, J., Goodman, M., Mitropoulou, V., Koenigsberg, H. W., and Silverman, J. M. (2001). Suicide, impulsive aggression, and HTR1B genotype. *Biological Psychiatry*, **50**: 62–5.

New, A. S., Hazlett, E. A., Buchsbaum, M. S. *et al.* (2002). Blunted prefrontal cortical 18fluorodeoxyglucose positron emission tomography response to meta-chlorophenylpiperazine in impulsive aggression. *Archives of General Psychiatry*, **59**: 621–9.

NICHD Early Child Care Research Network (1996). Characteristics of infant child care: Factors contributing to positive caregiving. *Early Childhood Research Quarterly*, **11**: 269–306.

Nickell, A. D., Waudby, C. J., and Trull, T. J. (2002). Attachment, parental bonding and borderline personality disorder features in young adults. *Journal of Personality Disorders*, **16**: 148–59.

Nielsen, T. A. and Powell, R. A. (1992). The day-residue and dream-lag effects: A literature review and limited replication of two temporal effects in dream formation. *Dreaming: Journal of the Association for the Study of Dreams*, **2**: 67–77.

Nigg, J. T. and Goldsmith, H. H. (1994). Genetics of personality disorders: perspectives from personality and psychopathology research. *Psychology Bulletin*, **115**: 346–80.

Normandin, L., Ensink, K., and Kernberg, P. (2002). The role of trauma in the development of borderline personality disturbance in children. In: *Transference Focused Psychotherapy for Borderline Personality Disorder Symposium.* New York.

Norton, K. (1992). A culture of enquiry—its preservation or loss. *Therapeutic Communities*, **13 (1)**: 3–25.

Ogata, S. N., Silk, K. R., Goodrich, S., Lohr, N. E., Westen, D., and Hill, E. (1990). Childhood sexual and physical abuse in adult patients with borderline personality disorder. *The American Journal of Psychiatry*, **147**: 1008–13.

O'Keane, V., Moloney, E., O'Neill, H., O'Connor, A., Smith, C., and Dinan, T. (1992). Blunted prolactin responses to d-fenfluramine in sociopathy. Evidence for subsensitivity of central serotonergic function. *British Journal of Psychiatry*, **160**: 643–6.

Oldham, J., Phillips, K., Gabbard, G., and Soloff, P. (2001). Practice guideline for the treatment of patients with borderline personality disorder. *American Psychiatric Association Practice Guidelines.*

Olio, K. A. (1989). Memory retrieval in the treatment of adult survivors of sexual abuse. *Transactional Analysis Journal*, **19**: 93–100.

Olson, S. L., Bates, J. E., and Bayles, K. (1990). Early antecedents of childhood impulsivity: the role of parent-child interaction, cognitive competence, and temperament. *Journal of Abnormal Child Psychology*, **18**: 317–34.

Panksepp, J., Nelson, E., and Bekkedal, M. (1999). Brain systems for the mediation of social separation-distress and social–reward: Evolutionary antecedents and neuropeptide intermediaries. In: *The Integrative Neurobiology of Affiliation* (ed. C. S. Carter, II Lederhendler and B. Kirkpatrick), pp. 221–43. Cambridge, MA: MIT Press.

Papousek, H. and Papousek, M. (1974). Mirror-image and self recognition in young human infants: A new method of experimental analysis. *Developmental Psychobiology*, **7**: 149–57.

Papousek, H. and Papousek, M. (1987). Intuitive parenting: a dialectic counterpart to the infant's integrative competence. In: *Handbook of Infant Development* (ed. J. D. Osofsky), pp. 669–720. New York: Wiley.

Paris, J., Brown, R., and Nowlis, D. (1987). Longterm follow-up of borderline patients in a general hospital. *Comprehensive Psychiatry*, **28**: 530–5.

Paris, J. and Frank, H. (1989). Perceptions of parental bonding in borderline patients. *The American Journal of Psychiatry*, **146**: 1498–9.

Paris, J., Zweig-Frank, H., and Guzder, H. (1993). The role of psychological risk factors in recovery from borderline personality disorder. *Comprehensive Psychiatry*, **34**: 410–3.

Paris, J., Zweig-Frank, H., and Guzder, J. (1994*a*). Psychological risk factors for borderline personality disorder in female patients. *Comprehensive Psychiatry*, **35**: 301–5.

Paris, J., Zweig-Frank, H., and Guzder, J. (1994*b*). Risk factors for borderline personality disorder in male outpatients. *Journal of Nervous and Mental Disease*, **182**: 375–413.

Paris, J. (1998*a*). Follow-up studies of BPD: A critical review. *Journal of Personality Disorders*, **2**: 189–97.

Paris, J. (1998*b*). Personality disorders in sociocultural perspective. *Journal of Personality Disorders*, **12**: 289–301.

Paris, J. (2000). Childhood precursors of borderline personality disorder. *The Psychiatric Clinic of North America*, **23**: 77–88.

Paris, J. and Zweig-Frank, H. (2001). A 27-year follow-up of patients with borderline personality disorder. *Comprehensive Psychiatry*, **42**: 482–7.

Paris, J. (2002). Commentary on the American Psychiatric Association guidelines for treatment of borderline personality disorder: evidence-based psychiatry and the quality of evidence. *Journal of Personality Disorders*, **16**: 130–4.

Parker, G., Barrett, E., and Hickie, I. B. (1992). From nurture to network: Examining links between perceptions of parenting received in childhood and social bonds in adulthood. *The American Journal of Psychiatry*, **149**: 877–85.

Patrick, M., Hobson, R. P., Castle, D., Howard, R., and Maughan, B. (1994). Personality disorder and the mental representation of early social experience. *Developmental Psychopathology*, **6**: 375–88.

Perez, C. and Widom, C. S. (1994). Childhood victimization and long-term intellectual and academic outcomes. *Child Abuse and Neglect*, **18**: 617–33.

Perner, J. (1991). *Understanding the Representational Mind.* Cambridge, Mass: MIT Press.

Perner, J., Ruffman, T., and Leekman, S. R. (1994). Theory of mind is contagious: You catch it from your sibs. *Child Development*, **65**: 1228–38.

Perner, J. and Lang, B. (2000). Theory of mind and executive function: Is there a developmental relationship? In: *Understanding Other Minds: Perspectives from Developmental Cognitive Neuroscience* (ed. S. Baron-Cohen, H. Tager–Flusberg, and D. J. Cohen), pp. 150–81. New York: Oxford University Press.

Perry, J. C. and Cooper, S. H. (1986). A preliminary report on defenses and conflicts associated with borderline personality disorder. *Journal of the American Psychoanalytic Association*, **34**: 863–93.

Perry, J. C., Banon, E., and Ianni, F. (1999). Effectiveness of psychotherapy for personality disorder. *The American Journal of Psychiatry*, **156**: 1312–21.

Peterson, C. C. and Siegal, M. (2000). Insights into theory of mind from deafness and autism. *Mind & Language*, **15**: 123–45.

Pfohl, B., Blum, N., and Zimmerman, M. (1997). *Structured Interview for DSM-IV Personality.* Washington, DC: American Psychiatric Press.

Piaget, J. (1936). *The Origins of Intelligence in Children.* New York: International Universities Press, 1952.

Pilkonis, P. (1988). Personality prototypes among depressives. *Journal of Personality Disorders,* **2**: 144–52.

Pilkonis, P. A., Blehar, M. C., and Prien, R. F. (1997). Introduction to the special feature: Research directions for the personality disorders. *Journal of Personality Disorders,* **11**: 201–4.

Pines, M. (1982). Reflections on mirroring. *Group Analysis*, **15 (supplement)**.

Piper, W. E., Rosie, J. S., Azim, H. F. A., and Joyce, A. S. (1993). A randomised trial of psychiatric day treatment for patients with affective and personality disorders. *Hospital and Community Psychiatry*, **44**: 757–63.

Plomin, R., DeFries, J. C., McLearn, G. E., and Rutter, R. (1997). *Behavioral Genetics.* New York: W.H. Freeman.

Pollak, S. D., Cicchetti, D., Hornung, K., and Reed, A. (2000). Recognizing emotion in faces: developmental effects of child abuse and neglect. *Developmental Psychology*, **36**: 679–88.

Posner, M. I. and Petersen, S. E. (1990). The attention system of the human brain. *Annual Review of Neuroscience*, **13**: 25–42.

Posner, M. I. and Rothbart, M. K. (1998). Attention, self regulation and consciousness. *Philosophical Transactions of the Royal Society of London, B.* **353**: 1915–27.

Posner, M. I. and Rothbart, M. K. (2000). Developing mechanisms of self-regulation. *Development and Psychopathology*, **12**: 427–41.

Povinelli, D. J. and Eddy, T. J. (1995). The unduplicated self. In: *The Self in Infancy: Theory and Research* (ed. P. Rochat), pp. 161–92. Elsevier: Amsterdam.

Pugh, G. (2002). Freud's "problem". *The International Journal of Psychoanalysis*, **83**: 1375–94.

Putnam, F. W., Trickett, P. K., Helmers, K., Dorn, L., and Everett, B. (1991). Cortisol abnormalities in sexually abused girls. Poster presented at the *144th Annual Meeting of the American Psychiatric Association*, Washington.

Putnam, F. W. (1997). *Dissociation in Children and Adolescents: A Developmental Perspective.* New York: Guilford Press.

Pynoos, R. S. and Nader, K. (1989). Children's memory and proximity to violence. *Journal of the American Academy of Child and Adolescent Psychiatry*, **28**: 236–341.

Pynoos, R., Steinberg, A., and Wraith, R. (1995). A developmental model of childhood traumatic stress. In: *Developmental Psychopathology (vol. 2)* (ed. D. Cicchetti and D. J. Cohen), pp. 72–95. New York: Wiley.

Racker, H. (1968). *Transference and Countertransference.* London: Hogarth Press.

Raine, A., Phil, D., Stoddard, J., Bihrle, S., and Buchsbaum, M. (1998). Prefrontal glucose deficits in murderers lacking psychosocial deprivation. *Neuropsychiatry, Neuropsychology and Behavioural Neurology*, **11**: 1–7.

Raine, A., Lencz, T., Bihrle, S., LaCasse, L., and Colletti, P. (2000). Reduced prefrontal gray matter volume and reduced autonomic activity in antisocial personality disorder. *Archives of General Psychiatry*, **57**: 119–27.

Rapaport, J. L. (ed.) (1999). *Child Onset of Adult Psychopathology.* Washington, DC: American Psychiatric Press.

Rauch, S. L., van der Kolk, B. A., Fisler, R. E. *et al.* (1996). A symptom provocation study of posttraumatic stress disorder using positron emission tomography and script-driven imagery. *Archives of General Psychiatry*, **53**: 380–7.

Reich, J., Yates, W., and Nduaguba, M. (1989). Prevalence of DSM-III personality disorders in the community. *Social Psychiatry and Psychiatric Epidemiology*, **24**: 12–6.

Reiss, D., Plomin, R., and Hetherington, E. M. (1991). Genetics and psychiatry: an unheralded window on the environment. *The American Journal of Psychiatry*, **148**: 283–91.

Repacholi, B. M. and Gopnik, A. (1997). Early reasoning about desires: Evidence from 14- and 18-month-olds. *Developmental Psychology*, **33**: 12–21.

Repo-Tiihonen, E., Halonen, P., Tiihonen, J., and Virkkunen, M. (2002). Total serum cholesterol level, violent criminal offences, suicidal behavior, mortality and the appearance of conduct disorder in Finnish male criminal offenders with antisocial personality disorder. *European Archives of Psychiatry and Clinical Neuroscience*, **252**: 8–11.

Rey, J. H. (1979). Schizoid phenomena in the borderline. In: *Advances in the Psychotherapy of the Borderline Patient* (ed. A. Capponi), pp. 449–84. New York: Jason Aronson.

Rey, J. M., Morris-Yates, A., Singh, M., Andrews, G., and Stewart, G. W. (1995). Continuities between psychiatric disorders in adolescents and personality disorders in young adults. *The American Journal of Psychiatry*, **152**: 895–900.

Rhee, S. H. and Waldman, I. D. (2002). Genetic and environmental influences on antisocial behavior: A metaanalysis of twin and adoption studies. *Psychological Bulletin*, **128**: 490–529.

Riccio, D. C., Rabinowitz, V. C., and Axelrod, S. (1994). Memory: When less is more. *American Psychologist*, **49**: 917–26.

Rinne, T., Westenberg, H. G., den Boer, J. A., and van den Brink, W. (2000). Serotonergic blunting to meta-chlorophenylpiperazine (m-CPP) highly correlates with sustained childhood abuse in impulsive and autoaggressive female borderline patients. *Biological Psychiatry*, **47**: 548–56.

Robinson, L. A., Berman, J. S., and Neimeyer, R. A. (1990). Psychotherapy for the treatment of depression: A comprehensive review of controlled outcome research. *Psychological Bulletin*, **108**: 30–49.

Rochat, P. and Morgan, R. (1995). Spatial determinants in the perception of self-produced leg movements in 3- to 5-month-old infants. *Developmental Psychology*, **31**: 626–36.

Roediger, H. L., Wheeler, M. A., and Rajaram, S. (1993). Remembering, knowing, and reconstructing the past. In: *The Psychology of Learning and Motivation: Advances in Theory and Research* (ed. D. L. Medin), pp. 97–134. New York: Academic Press.

Rogers, R. D., Owen, A. M., Middleton, H. C. *et al.* (1999). Choosing between small, likely rewards and large, unlikely rewards activates inferior and orbital prefrontal cortex. *The Journal of Neuroscience*, **19**: 9029–38.

Rogosch, F. A., Cicchetti, D., and Aber, J. L. (1995). The role of child maltreatment in early deviations in cognitive and affective processing abilities and later peer relationship problems. *Development and Psychopathology*, **7**: 591–609.

Rolls, E. T. (1999). *The Brain and Emotion.* New York: Oxford University Press.

Rosenberg, P. H. and Miller, G. A. (1989). Comparing borderline definitions: DSM-III borderline and schizotypal personality disorders. *Journal of Abnormal Psychology*, **98**: 161–9.

Rosenkrantz, J. and Morrison, T. L. (1992). Psychotherapist personality characteristics and the perception of the self and patients in the treatment of borderline personality disorder. *Journal of Clinical Psychology*, **48**: 544–53.

Rosenstein, D. S. and Horowitz, H. A. (1996). Adolescent attachment and psychopathology. *Journal of Consulting and Clinical Psychology.*, **64**: 244–53.

Rosser, R., Birch, S., Bond, H., Denford, J., and Schachter, J. (1987). Five year follow-up of patients treated with in-patient psychotherapy at the Cassel Hospital for Nervous Diseases. *Journal of the Royal Society of Medicine*, **80**: 549–55.

Roth, A. and Fonagy, P. (1996). *What Works for Whom? A Critical Review of Psychotherapy Research.* New York: Guilford Press.

Roth, A., Ostroff, R., and Hoffman, M. (1996). Naltrexone as a treatment for repetitive self-injurious behaviour: an open label trial. *Journal of Clinical Psychiatry*, **57**: 233–7.

Rothbart, M. K., Ahadi, S. A., and Evans, D. E. (2000). Temperament and personality: Origins and outcomes. *Journal of Personality and Social Psychology*, **78**: 122–35.

Rowe, A. D., Bullock, P. R., Polkey, C. E., and Morris, R. G. (2001). "Theory of mind" impairments and their relationship to executive functioning following frontal lobe excisions. *Brain*, **124**: 600–16.

Rubino, G., Barker, C., Roth, T., and Fearon, P. (2000). Therapist empathy and depth of interpretation in response to potential alliance ruptures: the role of therapist and patient attachment styles. *Psychotherapy Research*, **10**: 408–20.

Ruffman, T., Perner, J., Naito, M., Parkin, L., and Clements, W. (1998). Older (but not younger) siblings facilitate false belief understanding. *Developmental Psychology*, **34**: 161–74.

Ruffman, T., Slade, L., and Crowe, E. (2002). The relation between children's and mothers' mental state language and theory-of-mind understanding. *Child Development*, **73**: 734–51.

Ruiter, C. and Greeven, P. (2000). Personality disorders in a Dutch forensic psychiatric sample: convergence of interview and self-report measures. *Journal of Personality Disorders*, **14**: 162–70.

Russell, D. E. H. (1986). *The Secret Trauma: Incest in the Lives of Girls and Women.* New York: Basic Books.

Rutter, M. (1987). Temperament, personality and personality disorder. *British Journal of Psychiatry*, **150**: 443–58.

Rutter, M. (2000). Psychosocial influences: Critiques, findings and research needs. *Development and Psychopathology*, **12**: 375–405.

Ryle, A. (1990). *Cognitive Analytic Therapy: Active Participation in Change.* Chichester: Wiley.

Ryle, A. (1997). *Cognitive Analytic Therapy and Borderline Personality Disorder: The Model and the Method.* Chichester, UK: John Wiley & Sons.

Ryle, A. and Golynkina, K. (2000). Effectiveness of time-limited cognitive analytic therapy of borderline personality disorder: factors associated with outcome. *British Journal of Medical Psychology*, **73**: 197–210.

Sabbagh, M. A. and Callanan, M. A. (1998). Metarepresentation in action: 3-, 4-, and 5-year-olds' developing theories of mind in parent-child conversations. *Developmental Psychology*, **34**: 491–502.

Sack, A., Sperling, M. B., Fagen, G., and Foelsch, P. (1996). Attachment style, history, and behavioral contrasts for a borderline and normal sample. *Journal of Personality Disorders*, **10**: 88–102.

Safran, J. D., Crocker, P., McMain, S., and Murray, P. (1990). The therapeutic alliance rupture as a therapy event for empirical investigation. *Psychotherapy*, **27**: 154–65.

Safran, J. D. and Segal, Z. V. (1990). *Interpersonal Process in Cognitive Therapy.* New York: Basic Books.

Salzman, J., Salzman, C., and Wolfson, A. N. (1997). Relationship of childhood abuse and maternal attachment to the development of borderline personality disorder. In: *Role of Sexual Abuse in the Etiology of Borderline Personality Disorder* (ed. M. C. Zanarini). Washington, DC: American Psychiatric Press.

Sander, L. W. (1970). Regulation and organization of behavior in the early infant-caretaker system. In: *Brain and Early Behavior* (ed. R. Robinson), London: Academic Press.

Sanderson, C., Swenson, C., and Bohus, M. (2002). A critique of the American Psychiatric practice guideline for the treatment of patients with borderline personality disorder. *Journal of Personality Disorders*, **16**: 122–9.

Sandler, J. and Rosenblatt, B. (1962). The concept of the representational world. *The Psychoanalytic Study of the Child*, **17**: 128–45.

Sandler, J. (1976). Countertransference and role-responsiveness. *International Review of Psychoanalysis*, **3**: 43–7.

Sandler, J. (1987*a*). *From Safety to the Superego: Selected Papers of Joseph Sandler.* New York: Guilford Press.

Sandler, J. (1987*b*). *Projection, Identification, Projective Identification.* London: Karnac Books.

Sandler, J. (1993). Communication from patient to analyst: Not everything is projective identification. *British Psycho-Analytical Society Bulletin*, **29**: 8–16.

Sanislow, C. A., Grilow, C. M., and McGlashan, T. H. (2000). Factor analysis of DSM-III-R borderline personality criteria in psychiatric inpatients. *The American Journal of Psychiatry*, **157**: 1629–33.

Sansone, R. A., Gaither, G. A., and Songer, D. A. (2002). The relationships among childhood abuse, borderline personality, and self-harm behavior in psychiatric inpatients. *Violence and Victims*, **17**: 49–55.

Sapolsky, R. M. (1997). Why is stress so bad for your brain. *Science*, **273**: 749–50.

Sargant, W. (1967). *The Unquiet Mind.* London: Heinemann.

Sayar, K., Ebrinc, S., and Ak, I. (2001). Alexithymia in patients with antisocial personality disorder in a military hospital setting. *The Israel Journal of Psychiatry and Related Sciences*, **38**: 81–7.

Schacter, D. L., Norman, K. A., and Koutstaal, W. (2000). The cognitive neuroscience of constructive memory. In: *False-Memory Creation in Children and Adults: Theory, Research and Implications* (ed. D. F. Bjorklund), pp. 129–68. Mahwah, NJ: Lawrence Erlbaum Associates.

Schafer, R. (1980). Narration in the psychoanalytic dialogue. *Critical Inquiry*, **7**: 29–53.

Schmuckler, M. A. (1996). Visual-proprioceptive intermodal perception in infancy. *Infant Behavior and Development*, **19**: 221–32.

Schneider-Rosen, K. and Cicchetti, D. (1991). Early self-knowledge and emotional development: Visual self-recognition and affective reactions to mirror self-image in maltreated and non-maltreated toddlers. *Developmental Psychology*, **27**: 481–8.

Schölmerich, A., Lamb, M. E., Leyendecker, B., and Fracasso, M. P. (1997). Mother-infant teaching interactions and attachment security in Euro-American and Central-American immigrant families. *Infant Behavior and Development*, **20**: 165–74.

Schore, A. N. (2001). Effects of a secure attachment relationship on right brain development, affect regulation, and infant mental health. *Infant Mental Health Journal*, **22**: 7–66.

Schore, A. N. (2003). *Affect Regulation and the Repair of the Self.* New York: Norton.

Schuengel, C., Bakermans-Kranenburg, M. J., van IJzendoorn, M. H., and Blom, M. (1999). Unresolved loss and infant disorganisation: Links to frightening maternal behavior. In: *Attachment Disorganization* (ed. J. Solomon and C. George), pp. 71–94. New York: Guilford.

Schuker, E. (1979). Psychodynamics and treatment of sexual assault victims. *Journal of the American Academy of Psychoanalysis*, **7**: 553–73.

Schultz, P. M., Soloff, P. H., Kelley, T., Morgenstern, M., Di Franco, R., and Schultz, S. C. (1989). A family history study of borderline subtypes. *Journal of Personality Disorders*, **3**: 217–29.

Schulz, S. C., Cornelius, J., Schultz, P. M., and Soloff, P. H. (1988). The amphetamine challenge test in patients with borderline disorder. *The American Journal of Psychiatry*, **145**: 809–14.

Schulz, S. C., Camlin, K., Berry, S., and Jesberger, J. (1999*a*). Olanzapine safety and efficacy in patients with borderline personality disorder and comorbid dysthymia. *Biological Psychiatry*, **46**: 1429–35.

Schulz, S. C., Camlin, K. L., Berry, S. A., and Jesberger, J. A. (1999*b*). A controlled study of Risperidone for borderline personality disorder. Paper presented at the *7th International Congress on Schizophrenia Research*, Santa Fe, New Mexico.

Segal, H. (1964). *Introduction to the Work of Melanie Klein.* New York: Basic Books.

Shachnow, J., Clarkin, J., DiPalma, C. S., Thurston, F., Hull, J., and Shearin, E. (1997). Biparental psychopathology and borderline personality disorder. *Psychiatry*, **60**: 171–81.

Shapiro, D. and Firth-Cozens, J. (1987). Prescriptive v. exploratory therapy: outcomes of the Sheffield psychotherapy project. *British Journal of Psychiatry*, **151**: 790–9.

Shapiro, D. A., Rees, A., Barkham, M., Hardy, G., Reynolds, S., and Startup, M. (1995). Effects of treatment duration and severity of depression on the maintenance of gains after cognitive-behavioral and psychodynamic-interpersonal psychotherapy. *Journal of Consulting and Clinical Psychology*, **63**: 378–87.

Shea, M. T., Pilkonis, P. A., Beckham, E. *et al.* (1990). Personality disorders and treatment outcome in the NIMH Treatment of Depression Collaborative Research Program. *The American Journal of Psychiatry*, **147**: 711–8.

Shearin, E. and Linehan, M. M. (1992). Patient-therapist ratings and relationship to progress in dialectical behaviour therapy for borderline personality disorder. *Behaviour Therapy*, **23**: 730–41.

Shedler, J. (2002). A new language for psychoanalytic diagnosis. *Journal of the American Psychoanalytic Association*, **50**: 429–56.

Shields, A. M., Cicchetti, D., and Ryan, R. M. (1994). The development of emotional and behavioural self-regulation and social competence among maltreated school-aged children. *Development and Psychopathology*, **6**: 57–75.

Shields, A. M. and Cicchetti, D. (1997). Emotion regulation among school-age children: The development and validation of a new criterion Q-sort scale. *Developmental Psychology*, **33**: 906–16.

Shin, L. M., McNally, R. J., Kosslyn, S. M. *et al.* (1999). Regional cerebral blood flow during script-driven imagery in childhood sexual abuse-related PTSD: A PET investigation. *The American Journal of Psychiatry*, **156**: 575–84.

Shin, L. M., Whalen, P. J., Pitman, R. K. *et al.* (2001). An fMRI study of anterior cingulate function in posttraumatic stress disorder. *Biological Psychiatry*, **50**: 932–42.

Shipman, K. L. and Zeman, J. (1999). Emotional understanding: a comparison of physically maltreating and nonmaltreating mother-child dyads. *Journal of Clinical Child Psychol*, **28**: 407–17.

Shipman, K., Zeman, J., Penza, S., and Champion, K. (2000). Emotion management skills in sexually maltreated and nonmaltreated girls: a developmental psychopathology perspective. *Development and Psychopathology*, **12**: 47–62.

Shipman, K. L. and Zeman, J. (2001). Socialization of children's emotion regulation in mother-child dyads: A developmental psychopathology. *Development and Psychopathology*, **13**: 317–36.

Siegal, M. and Varley, R. (2002). Neural systems involved in "theory of mind". *Natural Reviews Neuroscience*, **3**: 463–71.

Siegel, D. J. (1999). *The Developing Mind: Toward a Neurobiology of Interpersonal Experience.* New York: Guilford.

Siever, L. J. and Davis, K. L. (1991). A psychobiological perspective on the personality disorders. *The American Journal of Psychiatry*, **148**: 1647–58.

Siever, L. and Trestman, R. L. (1993). The serotonin system and aggressive personality disorder. *International Clinical Psychopharmacology*, **8 Suppl 2**: 33–9.

Siever, L. J., Buchsbaum, M. S., New, A. S. *et al.* (1999). d,l-fenfluramine response in impulsive personality disorder assessed with [18F]fluorodeoxyglucose positron emission tomography. *Neuropsychopharmacology*, **20**: 413–23.

Silk, K. R. (2000). Borderline personality disorder. Overview of biologic factors. *The Psychiatric Clinics of North America*, **23**: 61–75.

Silverman, A. B., Reinherz, H. Z., and Giaconia, R. M. (1996). The long-term sequelae of child and adolescent abuse: A longitudinal community study. *Child Abuse and Neglect*, **20**: 709–23.

Silverman, I. W. and Ragusa, D. M. (1990). Child and maternal correlates of impulse control in 24-month-old children. *Genetic, Social, and General Psychology Monographs*, **116**: 435–73.

Skodol, A. E., Buckley, P., and Charles, E. (1983). Is there a characteristic pattern to the treatment history of clinic patients with borderline personality? *Journal of Nervous and Mental Disorders*, **171**: 405–10.

Skodol, A. E., Stout, R. L., McGlashan, T. H., Grilo, C. M., Gunderson, J. G., and Shea, M. T. (1999). Co-occurrence of mood and personality disorders: A report from the Collaborative Longitudinal Personality Disorders Study (CLPS). *Depression and Anxiety*, **10**: 175–82.

Skodol, A. E., Gunderson, J. G., McGlashan, T. H. *et al.* (2002*a*). Functional impairment in patients with schizotypal, borderline, avoidant, or obsessive-compulsive personality disorder. *The American Journal of Psychiatry*, **159**: 276–83.

Skodol, A. E., Gunderson, J. G., Pfohl, B., Widiger, T. A., Livesley, W. J., and Siever, L. J. (2002*b*). The borderline diagnosis I: psychopathology, comorbidity and personality and personality structure. *Biological Psychiatry*, **51**: 936–50.

Skodol, A. E., Siever, L. J., Livesley, W. J., Gunderson, J. G., Pfohl, B., and Widiger, T. A. (2002*c*). The borderline diagnosis II: biology, genetics, and clinical course. *Biological Psychiatry*, **51**: 951–63.

Slade, A., Belsky, J., Aber, L., and Phelps, J. L. (1999). Mothers' representations of their relationships with their toddlers: Links to adult attachment and observed mothering. *Developmental Psychology*, **35**: 611–19.

Slade, A., Grienenberger, J., Bernbach, E., Levy, D., and Locker, A. (2001). Maternal reflective functioning: Considering the transmission gap. Paper presented at the *Biennial Meetings of the Society for Research in Child Development*. Minneapolis, MN.

Smith, T. E., Koenigsberg, H. W., Yeomans, F. E., Clarkin, J. F. *et al.* (1995). Predictors of dropout in psychodynamic psychotherapy of borderline personality disorder. *Journal of Psychotherapy Practice and Research*, **4**: 205–13.

Smythies, J. R. (1997). Oxidative reactions and schizophrenia: A review-discussion. *Schizophrenia Research*, **24**: 357–64.

Soldz, S., Budman, S., Demby, A. *et al.* (1993). Representation of personality disorders in circumplex and five-factor space: Explorations with a clinical sample. *Psychological Assessment*, **5**: 41–52.

Soloff, P. and Millward, J. (1983). Developmental histories of borderline patients. *Comprehensive Psychiatry*, **24**: 574–88.

Soloff, P. H., George, A., Nathan, R. S., *et al.* (1986*a*). Progress in pharmacotherapy of borderline disorders. A double-blind study of amitriptyline, haloperidol, and placebo. *Arch Gen Psychiatry*, **43**(7): 691–7.

Soloff, P. H., George, A., Nathan, S., *et al.* (1986*b*). Amitriptyline and haloperidol in unstable and schizotypal borderline disorders. *Psychopharmacol Bull*, **22**(1): 177–82.

Soloff, P., Cornelius, J., and George, A. (1993). Efficacy of phenelzine and haloperidol in borderline personality disorder. *Archives of General Psychiatry*, **50**: 377–85.

Soloff, P. (1998). Algorithms for psychopharmacological treatment of personality dimensions: Symptom-specific treatments for cognitive-perceptual, affective, and impulsive-behavioural dysregulation. *Bulletin of the Menninger Clinic*, **62**: 195–214.

Soloff, P., Meltzer, C. C., Greer, P. J., Constantine, D., and Kelly, T. M. (2000). A fenfluramine-activated FDG-PET study of borderline personality disorder. *Biological Psychiatry*, **47**: 540–7.

Solomon, J. and George, C. (1999). *Attachment Disorganization*. New York: Guilford.

Southwick, S., Krystal, J. H., Johnson, D., and Charney, D. (1992). Neurobiology of posttraumatic stress disorder. In *Review of Psychiatry* (ed. A. Tasman and M. Riba), pp. 347–67. Washington, DC: American Psychiatric Press.

Spence, D. P. (1994). Narrative truth and putative child abuse. *International Journal of Clinical and Experimental Hypnosis. Special Issue: Hypnosis and Delayed Recall—I*, **42**: 289–303.

Spillius, E. B. (1994). Developments in Kleinian thought: Overview and personal view. *Psychoanalytic Inquiry*, **14**: 324–64.

Springer, T., Lohr, N., Buchtel, H., *et al.* (1996). A preliminary report of short-term cognitive-behavioral group therapy for inpatients with personality disorders. *Journal of Psychotherapy Practice and Research*, **5**: 57–71.

Sprock, J., Rader, T. J., Kendall, J. P., and Yoder, C. Y. (2000). Neuropsychological functioning in patients with borderline personality disorder. *Journal of Clinical Psychology*, **56**: 1587–600.

Sroufe, L. A. (1990). An organizational perspective on the self. In: *The Self in Transition: Infancy to Childhood* (ed. D. Cicchetti and M. Beeghly), pp. 281–307. Chicago: University of Chicago Press.

Sroufe, L. A. (1996). *Emotional Development: The Organization of Emotional Life in the Early Years*. New York: Cambridge University Press.

Stalker, C. A. and Davies, F. (1995). Attachment organization and adaptation in sexually-abused women. *Canadian Journal of Psychiatry*, **40**: 234–40.

Stanley, B., Winchel, R., Molcho, A., Simeon, D., and Stanley, M. (1992). Suicide and the self-harm continuum: Phenomenological and biochemical evidence. *International Review of Psychiatry*, **4**: 149–55.

Stanley, B., Gameroff, M. J., Michalsen, V., and Mann, J. J. (2001). Are suicide attempters who self-mutilate a unique population? *The American Journal of Psychiatry*, **158**: 427–32.

Startup, M., Heard, H., Swales, M., Jones, B., Williams, J. M., and Jones, R. S. (2001). Autobiographical memory and parasuicide in borderline personality disorder. *British Journal of Clinical Psychology*, **40**: 113–20.

Steele, M., Steele, H., Croft, C., and Fonagy, P. (1999). Infant-mother attachment at one year predicts children's understanding of mixed emotions at 6 years. *Social Development*.

Stein, M. B. (1997). Hippocampal volume in women victimised by childhood sexual abuse. *Psychological Medicine*, **27**: 951–9.

Steiner, J. (1992). The equilibrium between the paranoid-schizoid and the depressive positions. In: *Clinical Lectures on Klein and Bion* (ed. R. Anderson), pp. 46–58. London: Routledge.

Steiner, J. (1993). *Psychic Retreats: Pathological Organisations in Psychotic, Neurotic and Borderline Patients*. London: Routledge.

Stern, A. (1938). Psychoanalytic investigation and therapy in borderline group of neuroses. *Psychoanalytic Quarterly*, **7**: 467–89.

Stern, D. N. (1977). *The First Relationship: Mother and Infant.* Cambridge: Harvard University Press.

Stern, D. N. (1985). *The Interpersonal World of the Infant: A View from Psychoanalysis and Developmental Psychology.* New York: Basic Books.

Stevenson, J. and Meares, R. (1992). An outcome study of psychotherapy for patients with borderline personality disorder. *The American Journal of Psychiatry*, **149**: 358–62.

Stevenson, J. and Meares, R. (1999). Psychotherapy with borderline patients: II. A preliminary cost benefit study. *Australian and New Zealand Journal of Psychiatry*, **33**: 473–7.

Stiles, W. B., Agnew-Davies, R., Hardy, G.E., Barkham, M., and Shapiro, D.A. (1998). Relations of the alliance with psychotherapy outcome: Findings in the second Sheffield Psychotherapy Project. *Journal of Consulting and Clinical Psychology*, **66**: 791–802.

Stone, M. H. (1980). *The Borderline Syndromes: Constitution, Personality and Adaptation.* New York: McGraw-Hill.

Stone, M. H., Kahn, E., and Flye, B. (1981). Psychiatrically ill relatives of borderline patients: a family study. *The Psychiatric Quarterly.* **53**: 71–84.

Stone, M. H., Hurt, S. W., and Stone, D. K. (1987). The PI 500: Long-term follow-up of borderline inpatients meeting DSM-III criteria: I. Global outcome. *Journal of Personality Disorders*, **1**: 291–8.

Stone, M. H. (1990). *The Fate of Borderline Patients: Successful Outcome and Psychiatric Practice.* New York: Guilford Press.

Stone, M. (1993). Long-term outcome in personality disorders. *British Journal of Psychiatry*, **162**: 299–313.

Stone, M. H. (2002). Prediction of violent recidivism. *Acta Psychiatrica Scandinavica Suppl*, **412**: 44–6.

Stone, V. E. (2000). The role of the frontal lobes and the amygdala in theory of mind. In: *Understanding Other Minds: Perspectives from Developmental Cognitive Neuroscience (2nd edition)* (ed. S. Baron-Cohen, H. Tager-Flusberg, and D.J. Cohen), pp. 253–73. New York: Oxford University Press.

Strayhorn, J. M. (2002). Self-control: towards systematic training programmes. *Journal of the American Academy of Child and Adolescent Psychiatry*, **41**: 17–27.

Stuss, D. T. and Alexander, M. P. (2000). Executive functions and the frontal lobes: A conceptual review. *Psychological Research*, **63**: 289–98.

Stuss, D. T., Gallup, G., G. Jr., and Alexander, M. P. (2001). The frontal lobes are necessary for 'theory of mind'. *Brain*, **124**: 279–86.

Svrakic, D. M., Whitehead, C., Przybeck, T. R., and Cloninger, C. R. (1993). Differential diagnosis of personality disorders by the seven-factor model of temperament and character. *Archives of General Psychiatry*, **50**: 991–9.

Swartz, M., Blazer, D., George, L., and Winfield, I. (1990). Estimating the prevalence of borderline personality disorder in the community. *Journal of Personality Disorders*, **4**: 257–72.

Swenson, C. (1989). Kernberg and Linehan: two approaches to the borderline patient. *Journal of Personality Disorders*, **3**: 26–35.

Swirsky-Sacchetti, T. Gorton, G. Samuel, S. Sobel, R. Genetta-Wadley, A., and Burleigh, B. (1993). Neuropsychological function in borderline personality disorder. *Journal of Clinical Psychology*, **49**: 385–96.

Symons, D. K. and Clark, S. E. (2000). A longitudinal study of mother-child relationships and theory of mind during the preschool period. *Social Development*, **9**: 3–23.

Target, M. and Fonagy, P. (1996). Playing with reality II: The development of psychic reality from a theoretical perspective. *International Journal of Psychoanalysis*, **77**: 459–79.

Target, M., Shmueli-Goetz, Y., and Fonagy, P. (in press). Attachment representations in school-age children: The early development of the Child Attachment Interview (CAI). *Journal of Infant, Child and Adolescent Psychotherapy.*

Teasdale, J. D., Segal, Z. V., Williams, J. M. G., *et al.* (2000). Prevention of relapse/recurrence in major depression by Mindfulness-Based Cognitive Therapy. *Journal of Consulting and Clinical Psychology*, **68**: 615–23.

Teicher, M. H., Ito, Y., Glod, C. A., Schiffer, F., and Gelbard, H. A. (1994). Early abuse, limbic system dysfunction, and borderline personality disorder. In: *Biological and Neurobehavioral Studies of Borderline Personality Disorder* (ed. K. R. Silk), pp. 177–207. Washington, DC: American Psychiatric Press.

Teicher, M. H., Andersen, S. L., Polcari, A., Anderson, C. M., and Navalta, C. P. (2002). Developmental neurobiology of childhood stress and trauma. *The Psychiatric Clinics of North America*, **25**: 397–426, vii–viii.

Teicher, M. H., Andersen, S. L., Polcari, A., Anderson, C. M., Navalta, C. P., and Kim, D. M. (2003*a*). The neurobiological consequences of early stress and childhood maltreatment. *Neuroscience and Biobehavioral Reviews*, **27**: 33–44.

Teicher, M. H., Polcari, A., Andersen, S. L., Anderson, C. M., and Navalta, C. P. (2003*b*). Neurobiological effects of childhood stress and trauma. In: *September 11: Trauma and Human Bonds* (ed. S. Coates, J. L. Rosenthal, and D. S. Schechter), pp. 211–38. Hillsdale, NJ: Analytic Press.

Terr, L. (1994). *Unchained Memories: True Stories of Traumatic Memories, Lost and Found.* New York: Basic Books.

Terr, L. C. (1991). Childhood traumas: An outline and overview. *The American Journal of Psychiatry*, **148**: 10–20.

Thompson, P. M., Giedd, J. N., Woods, R. P., MacDonald, D., Evans, A. C., and Toga, A. W. (2000). Growth patterns in the developing brain detected by using continuum mechanical tensor maps. *Nature*, **404**: 190–3.

Thompson, R. and Calkins, S. (1996). The double-edged sword: Emotion regulation for children at risk. *Development and Psychopathology*, **8**: 163–82.

Tomasello, M. (1999). *The Cultural Origins of Human Cognition.* Cambridge, MA: Harvard University Press.

Torgersen, S. and Alnaes, R. (1992). Differential perception of parental bonding in schizotypal and borderline personality disorder patients. *Comprehensive Psychiatry*, **33**: 34–8.

Torgersen, S., Lygren, S., Oien, P. A. *et al.* (2000). A twin study of personality disorders. *Comprehensive Psychiatry*, **41**: 416–25.

Torgersen, S., Kringlen, E., and Cramer, V. (2001). The prevalence of personality disorders in a community sample. *Archives of General Psychiatry*, **58**: 590–6.

Trevarthen, C. (1979). Communication and cooperation in early infancy: A description of primary intersubjectivity. In: *Before Speech: The Beginning of Interpersonal Communication* (ed. M. M. Bullowa). New York: Cambridge University Press.

Trickett, P. and McBride-Chang, C. (1995). The developmental impact of different forms of child abuse and neglect. *Developmental Review*, **15**: 311–37.

Tronick, E. Z. and Gianino, A. F. (1986). The transmission of maternal disturbance to the infant. In: *Maternal Depression and Infant Disturbance* (ed. E. Z. Tronick and T. Field), pp. 5–11. San Francisco: Jossey Bass.

Tronick, E. Z. (1989). Emotions and emotional communication in infants. *American Psychologist*, **44**: 112–9.

True, W. R., Rice, J., Eisen, S. A. *et al.* (1993). A twin study of genetic and environmental contributions to liability for posttraumatic stress symptoms. *Archives of General Psychiatry*, **50**: 257–64.

Trull, T. J. (1993). DSM-III-R personality disorders and the five-factor model of personality: an empirical comparison. *Journal of Abnormal Psychology*, **101**: 553–60.

Trull, T. J., Useda, J. D., Doan, B. T. *et al.* (1998). Two-year stability of borderline personality measures. *Journal of Personality Disorders*, **12**: 187–97.

Trull, T. J., Sher, K. J., Minks–Brown, C., Durbin, J., and Burr, R. (2000). Borderline personality disorder and substance use disorders: a review and integration. *Clinical Psychological Review*, **20**: 235–53.

Trull, T. J. (2001*a*). Relationships of borderline features to parental mental illness, childhood abuse, Axis I disorder, and current functioning. *Journal of Personality Disorders*, **15**: 19–32.

Trull, T. J. (2001*b*). Structural relations between borderline personality disorder features and putative etiological correlates. *Journal of Abnormal Psychology*, **110**: 471–81.

Tucker, L., Bauer, S. F., Wagner, S., Harlam, D., and Sher, I. (1987). Long-term hospital treatment of borderline patients: A descriptive outcome study. *The American Journal of Psychiatry*, **144**: 1443–8.

Twemlow, S. W. (2001*a*). Training psychotherapists in attributes of "mind" from Zen and psychoanalytic perspectives, Part I: Core principles, emptiness, impermanence, and paradox. *American Journal of Psychotherapy*, **55**(1): 1–21.

Twemlow, S. W. (2001*b*). Training psychotherapists in attributes of "mind" from Zen and psychoanalytic perspectives, Part II: Attention, here and now, nonattachment, and compassion. *American Journal of Psychotherapy*, **55**(1): 22–39.

Tyrer, P. and Ferguson, B. (1988). Development of the concept of abnormal personality. In: *Personality Disorders: Diagnosis, Management and Course* (ed. P. Tyrer), pp. 1–11. London: Wright.

Tyrer, P., Seivewright, N., Ferguson, B. *et al.* (1990). The Nottingham Study of Neurotic Disorder: relationship between personality status and symptoms. *Psychological Medicine*, **20**: 423–31.

Tyrer, P. (2002*a*). Nidotherapy: a new approach to the treatment of personality disorder. *Acta Psychiatrica Scandinavica*, **105**: 469–72.

Tyrer, P. (2002*b*). Practice guideline for the treatment of borderline personality disorder: a bridge too far. *Journal of Personality Disorders*, **16**: 113–8.

Tyrer, P., Thompson, S., Schmidt, U., *et al.* (2003). Randomized controlled trial of brief cognitive behaviour therapy versus treatment as usual in recurrent deliberate self-harm: the POPMACT study. *Psychological Medicine*, **33**(6): 969–76.

Tyrrell, C., Dozier, M., Teague, G., *et al.* (1999). Effective treatment relationships for persons with serious psychiatric disorders: the importance of attachment states of mind. *Journal of Consulting and Clinical Psychology*, **67**(5): 725–33.

Tyson, P. and Tyson, R. L. (1990). *Psychoanalytic theories of development: An integration.* New Haven and London: Yale University Press.

Usher, J. A. and Neisser, U. (1993). Childhood amnesia and the beginnings of memory for four early life events. *Journal of Experimental Psychology: General*, **122**: 155–165.

van Elst, L. T., Woermann, F. G., Lemieux, L., Thompson, P. J., and Trimble, M. R. (2000). Affective aggression in patients with temporal lobe epilepsy: a quantitative MRI study of the amygdala. *Brain*, **123 (Pt 2)**: 234–43.

van IJzendoorn, M. H., Moran, G., Belsky, J., Pederson, D., Bakermans-Kranenburg, M. J., and Kneppers, K. (2000). The similarity of siblings attachments to their mothers. *Child Development*, **71**: 1086–98.

van Reekum, R., Links, P. S., Finlayson, M. A. *et al.* (1993). Repeat neurobehavioral study of borderline personality disorder. *Journal of Psychiatry and Neuroscience*, **21**: 13–20.

van Reekum, R., Conway, C. A., Gansler, D., White, R., and Bachman, D. L. (1996). Neurobehavioral study of borderline personality disorder. *Journal of Psychiatry and Neuroscience*, **18**: 121–9.

Veen, G. and Arntz, A. (2000). Multidimensional dichotomous thinking characterizes borderline personality disorder. *Cognitive Therapy and Research*, **24**: 23–45.

Verheul, R., Van Den Bosch, L. M., Koeter, M. W,. De Ridder, M. A., Stijnen, T. and Van Den Brink, W. (2003). Dialectical behaviour therapy for women with borderline personality disorder: 12-month, randomised clinical trial in The Netherlands. *British Journal of Psychiatry*, **182**: 135–40.

Vermote, R., Vertommen, H., Corveleyn, J., Verhaest, Y., Franssen, M., and Peuskens, J. (2003). The Kortenberg-Leuven Process-Outcome Study. Paper presented at the *IPA Congress.* Toronto.

Vinden, P. G. (2001). Parenting attitudes and children's understanding of mind: A comparison of Korean American and Anglo-American families. *Cognitive Development*, **16**: 793–809.

Vitiello, B. and Stoff, D. M. (1997). Subtypes of aggression and their relevance to child psychiatry. *Journal of the American Academy of Child and Adolescent Psychiatry*, **36**: 307–15.

Wallerstein, R. S. (1986). *Forty-two Lives in Treatment: A Study of Psychoanalysis and Psychotherapy.* New York: Guildford Press.

Walsh, F. (1977). The family of the borderline patient. In: *The Borderline Patient* (ed. R.Grinker and B.Werble), pp. 149–77. New York: Aronson.

Watson, J. S. (1972). Smiling, cooing, and "the game". *Merrill-Palmer Quarterly*, **18**: 323–39.

Watson, J. S. (1979). Perception of contingency as a determinant of social responsiveness. In: *The Origins of Social Responsiveness* (ed. E.B.Thoman), pp. 33–64. New York: Lawrence Erlbaum.

Watson, J. S. (1985). Contingency perception in early social development. In: *Social Perception in Infants* (ed. T. M. Field and N. A. Fox), pp. 157–76. Norwood, NJ: Ablex.

Watson, J. S. (1994). Detection of self: The perfect algorithm. In: *Self-Awareness in Animals and Humans: Developmental Perspectives* (ed. S. Parker, R. Mitchell, and M. Boccia), pp. 131–49. Cambridge: Cambridge University Press.

Watson, J. S. (1995). Self-orientation in early infancy: The general role of contingency and the specific case of reaching to the mouth. In: *The Self in Infancy: Theory and Research* (ed. P. Rochat,), pp. 375–93. Amsterdam: Elsevier.

Wellman, H. (1990). *The Child's Theory of Mind.* Cambridge, Mass: Bradford Books/ MIT Press.

Wellman, H. M. and Phillips, A. T. (2000). Developing intentional understandings. In: *Intentionality: A Key to Human Understanding* (ed. B. Malle, L. Moses, and D. Baldwin) pp. 125–48. Cambridge, MA: MIT Press.

Westen, D., Ludolph, P., Misle, B., Ruffins, S., and Block, J. (1990). Physical and sexual abuse in adolescent girls with borderline personality disorder. *American Journal of Orthopsychiatry*, **60**: 55–66.

Westen, D. (1998). Refining the measurment of Axis II: A Q-sort procedure for assessing personality pathology. *Assessment*, **5**: 335–55.

Westen, D. and Shedler, J. (1999*a*). Revising and Assessing Axis-II, Part II: Toward an empirically based and clinically useful classification of personality disorders. *American Journal of Psychiatry*, **156**: 273–85.

Westen, D. and Shedler, J. (1999*b*). Revising and Assessing Axis-II: Part I: Developng a clinical and empirically valid assessment method. *American Journal of Psychiatry*, **156**: 258–72.

Whiten, A. (1991). *Natural Theories of Mind.* Oxford: Basil Blackwell.

Widiger, T. and Trull, T. (1992). Borderline and narcissistic personality disorders. In: *Comprehensive Handbook of Psychopathology* (ed. P. Surker and H. Adams), pp. 467–573. New York: Plenum Press.

Widom, C. S. (1989). Does violence beget violence? A critical examination of the literature. *Psychological Bulletin*, **106**: 3–28.

Widom, C. S. (1999). Posttraumatic stress disorder in abused and neglected children grown up. *The American Journal of Psychiatry*, **156**: 1223–9.

Wildgoose, A., Clarke, S., and Waller, G. (2001). Treating personality fragmentation and dissociation in borderline personality disorder: a pilot study of the impact of cognitive analytic therapy. *The British Journal of Medical Psychology*, **74**: 47–55.

Williams, M. (1987). Reconstruction of early seduction and its aftereffects. *Journal of the American Psychoanalytic Association*, **35**: 145–63.

Wimmer, H. and Perner, J. (1983). Beliefs about beliefs: Representation and constraining function of wrong beliefs in young children's understanding of deception. *Cognition*, **13**: 103–28.

Winnicott, D. W. (1967). Mirror-role of the mother and family in child development. In: *The Predicament of the Family: A Psycho-Analytical Symposium* (ed. P. Lomas), pp. 26–33. London: Hogarth Press.

Winnicott, D. W. (1971). Transitional objects and transitional phenomena. In: *Playing and Reality* (ed. D. W. Winnicott), pp. 1–25. London: Tavistock.

Winston, A. Pollack, J. McCullough, L. Flegenheimer, W. Kestenbaum, R., and Trujillo, M. (1991). Brief psychotherapy of personality disorders. *Journal of Nervous and Mental Disease*, **179**: 188–93.

Winston, A., Laikin, M., Pollack, J., Samstag, L. W., McCullough, L., and Muran, J. C. (1994). Short-term dynamic psychotherapy of personality disorders. *The American Journal of Psychiatry*, **15**: 190–4.

Woolfe, T., Want, S. C., and Siegal, M. (2002). Signposts to development: Theory of mind in deaf children. *Child Development*, **73**: 768–78.

Work Group on Borderline Personality Disorder (2001). Practice guideline for the treatment of patients with borderline personality disorder. *The American Journal of Psychiatry*, **158 (suppl)**: 1–52.

Woyshville, M. J., Lackamp, J. M., Eisengart, J. A., and Gilliland, J. A. (1999). On the meaning and measurement of affective instability: clues from chaos theory. *Biological Psychiatry*, **45**: 261–9.

Yapko, M. (1993). The seductions of memory. *Networker*, **September/October**: 31–7.

Yeamans, F. E., Gutfreund, J., Selzer, M. A., and Clarkin, J. F. (1994). *Journal of Psychotherapy Practice and Research*, **3**: 16–24.

Yehuda, R., Kahana, B., Binder-Brynes, K., Southwick, S. M., Mason, J. W., and Giller, E. L. (1995*a*). Low urinary cortisol excretion in Holocaust survivors with posttraumatic stress disorder. *The American Journal of Psychiatry*, **152**: 982–6.

Yehuda, R., Kahana, B., Schmeidler, J., Southwick, S., Wilson, S., and Giller, E. (1995*b*). Impact of cumulative lifetime trauma and recent stress on current posttraumatic stress disorder symptoms in holocaust survivors. *The American Journal of Psychiatry*, **152**: 1815–8.

Yehuda, R. (1998). Psychoneuroendocrinology of post-traumatic stress disorder. *The Psychiatric Clinic of North America*, **21**: 359–79.

Yeomans, F. E., Selzer, M. A., and Clarkin, J. F. (1992). *Treating the Borderline Patient: A Contract-Based Approach*. New York: Basic Books.

Young, J. E. (1999). *Cognitive Therapy for Personality Disorders: A Schema-Focused Approach*. 3rd edition. Sarasota, Florida: Professional Resource Exchange.

Zanarini, M. C., Frankenburg, F. R., Chauncey, D. L., and Gunderson, J. G. (1987). The Diagnostic Interview for Personality Disorders: Interrater and test-retest reliability. *Comprehensive Psychiatry*, **28**: 467–80.

Zanarini, M. C. Gunderson, J. G. Marino, M. F. Schwartz, E. D., and Frankenburg, F. R. (1988). DSM–III disorders in the families of borderline outpatients. *Journal of Personality Disorders*, **2**: 292–302.

Zanarini, M. C., Gunderson, J., Frankenburg, F. R., and Chauncey, D. (1989). The revised Diagnostic Interview for Borderlines: Discriminating BPD from other Axis II disorders. *Journal of Personality Disorders*, **3**: 10–18.

Zanarini, M. C., Gunderson, J. G., Marino, M. F., Schwartz, E. O., and Frankenburg, F. R. (1989*c*). Childhood experiences of borderline patients. *Comprehensive Psychiatry*, **30**: 18–25.

Zanarini, M., Gunderson, J. G., and Frankenburg, F. R. (1990). Discriminating borderline personality disorder from other Axis II disorders. *The American Journal of Psychiatry*, **147**: 161–7.

Zanarini, M. C. and Frankenburg, F. R. (1994). Emotional hypochondriasis, hyperbole and the borderline patient. *Journal of Psychotherapy Practice and Research*, **3**: 25–36.

Zanarini, M. C., Dubo, E., Lewis, R., and Williams, A. (1996). Childhood factors associated with the development of borderline personality disorders. In: *Role of Sexual Abuse in the Etiology of Borderline Personality Disorder* (ed. M. C. Zanarini), pp. 29–44. Washington, DC: American Psychiatric Press.

Zanarini, M. C. and Frankenburg, F. R. (1997). Pathways to the development of borderline personality disorder. *Journal of Personality Disorders*, **11**: 93–104.

Zanarini, M. C., Williams, A. A., Lewis, R. E. *et al.* (1997). Reported pathological childhood experiences associated with the development of borderline personality disorder. *The American Journal of Psychiatry*, **154**: 1101–6.

Zanarini, M. C., Frankenburg, F. R., DeLuca, C. J., Hennen, J., Khera, G. S., and Gunderson, J. G. (1998). The pain of being borderline: Dysphoric states specific to borderline personality disorder. *The American Journal of Psychiatry*, **147**: 57–63.

Zanarini, M. C. (2000). Childhood experiences associated with the development of borderline personality disorder. *The Psychiatric Clinics of North America*, **23**: 89–101.

Zanarini, M. C., Frankenburg, F. R., Reich, D. B. *et al.* (2000*a*). Biparental failure in the childhood experiences of borderline patients. *Journal of Personality Disorders*, **14**: 264–73.

Zanarini, M. C., Skodol, A. E., Bender, D. *et al.* (2000*b*). The collaborative longitudinal personality disorders study: Reliability of Axis I and II diagnoses. *Journal of Personality Disorders*, **14**: 291–9.

Zanarini, M. C. and Frankenburg, F. R. (2001). Olanzapine treatment of borderline patients: a double-blind, placebo-controlled study. *The Journal of Clinical Psychiatry*.

Zanarini, M. C., Frankenburg, F. R., Hennen, J., and Silk, K. (2003). The Longitudinal Course of Borderline Psychopathology: 6-year prospective follow-up of the phenomenology of borderline personality disorder. *The American Journal of Psychiatry*, **160**: 274–83.

Zeanah, C. H. and Benoit, D. (1995). Clinical applications of a parent perception interview in infant mental health. *Child and Adolescent Psychiatric Clinics of North America*, **4**: 539–54.

Zelkowitz, P., Paris, J., Guzder, J., and Feldman, R. (2001). Diatheses and stressors in borderline pathology of childhood: the role of neuropsychological risk and trauma. *Journal of the American Academy of Child and Adolescent Psychiatry*, **40**: 100–5.

Zimmerman, M. and Mattia, J. I. (1999). Axis I diagnostic comorbidity and borderline personality disorder. *Comprehensive Psychiatry*, **40**: 245–52.

Zlotnick, C., Mattia, J., and Zimmerman, M. (2001). Clinical features of survivors of sexual abuse with major depression. *Child Abuse and Neglect*, **25**: 357–67.

Zubieta, J. K., Chinitz, J. A., Lombardi, U., Fig, L. M., Cameron, O. G., and Liberzon, I. (1999). Medial frontal cortex involvement in PTSD symptoms: a SPECT study. *Journal of Psychiatric Research*, **33**: 259–64.

Zweig-Frank, H. and Paris, J. (1991). Parents' emotional neglect and overprotection according to the recollections of patients with borderline personality disorder. *The American Journal of Psychiatry*, **148**: 648–51.

Zweig-Frank, H. and Paris, J. (1995). The five-factor model of personality in borderline and nonborderline personality disorders. *Canadian Journal of Psychiatry*, **40**: 523–6.

Zweig-Frank, H. and Paris, J. (2002). Predictors of outcome in a 27-year follow-up of patients with borderline personality disorder. *Journal of Psychiatric Research*, **43**: 103–7.

Index

addiction problems 18
adherence 180–1
admission 159–62
  feedback questionnaire 321–2
Adult Attachment Interview 35, 37, 56, 75–6, 78, 84, 92–3, 94
affect dysregulation 32–4
affect, identification and appropriate expression of 222–52
  aggression, passive 238–40
  coherent sense of self, formation of 260–3
  envy 240–2
  general principles 222–4, 233–8
  hate and contempt 247–50
  idealization 242–4
  impulse control 224–33
  love and attachment 250–2
  representational systems, stable 252–60
  secure relationships, development of capacity to form 263–6
  sexual attraction 244–7
affect representation, enfeebled 85–7
affect storms 311, 317
affective disorder 21
Affective Picture System 15
aggression 234–6
  passive 238–40
  violence
aggressive dementia 16
agoraphobia 7
alcohol 161–2
'alien self'
  establishment 88–90
  see also mentalization and 'alien self'
anterior cingulate dysfunction 31–2
antidepressant drugs 51
antipsychotic drugs 51, 199
antisocial personality disorder 47, 51, 93, 101, 235–6
  epidemiological and aetiological research 3, 5, 8, 10, 13, 16, 17, 18, 25, 29
anxiety 33
  paranoid 234–6
arousal 'switch', changes to 94–6
assessment 156–8
attachment 34–7, 75–9, 250–2
  disorganization 87–8
  model, simple 37
  rating scale 35, 36
  self-report measures 35–6
  style questionnaire 6, 36
  theory 20, 56
  see also attachment trauma; self-development, optimal in secure attachment context
attachment trauma, impact of 91–108
  arousal 'switch', changes to 94–6
  mentalization and 'alien self' 92–4, 97–104
  psychic equivalence, shame and teleological stance 96–7
  remembering trauma 104–8
attention 18–19
  deficit hyperactivity disorder 7, 17, 18
attentional control 85–7
audit of resources 272
Axis-I disorders 16, 17, 21, 23, 33, 35, 156
Axis-II disorders 23, 24, 33, 35, 43, 135, 156

behavioural dyscontrol 4
biological considerations 12–19

biological considerations *contd.*
- attention and self-control 18–19
- biological markers 12
- candidate genes 14–15
- cortical localization 15–18
- genetic studies 12–13
- neurostransmitter abnormality 14

biological pathways of impact of extreme stress 29–32
bipolar I disorder 7
bipolar II disorder 5, 7
borderline personality organization 5, 12, 112–14
boundary violations 184–6
brain development, adverse 29–30

Cambridge Neuropsychological Test Automated Battery 17
Canada 23, 136
candidate genes 14–15
carbamazepine 51
care
- individual approach to 194–5
- programme approach 179–80

Cassel Hospital (United Kingdom) 139
challenging behaviours 281
childhood
- attachment interviews 92
- trauma and maltreatment 23–6
- *see also* sexual abuse

clarity of treatment aims 274
clinical
- picture in BPD 3–9, 103–4

Clinical Practice Guidelines for the Treatment of Patients with BPD 147
Cloninger's trait dimensions 6
clozapine 51
cognitive analytic therapy 46, 111, 112, 117, 129–32, 140
cognitive behavioural therapy 39, 46–7, 117, 123, 126–8
- Manual Assisted 47

coherence of treatment 187–9
coherent sense of self, formation of 260–3
Collaborative Longitudinal Personality Disorder Study 4, 10
colour naming (Stroop) test 87
co-morbidity 7
conduct disorder 18, 29, 78
confidentiality 161
consistency of treatment 187–9, 274–5
constancy of treatment 187–9
contempt 247–50
context 270–1
contingency detection module 59, 60
cortical localization 15–18
countertransference 198, 211–12
course of BPD 10–12
crisis management
- plan 313–14
- telephone calls 309–10

current mental states, working with 304–5, 317
current practice, iatrogenic aspects of 278–9

day-hospital programme 148–50, 158
defence mechanisms 5
delinquency 78
dementia, aggressive 16
Denmark 49, 139
depression 12
- *see also* major depressive disorders

Descartes, R./Cartesian 55, 64
Dexamethasone Suppression Test 31
diagnosis
- stability of over time 9
- thresholds 2–3

Diagnostic Interview for Borderlines 2, 11, 23, 136, 137, 156
Diagnostic Interview for DSM-IV Personality Disorders 2
diagnostic procedures 2
dialectical behaviour therapy 47–9, 111, 117, 119–26, 139, 140
- dialectics 119–21
- emotional dysregulation 121–2
- mentalization and mindfulness 122–3
- practice 124–6

Dimensional Assessment of Personality Pathology Baseline Questionnaire 13
dimensional models of BPD 8–9
disturbed relatedness 4
drop-outs 174
drug treatments *see* medication
DSM criteria 3, 156
DSM-III 1, 135
DSM-III-R 43, 47
DSM-IV 1
Dunedin Prospective Longitudinal Cohort Study 29
dynamic formulation 169–72
dysregulation, emotional 121–2
dysthymia 7

Early Child Care Research Network 84
Early Maladaptive Schemas 127–8
eating disorders 18
empathy 167–9
empirical data 35–7, 43–4
endogenous opiate system 30
envy 240–2
epidemiological and aetiological research 1–38
  attachment and BPD 34–7
  clinical picture 3–9
  definition of the problem 1–3
  epidemiology 3
  mechanisms and aetiological factors 12–37
    biological considerations 12–19
    psychosocial influences 19–34
  natural history of BPD 9–12
  psychosocial influences 19–34
Europe 119, 139–40, 154
expressive therapies 172–4

family history 21–2
fears 257–60
Finland 12
flexibility 191–2
Francis Dixon Lodge (United Kingdom) 140
functional impairment 4

genetic studies 12–13
Germany 139, 147
goals, clear-agreed 163–4
group therapy 160–1, 232–3
  affect, identification and appropriate expression of 222–3
  capacity to form secure relationships 266
  challenging affect states, other 237–8
  coherent sense of self 262–3
  envy 241–2
  hate and contempt 249–50
  idealization 243–4
  impulse control 232–3
  love and attachment 251–2
  passive aggression 239–40
  sexual attraction 246–7
  stable representational systems 253–60
  wishes, hopes and fears 259–60

Halliwick Day Unit/model 145, 149, 283–4
haloperidol 197
Happe advanced theory of mind 78
hate 247–50
Health Maintenance Organizations 118
Henderson Hospital (United Kingdom) 139, 140
history taking 165–6
histrionic personality disorder 10
hopes 257–60
'how' skills 122
HPA axis 30–1

iatrogenic techniques 279–81
idealization 242–4

implementation pathway 269–85
  audit of resources 272
  challenging behaviours 281
  context 270–1
  iatrogenic aspects of current practice 278–9
  mentalization skill, increasing 279–81
  organizational principles 272–7
  patient experience and treatment 282–5
  skills 271–2
  systemic adherence 282
  therapy adherence 281–2
impulse control 224–33
  group therapy 232–3
  rationale 224–5
  self-harm 230–1
  strategic recommendations 225
  suicide 228–30
  therapy, individual 231–2
impulsivity 4
individual therapy
  affect, identification and appropriate expression of 222–3
  capacity to form secure relationships 265–6
  challenging affect states, other 236–7
  coherent sense of self 261–2
  envy 240–1
  hate and contempt 248–9
  idealization 242–3
  impulse control 231–2
  love and attachment 250–1
  passive aggression 238–9
  sexual attraction 245
  stable representational systems 253–60
  wishes, hopes and fears 258–9
infant sensitivity to social contingency 59–60
information provision 159–62
in-patient care 174–5
insecure base, impact of 82–91
  on affect representation 85–7
  'alien self', establishment of 88–90
  attachment, disorganization of 87–8
  on attentional control 85–7
  IWM, controlling 90–1
  mirroring, failure of 82–3
  playfulness, lack of 83–5
intensity 192–4, 276–7
Intensive Out-patient Programme 148–9, 153, 156, 180, 192, 319–20
intentional agent 62–8
internal working models 57, 58
  controlling 90–1
internalizing and externalizing disorder 7, 11
International Personality Disorder Examination 2
International Society for the Study of Personality Disorder 140
interpersonal
  group psychotherapy 138
  interpretive function 58, 74–5
  relating 99–100
interpretation 130–2
intimate relationships 165–6
Italy 139

Kernberg's Structural Interview 2
key problems, clarification of 160
key worker 153–4, 164
Kortenberg-Leuven Process Outcome Study 92–3

listening 169
lithium 51
Longitudinal Interval Follow-up Evaluation Interview 4
love 250–2

McLean Hospital 137
major depressive disorders 4, 7, 10, 16, 31
maltreatment 23–6
markedness 66–7
medical intervention 287–8, 297
medication 50–2, 161–2, 195–200, 277
memories, working with 217–18

Menninger project 40, 41, 94, 137
mental closeness 210–12
Mental Health Act (1983) 154, 164
mental state concepts 64–8
mentalization xvii-xviii, 70–5, 141–4, 302–3, 316
  and 'alien self' 97–104
    clinical illustration 103–4
    impulsive acts 101–3
    interpersonal relating and transference 99–100
    self-harm 100–1
    suicide 101
  enhancement 203–4
  failure 92–4
  hyperactive 218–20
  and mindfulness 122–3
  neurological basis 79–82
  skill 279–81
  see also mentalization-based treatment; mentalization-based understanding
mentalization-based treatment 43–4, 183–201
  adherence and competence rating 315–18
  care, individual approach to 194–5
  consistency, constancy and coherence 187–9
  current models of treatment 112, 117–19, 121, 123–6, 130–2, 134–5
  flexibility 191–2
  intensity 192–4
  medication 195–200
  relationship focus 189–91
  structure 183–73
  therapy, integration of modalities of 200–1
  treatment organization 153, 180–1
  treatment strategies 220
  treatment techniques 221
mentalization-based understanding of BPD 55–109
  attachment theory 56
  attachment trauma, impact of 91–108
  developmental roots 55
  insecure base, impact of 82–91
  self-development, optimal in secure attachment context 57–82
mindfulness 122–3
mirroring
  failure 82–3
  parental 64–8
mood 33
  disorder 7, 12
  stabilizers 51–2, 199
motivational states 257–60
multiple pathway model 28–9

narcissistic personality disorder 8, 13, 16, 235–6
National Health Service 118
National Institute for Mental Health in England 148
natural history of BPD 9–12
neglect 24–5, 26–34
Netherlands 3, 48, 139, 147
neurostransmitter abnormality 14
New York Children in the Community Study 25
Nidotherapy 139
night sedation 199
non-aggressive dementia 16
North America 3, 135–9
  see also Canada; United States
Norway 13, 139, 147
no-therapy therapy 138
nursing intervention 297

object relations 5–6, 111
  inventory 93
obsessive-compulsive disorder 4, 13
olanzapine 51
oppositional defiant disorder 29
organic brain disorders 17
organizational principles 272–7
  clarity 274
  consistency 274–5
  intensity 276–7
  medication 277

organizational principles *contd.*
relationship focus 275–6
structure 273
outcome *see* therapy research and outcome

panic disorder 7
paranoia 3, 4
Parent Development Interview 76, 88
Parental Bonding Instrument 6
parental mirroring 64–8
parenting 21–2
passive-aggressive personality disorder 10
patient
contact, assuring possibility of 162–3
experience and treatment 282–5
Partial Hospital (PH) programme 193–4
phenomenological picture 3–4
physical abuse 28
Psychodynamic Interpersonal 134
Manualized 42
Pilkonis's attachment prototype interview assessment 36–7
playfulness, lack of 83–5
Porteus Mazes task 17
post-traumatic stress disorder 23, 26–7, 30, 92, 95, 106
pretend mode 68–70, 218–20
primary affective disorder 7
primary beliefs, identification of 254–5
primary clinician 153–4
problems, common 174–5
professionals, roles of 164
projective identification 83
evocatory 90
psychic equivalence 68–70, 96–7
psychoanalytic psychotherapy 40–6, 111, 140
empirical evidence for mentalization-based treatment 43–4
results 44–6
psychodynamic therapy 39, 132–4
psychological pathways 32–4
psychological treatments 40–50
cognitive analytic therapy 46
cognitive therapy 46–7
dialectical behaviour therapy 47–9
drug treatments 50–2
psychoanalytic psychotherapy 40–6
therapeutic community treatments 49–50
psychopharmacological treatment 199–200
psychosis 4, 14
psychosocial influences 19–34
biological pathways of impact of extreme stress 29–32
childhood trauma and maltreatment 23–6
multiple pathway model 28–9
parenting 21–2
post-traumatic stress disorder model 26–7
psychological pathways and impact of extreme stress 32–4
stress-diathesis model 27–8
theoretical considerations 19–21
psychotic personality organization 112–13

randomization 52–3
rationale
affect, identification and appropriate expression of 222
capacity to form secure relationships 263–4
challenging affect states, other 233–4
coherent sense of self 260–1
impulse control 224–5
stable representational systems 252–3
reasonable mind 122
reciprocal roles 129–30
reflective function 74–9, 88, 92, 93, 94
reformulation 130–2
relational alliance 167–9
Relationship Attachment Questionnaire 36
relationship focus 189–91, 275–6
Relationship Questionnaire 35, 36
Relationship Scales Questionnaire 35
relationships, real 216–20
reliability 169
remembering trauma 104–8
representational agent 62–8
representational systems, stable 252–60
individual and group sessions 253–60
rationale 252–3
strategic recommendations 253

responsible medical officer 154–6, 164
risperidone 51
Romanian orphans 87

schizophrenia 4, 12, 14
second-order belief states 256–7
secure relationships, development of capacity to form 263–6
selective serotonin reuptake inhibitors 51, 199
self as intentional and representational agent 62–8
  parental mirroring and mental state concepts 64–8
self-control 18–19
self-development, optimal in secure attachment context 57–82
  early stages of self-development 59–62
  mentalization 70–5, 79–82
  psychic equivalence and pretend mode 68–70
  reflective function and attachment 75–9
  self as intentional and representational agent 62–8
self-harm 100–1, 230–1, 306–9
self-report measures 35–6
sensitivity, infant 59–60
separation-individuation phase 20
serotonin system 30
  see also selective serotonin reuptake inhibitors
service models 145–8
  divided functions 145
  one-team 146–7
sexual
  abuse 23–8, 31, 92, 108
  attraction 244–7
  relationships 162
shame 96–7
sibling effect 73
simple attachment model 37
skills 271–2
Social Adjustment Scale 50
social aspects of care, stabilization of 162
social contingency 59–60
sodium valproate 51, 52
Spain 139
staff 150–6
  key worker or primary clinician 153–4
  responsible medical officer 154–6
  selection 150–1
  team 152–3
  training characteristics 152
strategic recommendations
  affect, identification and appropriate expression of 222
  capacity to form secure relationships 265
  challenging affect states, other 234
  coherent sense of self 261
  impulse control 225
  stable representational systems 253
stress
  -diathesis model 27–8
  extreme 29–34
Stroop test 87
structure 273
Structured Clinical Interview 2, 93, 156
substance abuse 7, 17, 33
suicide 3, 101, 228–30, 306–9
  see also suicide and self-harm inventory
suicide and self-harm inventory 287–300
  acts of self-harm 297–300
  attempted suicide 288–96
  criteria for acts of self-harm 296–7
  criteria for suicidal acts 287–8
supervision 177–8
supportive psychotherapy 140
Sweden 3
Symptom Check-List-90-R 50
systemic adherence 282

team 152–3
  morale 175–7
  support 175–8
teleological stance 61–2, 96–7
telephone calls 309–10
Temperament and Character Inventory 6, 8
theoretical considerations 19–21, 34
'theory of mind' 72

therapeutic communities 49–50, 134–5
therapist techniques 303, 304–5
therapy
  adherence 281–2
  integration of modalities 200–1
  research and outcome 39–53
    drug treatments 50–2
    problems 52–3
    psychological treatments 40–50
  see also group; individual 231–2
tissue damage, visible 297
Toronto Alexithymia Scale 93
Tower of London task 17
training characteristics 152
training materials 301–11
  affect storms 311
  bridging gaps 305
  crisis telephone calls 309–10
  current mental states 304–5
  framework of treatment 301–2
  mentalization 302–3
  suicide and self-harm 306–9
  transference 306
transference 99–100, 198, 207–10, 306, 318
  -focused psychotherapy 42, 99–100, 112–19
trauma 23–34
treatment
  context 147
  framework 160, 301–2 , 315–316
  guidelines 147–8
  previous 166
  techniques 221–67
    see also affect, identification and appropriate expression of
  see also treatment, current models for; treatment, engagement in; treatment organization; treatment strategies
treatment, current models for 111–44
  cognitive analytic therapy 129–32
  cognitive behavioural therapy 126–8
  dialectical behaviour therapy 119–26
  European approaches, other 139–40
  mentalization 141–4
  North American approaches, other 135–9
  psychodyamic-interpersonal therapy 132–4
  therapeutic communities 134–5
  transference-focused psychotherapy 112–19
treatment, engagement in 158–75
  admission 159–62
  common problems 174–5
  dynamic formulation 169–72
  expressive therapies 172–4
  goals, clear-agreed 163–4
  history taking 165–6
  patient contact, assuring possibility of 162–3
  professionals, roles of 164
  relational and working alliance 167–9
  social aspects of care, stabilization of 162
treatment organization 145–81
  adherence 180–1
  assessment 156–8
  care programme approach 179–80
  service models 145–8
  staff 150–6
  team support 175–8
  treatment, engagement in 158–75
  treatment programmes 148–50
treatment strategies 203–20
  bridging gaps 205–7
  current mental states, working with 212–14
  deficits 214–16
  mental closeness retention 210–12
  mentalization enhancement 203–4
  relationships, real 216–20
  transference 207–10

United Kingdom 3, 40, 49, 84–5, 139, 140
  treatment organization 147, 154, 156, 179
United States 49, 135, 147, 148

validation 167–9
venlafaxine 51
Vietnam Veterans 28, 92
violence 101–3, 161

'what' skills 122
Winterbourne House
(United Kingdom) 140
wise mind 122–3
wishes 257–60
working alliance 167–9
Working Model of the Child
Interview 76–7

Zen spiritual practices 122–3

Lightning Source UK Ltd.
Milton Keynes UK
13 February 2010

149993UK00002B/6/P